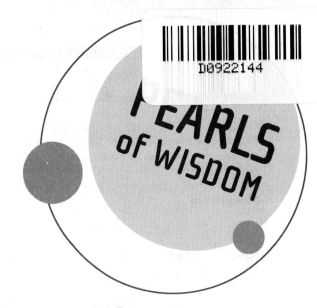

PEARLS of WISDOM

Obstetrics and Gynecology
BOARD REVIEW

Third Edition

Stephen G. Somkuti, MD, PhD
Associate Professor
Department of Obstetrics and Gynecology and Reproductive Sciences
Temple University School of Medicine School
Philadelphia, Pennsylvania
Director, The Toll Center for Reproductive Sciences
Division of Reproductive Endocrinology
Department of Obstetrics and Gynecology
Abington Memorial Hospital
Abington Reproductive Medicine
Abington, Pennsylvania

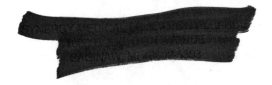

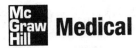 **Medical**

New York Chicago San Francisco Lisbon London   Madrid Mexico City Milan
New Delhi   San Juan Seoul Singapore   Sydney Toronto

Obstetrics and Gynecology Board Review: Pearls of Wisdom, Third Edition

1 2 3 4 5 6 7 8 9 0   QPD/QPD   12 11 10 9 8

ISBN: 978-0-07-149703-9
MHID: 0-07-149703-X

This book was set in Adobe Garamond by Aptara®, Inc.
The editors were Catherine A. Johnson, Kirsten Funk, and Peter J. Boyle.
The production supervisor was Sherri Souffrance.
Project management was provided by Sandhya Joshi, Aptara, Inc.
The cover designer was Handel Low.
The text designer was Eve Siegel.
Québecor Dubuque was printer and binder.

This book is printed on acid-free paper.

Library of Congress Cataloging-in-Publication Data

Obstetrics and gynecology board review / [editor] Stephen G. Somkuti. —3rd ed.
    p. ; cm. – (Pearls of wisdom)
    Includes bibliographical references and index.
    ISBN-13: 978-0-07-149703-9 (pbk. : alk. paper)
    ISBN-10: 0-07-149703-X (pbk. : alk. paper)   1. Obstetrics–Examinations, questions, etc.
2. Gynecology–Examinations, questions, etc.   I. Somkuti, Stephen G.   II. Series.
    [DNLM: 1. Obstetrics–methods–Examination Questions.   2. Gynecology–methods–
Examination Questions. WQ 18.2 O143 2008]
    RG111.O32 2008
    618.076–dc22

                                                        2008008605

DEDICATION

To my loving family
Andrea my wife, Fiva and Michael our children.

CONTENTS

CONTRIBUTORS

Oren Azulay, MD
Department of Obstetrics and Gynecology
Kaiser Permanente
Fontana, California
Genital Prolapse

Julie A. Braga, MD
Department of Obstetrics and Gynecology
Dartmouth Hitchcock Medical Center
Lebanon, New Hampshire
Primary and Preventative Care

Miki Chiguchi, MD
Division of Obstetrics and Gynecology
Department of Obstetrics and Gynecology
Abington Memorial Hospital
Abington, Pennsylvania
Anatomy of the Pelvis and Reproductive Tract
Dysmenorrhea and Premenstrual Syndrome

Jerry Cohen, MPH
Research Consultant
Residency Training Program
Department of Obstetrics and Gynecology
Abington Memorial Hospital
Abington, Pennsylvania
Epidemiology and Clinical Biostatistics

Rachel Cohen, DO
Department of Obstetrics and Gynecology
Mercy Suburban Hospital
Norristown, Pennsylvania
Embryology of the Genital Tract
Physiology of Normal Pregnancy
Breech
Primary and Preventative Care
Family Planning and Sterilization

Frank Craparo, MD
Division Director
Maternal Fetal Medicine
Abington Memorial Hospital
Abington, Pennsylvania
Labor and Delivery
Rh Isoimmunization

Hipolito Custodio III, MD, MS
Department of Obstetrics and Gynecology
Albert Einstein Medical Center
Philadelphia, Pennsylvania
Gastrointestinal Disorders in Pregnancy
Pediatric and Adolescent Gynecology
Ethics and Psychiatric Pearls

Darnelle L. Dorsainville, MS, CGC
Board Certified Genetic Counselor
Division of Genetics
Department of Pediatrics
Albert Einstein Medical Center
Philadelphia, Pennsylvania
Genetics for the Obstetrician

Mitchell I. Edelson, MD
Gynecologic Oncology Institute
Abington Memorial Hospital
Abington, Pennsylvania
Uterine Sacromas
Epithelial and Nonepithelial Ovarian Cancer
Fallopian Tube Neoplasms
Vulvar and Vaginal Carcinoma
Radiation Therapy, Chemotherapy, Immunotherapy,
  and Tumor Markers
Gestational Trophoblastic Disease
Gynecologic Pathology

Stephanie J. Estes, MD
Assistant Professor
Division of Reproductive Endocrinology and
  Infertility
Department of Obstetrics and Gynecology
Penn State Milton S. Hershey Medical Center
Hershey, Pennsylvania
Amenorrhea
Disorders of Prolactin Secretion

Gretchen E. Glaser, MD
Department of Obstetrics and Gynecology
Abington Memorial Hospital
Abington, Pennsylvania
Rh Isoimmunization
Lactation
Benign Disorders of the Upper Genital Tract

Abby M. Gonik, MD
Department of Obstetrics and Gynecology
Abington Memorial Hospital
Abington, Pennsylvania
Cervical Lesions and Cancer
Endometrial Hyperplasia and Carcinoma

Karen Hancock, MD
Department of Obstetrics and Gynecology
Mercy Suburban Hospital
Norristown, Pennsylvania
Menopause
Osteoporosis

Denise Hartman, MD
Adjunct Assistant Professor
Division of Gynecology
Department of Obstetrics and Gynecology
Temple University School of Medicine
Philadelphia, Pennsylvania
Obstetrician and Gynecologist
and
Division of Gynecology
Department of Obstetrics and Gynecology
Abington Memorial Hospital
Abington, Pennsylvania
Benign Vulvar and Vaginal Lesions
Preoperative Evaluation and Preparation for
   Gynecologic Surgery
Postoperative Care of the Gynecologic Patient

Maria A. Giraldo-Isaza, MD
Department of Obstetrics and Gynecology
Albert Einstein Medical Center
Philadelphia, Pennsylvania
The Puerperium
Genital Tract Infections and Pelvic
   Inflammatory Disease

Namita Kattal, MD
Department of Obstetrics and Gynecology
Albert Einstein Medical Center
Philadelphia, Pennsylvania
Miscarriage, Recurrent Miscarriage, and Pregnancy
   Termination
Family Planning and Sterilization

Radmilla Kazanegra, MD
Gynecologic Endoscopy Fellow
Center for Minimally Invasive Surgery
Stanford University
Palo Alto, California
Ectopic Pregnancy
Hyperandrogenism

Rosanne B. Keep, MS, CGC
Abington Reproductive Medicine, P.C.
Abington IVF & Genetics, LP
Abington, Pennsylvania
Genetics for the Obstetrician

John S. Kukora, MD
Professor of Surgery
Department of Surgery
Drexel University College of Medicine
Philadelphia, Pennsylvania
Chairman
Department of Surgery
Abington Memorial Hospital
Abington, Pennsylvania
Breast Disorders

Richard Latta, MD
Division Director
Maternal Fetal Medicine
Abington Memorial Hospital
Abington, Pennsylvania
Operative Obstetrics

Annette Lee, MD, FACOG
Reproductive Endocrinologist
Abington Reproductive Medicine
Abington, Pennsylvania
Assisted Reproductive Technology

Michael S. Lempel, DO
Obstetrician/Gynecologist
Department of Obstetrics and Gynecology
Potomac Hospital
Woodbridge, Virginia
Antepartum Fetal Monitoring and Fetal Surveillance
Adenomyosis and Endometriosis

Vincent Lucente MD, MBA
Clinical Professor of Obstetrics and Gynecology
Division of Gynecology
Department of Obstetrics and Gynecology
Temple University College of Medicine
Philadelphia, Pennsylvania
Chief of Gynecology
Division of Urogynecology
Department of Obstetrics and Gynecology
St. Luke's Hosptial
Allentown, Pennsylvania
Urinary Tract Injuries
Urinary Incontinence and Urodynamics

Amy Mackey, MD
Department of Obstetrics and Gynecology
Abington Memorial Hospital
Abington, Pennsylvania
Obstetric Complications

Julio Mateus, MD
Maternal Fetal Medicine Fellow
Division of Maternal Fetal Medicine
Department of Obstetrics and Gynecology
University of Texas Medical Branch at Galveston
Galveston, Texas
Breech

Vasiliki A. Moragianni, MD, MSc
Department of Obstetrics and Gynecology
Abington Memorial Hospital
Abington, Pennsylvania
Infertility
GnRH and GnRH Analogs
Laparoscopy and Infertility Surgery

Diane M. Opatt, MD
Clinical Assistant Professor of Surgery
Department of Surgery
Drexel University College of Medicine
Philadelphia, Pennsylvania
Assistant Surgeon
Department of Surgery
Abington Memorial Hospital
Abington, Pennsylvania
Breast Disorders

David Peleg, MD
Department of Obstetrics and Gynecology
Abington Memorial Hospital
Abington, Pennsylvania
First Trimester Ultrasound

Roberto Prieto-Harris, MD
Obstetrician/Gynecologist
Department of Obstetrics and Gynecology
Doctors Hospital at Renaissance
McAllen, Texas
Multiple Gestation

Shai Pri-Paz, MD
Department of Obstetrics and Gynecology
Albert Einstein Medical Center
Philadelphia, Pennsylvania
Hypertension and Pregnancy
Medical and Surgical Complications
    in Pregnancy

Kristen Quinn, MD, MS
Department of Obstetrics and Gynecology
Abington Memorial Hospital
Abington, Pennsylvania
Amniotic Fluid

Jeffrey Sellers, MD
Department of Obstetrics and Gynecology
Abington Memorial Hospital
Abington, Pennsylvania
Functional and Dysfunctional Uterine Bleeding

Dana Shanis, MD
Department of Obstetrics and Gynecology
University of Connecticut Health Center
Farmington, Connecticut
Hypothalamic-Pituitary-Ovarian-Uterine Axis

Ruby Shrestha, MD
Department of Obstetrics and Gynecology
Abington Memorial Hospital
Abington, Pennsylvania
The Placenta and Umbilical Cord

Stephen J. Smith, MD
Assistant Clinical Professor
Division of Maternal-Fetal Medicine
Department of Obstetrics and Gynecology
Abington Memorial Hospital
Abington, Pennsylvania
Postdates Pregnancy and Fetal Demise
Labor Abnormalities

Hima Bindu Tam Tam, MD
Maternal Fetal Medicine Fellow
North Shore University Hospital
Manhasset, New York
Obstetrical Ultrasound and Fetal Abnormalities

Chase M. White, MD
Department of Obstetrics and Gynecology
Albert Einstein Medical Center
Philadelphia, Pennsylvania
Hysterectomy

Emese Zsiros, MD
Department of Obstetrics and Gynecology
Northwestern University's Feinberg School of
    Medicine
Chicago, Illinois
Reproductive Toxicology

INTRODUCTION

Congratulations on your purchase of *Obstetrics and Gynecology Board Review: Pearls of Wisdom* will help you learn some medicine. Originally designed as a study aid to improve performance on the Ob/Gyn Inservice and Written Boards exams, this book is full of useful information. A few words are appropriate discussing intent, format, limitations, and use *Wisdom*, third edition.

Since *Obstetrics and Gynecology Board Review* is primarily intended as a study aid, the text is written in rapid-fire question/answer format. This way, readers receive immediate gratification. Moreover, misleading or confusing "foils" are not provided. This eliminates the risk of erroneously assimilating an incorrect piece of information that makes a big impression. Questions themselves often contain a "pearl" intended to reinforce the answer. Additional "hooks" may be attached to the answer in various forms, including mnemonics, visual imagery, repetition, and humor. Additional information not requested in the question may be included in the answer. Emphasis has been placed on distilling trivia and key facts that are easily overlooked, that are quickly forgotten, and that somehow seem to be needed on board examinations.

Many questions have answers without explanations. This enhances ease of reading and rate of learning. Explanations often occur in a later question/answer. Upon reading an answer, the reader may think, "Hmm, why is that?" or, "Are you sure?" If this happens to you, go check! Truly assimilating these disparate facts into a framework of knowledge absolutely requires further reading of the surrounding concepts. Information learned in response to seeking an answer to a particular question is retained much better than information that is passively observed. Take advantage of this! Use this book with your preferred source texts handy and open.

Obstetrics and Gynecology Board Review has limitations. We have found many conflicts between sources of information. We have tried to verify in several references the most accurate information. Some texts have internal discrepancies further confounding clarification.

Obstetrics and Gynecology Board Review risks accuracy by aggressively pruning complex concepts down to the simplest kernel—the dynamic knowledge base and clinical practice of medicine is not like that! Furthermore, new research and practice occasionally deviates from that which likely represents the right answer for test purposes. This text is designed to maximize your score on a test. Refer to your most current sources of information and mentors for direction for practice. *Obstetrics and Gynecology Board Review* is designed to be used, not just read. It is an *interactive* text. Use a 3 × 5 card and cover the answers; attempt all questions. A study method we recommend is oral, group study, preferably over an extended meal or pitchers. The mechanics of this method are simple and no one ever appears stupid. One person holds this book, with answers covered, and reads the question. Each person, including the reader, says "Check!" when he or she has an answer in mind. After everyone has "checked" in, someone states his/her answer. If this answer is correct, on to the next one; if not, another person says their answer or the answer can be read. Usually the person who "checks" in first receives the first shot at stating the answer. If this person is being a smarty-pants answer-hog, then others can take turns. Try it, it's almost fun!

Obstetrics and Gynecology Board Review is also designed to be re-used several times to allow, dare we use the word, memorization. A hollow bullet is provided for any scheme of keeping track of questions answered correctly or incorrectly.

We welcome your comments, suggestions and criticism. Great effort has been made to verify these questions and answers. Some answers may not be the answer you would prefer. Most often this is attributable to variance between original sources. Please make us aware of any errors you find. We hope to make continuous improvements and would greatly appreciate any input with regard to format, organization, content, presentation, or about specific questions. We look forward to hearing from you!

Study hard and good luck!

S.G.S.

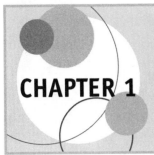

CHAPTER 1

Anatomy of the Pelvis and Reproductive Tract

Miki Chiguchi, MD

○ **Where are Gartner ducts located?**
In the lateral walls of the vagina.

○ **Gartner duct cysts are persistent portions of what embryonic structure?**
Mesonephric duct.

○ **The portion of the gubernaculum between the ovary and uterus becomes what structure?**
The ligament of the ovary (utero-ovarian ligament).

○ **The portion of the gubernaculum between the uterus and the labium majus becomes what structure?**
The round ligament.

○ **Failure of the development of adhesions between the uterus and what structure can result in the ovary migrating through the inguinal canal to the labium majus?**
The gubernaculum.

○ **What is the name of a pouch of peritoneum analogous to the saccus vaginalis in the male, which accompanies the gubernaculum in the inguinal canal?**
The canal of Nuck.

○ **Name the three coats of the ureter.**
Fibrous, muscular, mucosal.

○ **The epithelium lining the ureter is of what type?**
Transitional.

○ **Name the vessels that send branches to the ureter.**
Renal, ovarian, common iliac, hypogastric, uteric, vaginal, vesical middle hemorrhoidal, and superior gluteal arteries.

○   **Innervation of the ureter is derived from what nerve plexuses?**

Inferior mesenteric, ovarian, and pelvic.

○   **What are the attachments between the female bladder and the pubic bone called?**

The pubovesical ligaments.

○   **Name the four layers of the bladder.**

Serosa, muscular, submucosa, mucosa.

○   **What arteries supply the female bladder?**

Superior, middle and inferior vesicle, obturator, inferior gluteal, uterine, and vaginal arteries.

○   **Name the three layers of the urethra.**

Muscular, erectile, mucosa.

○   **What type of epithelium lines the urethra?**

Distal 1/2—stratified squamous epithelium, which becomes transitional near the bladder (proximal 2/3).

○   **The aorta lies at what spinal level?**

L4.

○   **What are the branches of the hypogastric (internal iliac) artery?**

Posterior branch: Iliolumbar, lateral sacral, superior gluteal

Anterior branch: Obturator, internal pudendal, inferior gluteal, umbilical, middle vesicle, inferior vesicle, middle hemorrhoidal, uterine, vaginal.

○   **Arterial blood supply to the uterus is derived from what arteries?**

Uterine and ovarian arteries. The uterine artery arises from the hypogastric. The ovarian artery directly from the aorta.

○   **Name the visceral branches of the internal iliac artery.**

Umbilical, inferior vesicle, middle vesicle, middle rectal, uterine, vaginal.

○   **What are the arcuate arteries?**

Branches of the uterine artery that unite with the opposite uterine artery. They supply the radial branches to the myometrium and basalis layer of endometrium. They also become the spiral arteries of the functional endometrium.

○   **What is the terminal branch of the hypogastric artery?**

Internal pudendal artery.

○ **What does the internal pudendal artery supply?**

The rectum, labia, clitoris, perineum.

○ **Name the parietal branches of the internal iliac artery.**

Obturator, internal pudendal, iliolumbar, lateral sacral, superior gluteal, inferior gluteal.

○ **Describe the anatomic relationship between the uterine artery and the ureter when they are at their closest position in relationship to the cervix.**

Approximately 2 cm from the cervix the uterine artery crosses above and in front of the ureter.

○ **Branches of the uterine and vaginal arteries anastomose forming median longitudinal vessels known as what arteries?**

Azygous arteries of the vagina.

○ **Name the artery from which the deep and dorsal arteries of the clitoris arise.**

Internal pudendal artery.

○ **The right ovarian vein opens into what structure?**

The inferior vena cava.

○ **The left ovarian vein flows into what structure?**

Left renal vein.

○ **Name the vein that begins near the upper part of the greater sciatic foramen and passes upward and backward in the pelvis.**

Internal iliac vein.

○ **Name the posterior branch of the hypogastric artery, which is responsible for gluteal ischemia at the time of hypogastric artery ligation.**

Superior gluteal artery.

○ **Name the main tributaries of the external iliac vein.**

Inferior epigastric, deep circumflex, and pubic veins.

○ **The ovarian arteries arise from what structure?**

The aorta.

○ **The inferior epigastric artery is one of the two main branches of what artery?**

The external iliac artery.

○ **The artery of the round ligament is a branch of what artery?**
Inferior epigastric artery.

○ **What structure crosses the obturator artery medially?**
Ureter.

○ **Where does the inferior mesenteric artery arise?**
3 cm above the aortic bifurcation.

○ **What does the inferior mesenteric artery supply?**
Parts of the transverse colon, descending colon, sigmoid, rectum, and it becomes the superior hemorrhoidal.

○ **The external iliac nodes receive afferent vessels from what regions?**
Lower extremity, lower anterior abdominal wall, perineum, pelvis.

○ **Where are the common iliac nodes located?**
Medial, lateral, and posterior to the common iliac vessels extending from the external iliac nodes to the bifurcation of the aorta.

○ **The internal iliac nodes receive lymphatics from what areas?**
Drainage corresponds to the branches of the internal iliac arteries.

○ **Efferent lymphatic vessels from the cervix course to what nodes?**
Laterally to the external iliac nodes, posteriolaterally to the internal iliac nodes, posteriorly to the common iliac and lateral sacral nodes.

○ **The majority of the lymphatic vessels of the fundal corpus of the uterus drain into what nodes?**
Internal iliac nodes primarily; also aortic, lumbar, pelvic.

○ **The upper vagina has lymphatic drainage to what nodes?**
External and internal iliac nodes.

○ **Lymphatic vessels from the middle region of the vagina terminate in what nodes?**
Internal iliac nodes.

○ **Lymphatic drainage from the vaginal orifice and vulva may terminate in what group of nodes?**
Superficial inguinal nodes.

○ **The superficial lymphatic vessels in the anal region course to what group of nodes?**
Superficial inguinal nodes.

○ **Lymphatic drainage deep in the ischiorectal fossa is to what group of nodes?**

Internal iliac nodes.

○ **Lymphatic drainage of the ovaries follows the course of the ovarian arteries to what groups of nodes?**

Lateral and preaortic lumbar nodes.

○ **Lymphatic drainage of the upper and middle portions of the fallopian tube is to what nodes?**

Lateral and preaortic lumbar nodes.

○ **Lymphatic drainage of the lower portion of the fallopian tube is to what nodes?**

Internal iliac and superficial inguinal nodes.

○ **Describe the autonomic innervations of the pelvis.**

The superior hypogastric plexus divided to form the two hypogastric nerves, which fan out to form the inferior hypogastric plexus.

○ **Name the three portions that the inferior hypogastric plexus (pelvic plexus) is divided into.**

The vesical plexus, uterovaginal plexus (Frankenhäuser ganglion), and the middle rectal plexus.

○ **What is Frankenhäuser plexus?**

An extensive concentration of both myelinated and nonmyelinated nerve fibers located in the uterosacral ligaments and supplying primarily the uterus and the cervix.

○ **Innervation of the urinary bladder is provided by what structures?**

Fibers from the third and the fourth sacral nerves and fibers from the hypogastric plexus.

○ **What is another name for the superior hypogastric plexus?**

Presacral nerve.

○ **Where is the presacral nerve located?**

It lies in the subserous fascia under the parietal peritoneum and extends from the level of the fourth lumbar to the first sacral vertebrae.

○ **Name the three supportive layers of the pelvic floor.**

Endopelvic fascia, levator ani muscles, and perineal membrane/external anal sphincter.

○ **Name the external genital muscles whose primary function appears to be sexual response.**

Ischiocavernosus, bulbocavernosus, and superficial transverse perineal muscles.

○ **What constitutes the pelvic diaphragm?**

Levator ani muscles and their superior and inferior fasciae.

○ **What is the anterior midline cleft in the pelvic diaphragm called?**

Urogenital hiatus.

○ **What structures pass through the urogenital hiatus?**

Urethra, vagina, and rectum.

○ **The broad sheet of endopelvic fascia that attaches the upper vagina, cervix, and uterus to the pelvic sidewalls is known by what name?**

Cardinal and uterosacral ligaments.

○ **What two muscles constitute the levator ani muscle?**

Pubococcygeus and iliococcygeus muscles.

○ **Innervation of the levator ani is from which nerves?**

Fourth sacral (sometimes, also, third or fifth sacral).

○ **Name five arteries that supply the rectum.**

1, superior hemorrhoidal artery; 2, two middle hemorrhoidal arteries; 3, two inferior hemorrhoidal arteries (see figure below).

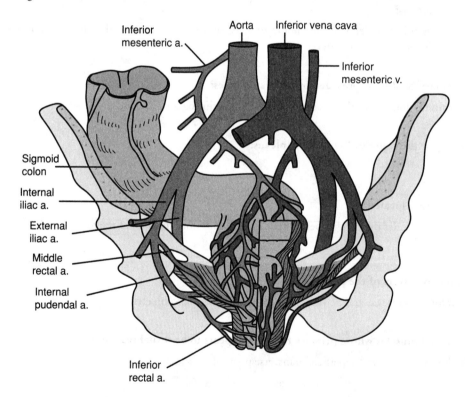

○ **Arterial blood supply to the female urethra arises from what structures?**

Inferior vesicle and internal pudendal arteries.

○ **Where does the innervation of the urethra develop?**

Pudendal nerves and pelvic plexuses.

○ **What is the name of the ovarian venous plexus?**

Pampiniform plexus.

○ **The whitish folded scar on the ovary resulting from regression of a corpus luteum is known as?**

Corpus albicans.

○ **A mass of cells on one side of a mature follicle protruding into the cavity is known by what term?**

Cumulus oophorus.

○ **The surface stroma of the ovary composed of short connective tissue fibers with fusiform cells between them is known by what name?**

Tunica albuginea.

○ **What name is given to the highest of the deep inguinal lymph nodes located in the lateral part of the femoral ring?**

Cloquet node.

○ **Where is the epoophoron (parovarian) located?**

In the mesosalpinx between the ovary and the tube.

○ **The greater vestibular glands are also known by what name?**

Bartholin glands.

○ **Where are Bartholin glands located?**

4 and 8 o'clock. They drain between the hymenal ring and labia minora.

○ **What structure is responsible for hemorrhage associated with removal of Bartholin cyst?**

The vestibular bulb.

○ **The Bartholin glands are the female homolog of what male structure?**

Cowper bulbourethral glands.

○ **Infected Bartholin glands may cause enlargement of what lymph nodes?**

Inguinal or external iliac nodes.

○ **What is the vestibule of the vagina?**

The cleft between the labia minora and the glans of the clitoris.

○   **In a virgin, the labia minora are usually joined across the midline by a fold of skin known by what term?**
Frenulum of the labia or fourchette.

○   **What is the normal weight of the non-gravid uterus?**
40 to 50 g.

○   **A retroflexed uterus is a normal variant found in what percentage of women?**
20% to 25%.

○   **Which nerve roots do the sensory fibers from the uterus enter?**
T11 and T12. Referred uterine pain is often located in the lower abdomen.

○   **Which nerve roots do the sensory fibers from the cervix enter?**
S2, S3, and S4. Referred pain from cervical inflammation is characterized as low back pain.

○   **What is the name of the slight constriction between the cervix and corpus of the uterus?**
Isthmus.

○   **Name the three portions of the fallopian tube external to the uterus.**
The proximal 1/3 is the isthmus, the medial 1/3 is the ampulla, the distal 1/3 is the infundibulum.

○   **Appendices vesiculosae of the tube are also known by what name?**
Hydatids of Morgagni.

○   **What covers the surfaces of the broad ligaments?**
Peritoneum.

○   **What structures are the boundaries of the cul-de-sac of Douglas?**
Ventrally, the supravaginal cervix and posterior fornix of the vagina; dorsally, the rectum; laterally, the uterosacral ligaments.

○   **What is the myometrium?**
The muscular wall of the uterus.

○   **What structures found in the labia majora are not found in the labia minora?**
Hair follicles.

○   **The primary tissue found in the mons pubis is what type of tissue?**
Adipose.

○   **Innervation of the uterus is primarily from where?**
Hypogastric and ovarian plexuses and the third and fourth sacral nerves.

○   **From where does the innervation of the vagina arise?**
Vaginal plexus and pudendal nerves.

○   **Name three branches of pudendal nerves and vessels.**
(1) Clitoral; (2) perineal; (3) inferior hemorrhoidal.

○   **What is the male homolog of the clitoris?**
Penis.

○   **By what cellular processes does the gravid uterus enlarge?**
Hypertrophy and hyperplasia.

○   **Skene glands are also known by what name?**
Paraurethral glands.

○   **Where are Skene glands located?**
Adjacent to the urethral opening.

○   **Skene glands are considered the homologs of what male structures?**
Prostatic glands.

○   **Which has a greater diameter, the abdominal portion or pelvic portion of the ureter?**
The abdominal (10 mm vs 5 mm).

○   **In the female bladder attachments directly between the bladder and pubic bone are known by what name?**
Pubovesical ligaments.

○   **The median umbilical ligament is the remnant of what structure?**
Urachus.

○   **The anterior angle of the trigone is formed by what?**
Internal orifices of the urethra.

○   **The posteriolateral angles of the trigone are formed by what?**
Orifices of the ureters.

○   **In the contracted bladder, the ureteral orifices are approximately how far apart?**
2.5 cm.

○   **Where in the female is the bulbospongiosus muscle located?**
Surrounding the lower end of the vagina.

○   **What is the blood supply to the vagina?**

It is an extensive network. The vaginal artery arises either directly from the uterine or from the internal iliac and also from the azygous arteries anastomosing from the cervical branch of the uterine.

○   **Name the four layers of the vagina.**

The mucosa—a stratified, nonkeratinized squamous epithelium.

The lamina tunica—a fibrous connective tissue.

The muscle layer—an inner circular layer and an outer longitudinal layer.

The cellular areolar connective tissue.

○   **What is the sensory innervation to the vagina?**

Pudendal nerve (S2–S4).

○   **Describe where the primary lymph drainage from the vagina goes to?**

Upper 1/3—external iliac.

Middle 1/3—common/internal iliac.

Lower 1/3—common iliac, superficial inguinal, perirectal.

○   **What is the average length of the endocervical canal?**

2.5 to 3 cm.

○   **What are the longitudinal folds in the mucous membrane of the endocervical canal called?**

Plicae palmatae.

○   **What is the arterial supply to the uterus?**

Cervical artery arises from the uterine artery. The cervical arteries approach the cervix at 3 and 9 o'clock.

○   **Name all the surgical cleavage spaces (7, 8, 9, 10, 11, and 12) that are filled with fatty or areolar connective tissue?**

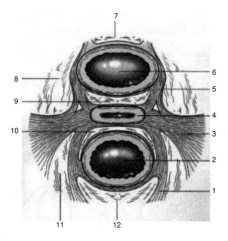

1	Uterosacral ligament
2	Rectum
3	Cardinal ligament
4	Vagina
5	Bladder pillar
6	Urinary bladder
7	
8	
9	
10	
11	
12	

7, prevesical space; 8, paravesical space; 9, vesicovaginal space; 10, rectovaginal space; 11, pararectal space; 12, retrorectal space.

○   **What is the name of the artery that supplies the round ligament?**

Sampson artery.

○   **How many oocytes are present in the human ovary at birth?**

1 to 2 million.

○   **How many oocytes eventually ovulate?**

Approximately 300 to 400.

○   **What is the venous drainage from the ovaries?**

The pampiniform plexus to the ovarian vein.

○   **Name the spinal segments on dermatome below.**

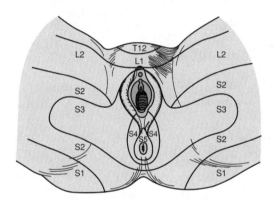

A, L2; B, S2; C, S3; D, S1.

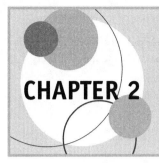

CHAPTER 2

Embryology of the Genital Tract

Rachael Cohen, DO

○ **At what gestational age are the gonadal ridges develop?**
Approximately 5 weeks.

○ **What are the direct precursors to the human sperm and ova?**
Germ cells.

○ **If the indifferent gonad is destined to become a testis, at what gestational age will differentiation occur?**
6 to 9 weeks gestation.

○ **Are primitive germ cells able to survive in any location other than the gonadal ridge?**
No.

○ **What are the three major anatomic parts of the ovary?**
The outer cortex, the medulla, and the hilum.

○ **Which portion of the ovary contains the oocytes?**
The inner portion of the cortex.

○ **What is the factor that determines if an indifferent gonad will become a testis?**
Testes-determining factor (TDF). TDF is a product of a gene located on the Y chromosome in the region of SRY.

○ **What is the function of anti-Müllerian hormone?**
Anti-Müllerian hormone inhibits the formation of Müllerian ducts. It is secreted at approximately 7 weeks gestation, when sertoli cell differentiation occurs.

○ **Name three functions of anti-Müllerian hormone (AMH)?**
AMH exerts an inhibitory effect on oocyte meiosis, helps to control the descent of the testes, and inhibits surfactant accumulation in the lungs.

○ **Is anti-Müllerian hormone completely absent in the female?**

No. AMH is not expressed prior to birth to ensure normal female differentiation. After puberty, AMH is produced and secreted by granulosa cells from small growing ovarian follicles and acts as a paracrine inhibitory factor.

○ **In which cells is inhibin produced?**

Sertoli cells.

○ **Which cells produce testosterone?**

Leydig cells.

○ **Do hCG levels remain constant in the fetus throughout gestation?**

No. hCG levels are similar in the fetus to levels in maternal circulation, peaking at 10 weeks and reaching a nadir at approximately 20 weeks.

○ **The loss of the Wolffian system in the female (including the epididymis, vas deferens, and seminal vesicle) is because of the lack of which hormone?**

Testosterone.

○ **Is the oogonal content of the ovary constant throughout gestation?**

No. Maximal oogonal content occurs during 16 to 20 weeks gestation, containing 6 to 7 million oogonia.

○ **What is the total cortical content of oogonia at the time of birth?**

Only 1 to 2 million as a result of the depletion of oocytes during fetal life.

○ **At which stage of meiosis I, do the oocytes arrest?**

Prophase.

○ **At what time is meiosis II complete, resulting in the haploid ovum?**

Fertilization.

○ **What is the mechanism of the loss of oocytes during the second half of pregnancy?**

Oocytes are lost after 20 weeks gestation as a result of follicular growth and subsequent atresia, as well as degeneration of oogonia not surrounded by granulosa cells. Also, germ cells that migrate to the surface of the ovary are lost in the peritoneal cavity.

○ **Is there any chromosome anomaly that accelerates the process of germ cell loss?**

Yes. Turner syndrome (45,X) is characterized by a fibrous streak of ovarian tissue, which lacks follicles.

○ **Do individuals with Turner syndrome (45,X) have germ cells, which undergo mitosis and meiosis?**

Turner syndrome patients have germ cells, which undergo mitosis, but oogonia do not undergo meiosis.

○ **Do individuals with Turner syndrome (45,X) have any follicles at birth?**

No.

○ **What are the characteristic findings in someone with Turner syndrome?**

The characteristic findings include short stature, streak gonads, webbed neck, high arched palate, cubitus valgus, shield-like chest with wide spaced nipples, low hairline on the neck, short 4th metacarpal bones, renal abnormalities, and coarctation of the aorta.

○ **What should one be suspicious for in an individual with 45,X karyotype with breast development or pubic/axillary hair development without exogenous therapy?**

Gonadoblastoma or dysgerminoma.

○ **What is the primordial follicle?**

An oocyte, which is arrested in prophase of meiosis, surrounded by a layer of pre-granulosa cells and a basement membrane.

○ **Does the development of a normal female phenotype require fetal estrogen production?**

No.

○ **What is the most common cause of an abdominal mass in a female fetus or newborn?**

Ovarian cysts.

○ **What are female infants FSH values up to a year of life?**

FSH levels in infants are higher than normal adult levels during a menstrual cycle. FSH levels then decrease to low levels by 1 year.

○ **Before puberty, is the ovary in the female quiescent?**

No. Follicles begin to grow and frequently reach the antral stage.

○ **What is the content of germ cells at the onset of puberty?**

300,000 to 500,000.

○ **Is the rate of follicular loss constant throughout adulthood?**

No. Loss is accelerated as adults approach menopause.

○ **The fusion of the Müllerian ducts by the tenth week of gestation is responsible for the formation of which portions of the female genital tract?**

The Müllerian duct fusion results in the uterus, tubes, and upper third of the vagina.

○ **What is the result if the germ cells fail to reach the genital ridges by the sixth week of gestation?**

Gonads will not develop, resulting in gonadal dysgenesis.

○ **What is the dense layer of tissue that separates the testicular cords from the surface epithelium?**

The tunica albigenea.

○ **What structure is formed when the Müllerian ducts reach the midline and form a broad transverse pelvic fold?**

The broad ligament of the uterus.

○ **What is the origin of a Gartner duct cyst?**

A Gartner duct cyst results from a Wolffian duct remnant, which may be seen in the wall of the vagina or the uterus.

○ **What is the name of the indifferent structure, which later divides into the anorectal canal and the urogenital sinus?**

The cloaca.

○ **What are the swellings on each side of the urethral fold that later develop into the scrotum in the male and labia majora in the female?**

Genital swellings.

○ **How does the phallus develop?**

Rapid elongation of the genital tubercle.

○ **Are the scrotal swellings in the male developed outside the abdominal cavity?**

No. The scrotal swellings are located initially in the inguinal region and then migrate caudally.

○ **What is the origin of the clitoris?**

The genital tubercle. In the female, the genital tubercle elongates only slightly resulting in the clitoris.

○ **What is the origin of the labia minora?**

Urethral folds.

○ **What is the gubernaculum testis?**

The gubernaculum testis is the column of mesenchyme that extends from the caudal pole of the testis to the genital swelling.

○ **Is the descent of the testis under any hormonal influence?**

Yes. The descent of the testis is influenced by androgens and gonadotropins.

○ **Describe complete androgen insensitivity (testicular feminization)?**

This condition is because of congenital insensitivity to androgens and is maternal X-linked recessive. People with this disorder have a female phenotype with a normal male karyotype (46,XY). The vagina is short and ends blindly, the uterus and tubes are absent, and the testes are normally developed but abnormally positioned.

○ **What percentage of primary amenorrhea is caused by androgen insensitivity?**

10%.

○ **Name the two conditions that present with a normal appearing female but an absent uterus? How are they differentiated?**

The two conditions are androgen insensitivity and Müllerian agenesis (Mayer-Rokitansky-Küster-Hauser syndrome). They are easily differentiated because the later condition is found to have a 46,XX karyotype with normal hair growth.

○ **Are the testes in patients with testicular feminization capable of spermatogenesis?**

No.

○ **Should the testes in patients with testicular feminization be surgically removed?**

Yes. The testes in these patients are at increased risk for developing tumors. The recommendation is for removal following puberty between 16 and 18 years.

○ **What is the diagnosis characterized by development of both active ovarian and testicular tissue?**

True hermaphroditism.

○ **What percentage of true hermaphrodites are genetic females?**

70%.

○ **What develops in the male if fusion of the urethral folds is incomplete, resulting in abnormal openings along the inferior aspect of the penis?**

Hypospadias.

○ **What is the result in the male if the gubernaculum fails to shorten and/or there is abnormal androgen production?**

Cryptorchism.

○ **If the caudal portions of the Müllerian ducts fail to fuse along the entire length, what uterine anomaly will result?**

Uterus didelphys.

○ **What condition is characterized by the uterus with two horns and a common vagina?**

Bicornuate uterus.

○ **At what gestational age does the fetus produce testosterone?**

8 weeks.

○ **What happens to excess genetic material as the oocytes progress through meiotic divisions during ovulation and later fertilization?**

Excess genetic material is extruded as polar bodies.

○ **What is the chromosomal content of the primary oocyte arrested in the diplotene stage prior to ovulation?**
46 chromosomes.

○ **What is the chromosomal content of a mature oocyte after completion of meiosis II?**
23 chromosomes.

○ **Does the cycle of follicle formation, ripening, and atresia occur in the fetus?**
Yes, however, ovulation does not occur.

○ **Does the Müllerian duct development depend on fetal gonadal steroid production?**
No. The Müllerian duct development is independent of the ovary.

○ **Is the fetal hypothalamic-pituitary portal circulation functional?**
Yes, the fetal hypothalamic-pituitary portal circulation is functional by the 12th week of gestation.

○ **Do both males and females have both the Wolffian ducts and Müllerian ducts present at any time?**
Yes. Both systems temporarily coexist until 8 weeks gestation.

○ **Name the three stages of renal development?**
Pronephric, mesonephric, metanephric.

○ **Are abnormalities in the development of tubes, uterus, and upper vagina associated with congenital abnormalities in any other organ system?**
Yes. These abnormalities are associated with abnormalities in the renal system, as they both require the appearance of the mesonephric ducts.

○ **In the absence of any gonad, what type of development will occur?**
Internal genitalia have intrinsic tendency to feminize, as Müllerian duct development will occur.

○ **The proliferation of the sinovaginal bulbs results in what portion of the female genital tract?**
Vagina.

○ **By what process do germ cells become oogonia?**
Mitosis.

○ **After mitosis, what is required for an oocyte to become a single ovum?**
Two meiotic divisions are required with the first at ovulation and the second at fertilization.

○ **Do male germ cells begin meiotic division prior to puberty?**
No.

○ **Do Leydig cell numbers remain constant throughout fetal life?**

No. Leydig cell numbers peak during 15 to 18 weeks.

○ **What is the tunica albigenea?**

The outermost portion of the ovarian cortex.

○ **What are the components of the urogenital ridge?**

Mesonephric duct and genital ridge.

○ **Do germ cells migrate from the yolk sac?**

Yes. Germ cells migrate through the hindgut to their gonadal sites between 4 and 6 weeks gestation.

○ **Do germ cells have the ability to proliferate during their migration?**

Yes. The germ cells multiply by mitosis during migration.

○ **What is the function of androgen binding protein?**

Androgen binding protein maintains the high androgen environment, necessary for spermatogenesis.

○ **How do fetal Leydig cells respond to high levels of hormones?**

Fetal Leydig cells respond to high levels of hCG and LH by increasing steroidogenesis and cell multiplication.

○ **Do adult Leydig cells respond to the same hormonal regulation as fetal cells?**

No. Adult Leydig cells are controlled by down regulation in response to high levels of hCG and LH.

○ **Which cells surround fetal spermatogonia?**

Sertoli cells.

○ **Does development of male external genitalia depend on testosterone?**

No. Development of the urogenital sinus and urogenital tubercle into male external genitalia, urethra, and prostate require conversion of testosterone to DHT.

○ **In females, androgen exposure at what gestation period may cause external ambiguity of the female phenotype?**

9 to 14 weeks gestation.

○ **Name the four enzymatic defects associated with congenital adrenal hyperplasia?**

21-hydroxylase, 3β-hydroxylase, 3β-hydroxysteroid dehydrogenase, and rarely 17α-hydroxylase.

○ **What is Swyer syndrome?**

Swyer syndrome is characterized by bilateral dysgenesis of the testes caused by a mutation of the SRY gene. They are found to have an XY karyotype with normal infantile female external and internal genitalia.

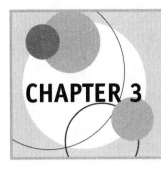

CHAPTER 3

Physiology of Normal Pregnancy

Rachael Cohen, DO

○ **What percentage of human chorionic gonadotropin (hCG) is carbohydrate?**

30%; it has the most CHO content of all human hormones.

○ **What is the plasma half-life of intact hCG?**

24 hours.

○ **hCG is structurally related to what three other glycoprotein hormones?**

LH, FSH, TSH.

○ **How are the four hormones—hCG, LH, FSH, and TSH—related?**

Each has an identical alpha subunit with a unique beta subunit.

○ **What chromosome codes for the alpha subunit of hCG?**

Chromosome 6 q12-q21 (a single gene).

○ **What chromosome codes for the beta subunit of hCG?**

Chromosome 19 (seven separate genes).

○ **What is the major source of hCG?**

Placenta-syncytiotrophoblast.

○ **At what gestational age does hCG peak?**

8 to 10 weeks.

○ **What is a blood pregnancy test measuring?**

The beta subunit of the intact hCG molecule.

○ **When is hCG detectable in plasma of pregnant women?**

8 to 9 days after ovulation. It is likely that it enters blood at the time of implantation.

○ **List four physiologic actions of hCG?**

(1) Maintenance of corpus luteum and continued progesterone production.

(2) Stimulation of fetal testicular testosterone secretion promoting male sexual differentiation.

(3) Stimulation of the maternal thyroid by binding to TSH receptors as its alpha subunit is identical.

(4) Promotion of relaxin secretion by the corpus luteum.

○ **Where can relaxin production be found other than by the corpus luteum?**

Relaxin is also produced by the placenta and myometrium.

○ **What is the most produced substance by the placenta?**

Human placental lactogen (hPL), otherwise known as human chorionic somatomammotropin (hCS) is produced in amounts as high as 1 to 4 g/d.

○ **What are the functions of human placental lactogen?**

(1) Lipolysis and an increase in the levels of circulating free fatty acids.

(2) Anti-insulin action leading to an increase in maternal levels of insulin providing mobilized sugars and amino acids.

○ **Is human placental lactogen required for successful pregnancy?**

No. Probably is a back up mechanism to ensure fetal nutrient supply.

○ **What other two hormones are homologous to hPL?**

Growth hormone (96% homology) and prolactin (67% homology).

○ **Where is hPL produced?**

Cytotrophoblast and syncytiotrophoblast.

○ **What is the biologic half-life of hPL?**

15 min.

○ **When does the corpus luteum stop producing progesterone in pregnancy?**

7 to 8 weeks of gestation.

○ **Name two consequences of excessive luteinization of the ovary?**

This may result in theca lutein cysts or a pregnancy luteoma.

○ **What is the daily rate of progesterone production in third trimester singleton pregnancy?**

250 mg/d.

○ **How is progesterone synthesized in the human placenta?**

Two step reaction. Cholesterol is converted to pregnenolone in mitochondria by cytochrome P450 side chain cleavage enzyme. Pregnenolone is converted to progesterone in microsomes by 3β-hydroxysteroid dehydrogenase, δ 5-4 isomerase.

○ **What is the primary source of cholesterol for placental progesterone synthesis?**

Maternal plasma LDL cholesterol (90%).

○ **What is the principal estrogen found in the plasma and urine of pregnant women?**

Estriol.

○ **Which hormone is decreased significantly after fetal death, umbilical cord ligation, and in anencephalic fetuses?**

Estrogen. However, measurements of estriol to predict fetuses at risk have not been shown to change perinatal morbidity or mortality.

○ **What is the average weight and volume of the nonpregnant uterus?**

Average weight is 40 to 70 g with a volume of 10 mL.

○ **What is the average weight and volume of the pregnant uterus at term?**

Average weight is 1100 to 1200 g with a volume of 5 L.

○ **What types of cellular changes occur during uterine enlargement in pregnancy?**

Hypertrophy and stretching of existing muscle. Hyperplasia is very limited. Hypertrophy results from the actions of estrogen and progesterone and occurs mostly before 12 weeks. The increase in uterine size after 12 weeks results from pressure from expanding products of conception.

○ **How many layers of muscle are in the uterus? Describe them.**

Three:
(1) An external layer that arches over the fundus to insert into the various ligaments.
(2) A middle layer of multidirectional interlacing muscle fibers between which extend blood vessels.
(3) An inner layer consisting of sphincter like fibers around the orifices of the tubes and internal os.

○ **What increased concentration of oxytocin receptors is found in the myometrium during pregnancy at term?**

They are found to increase 300-fold as compared to prepregnancy.

○ **At what gestational age does the uterus rise out of the pelvis?**

Approximately 12 weeks.

○ **During a term cesarian section you are examining the uterus before making the uterine incision. What direction of rotation are you most likely to see?**

Dextrorotation (to the right)—usually results from the presence of the rectosigmoid.

○ **In late pregnancy, what is the approximate rate of blood flow to the uterus?**

450 to 650 mL/min.

○ **What are the three substances thought to take part in the regulation of uterine blood flow during pregnancy and what are their effects on the uterine flow?**

(1) Estrogen—vasodilation.

(2) Catecholamines—increased sensitivity even when controlled for blood pressure.

(3) Angiotensin II—vascular refractoriness.

○ **At term, what percentage of uterine blood flow is directed toward the placenta?**

80% to 90%.

○ **What mechanism is responsible for the increased maternal-placental and fetal-placental blood flow in pregnancy?**

Maternal-placental is principally caused by vasodilation of existing vessels. Fetal-placental is principally caused by increasing numbers of placental vessels.

○ **During a strong contraction (50 mm Hg), by how much is uterine blood flow reduced?**

60%.

○ **What are the normal physical changes in the cervix during pregnancy?**

Softening and cyanosis. This is known as Goodell's sign.

○ **What is Chadwick's sign?**

This is described as a bluish discoloration of vagina.

○ **Microscopically, how are the cervical changes during pregnancy manifested?**

Increased vascularity and edema with hypertrophy and hyperplasia of cervical glands.

○ **What fraction of the cervical mass is composed of glands in the pregnant state?**

50%.

○ **What is the term for the normal eversion of the endocervical glands out to the ectocervix during pregnancy?**

Ectropion.

○ **What are the changes in cervical mucus that occur in pregnancy?**

Thick tenacious mucus forms a plug blocking the cervical canal, thus, preventing ascending infection (important in evaluating patients for pelvic inflammatory disease).

○ **What percentage of sodium chloride is necessary in the cervical mucus to develop a full ferning (arborization) pattern when dried on a slide?**

1%.

○ **What pattern is most likely seen on a slide of dried cervical mucus during pregnancy?**

Fragmentary crystallization or beading typical of the effect of progesterone-sodium chloride concentration, which is usually less than 1% during pregnancy.

○ **Does the strength of the cervix decrease during pregnancy?**

Yes, collagen is rearranged to produce a 12-fold reduction in mechanical strength.

○ **Describe the changes in vaginal secretions in pregnancy?**

Increased cervical and vaginal secretions result in thick, white, odorless discharge. The pH is between 3.5 and 6.0 resulting from increased production of lactic acid from the action of *Lactobacillus acidophilus*.

○ **What is the proposed mechanism for the increased pigmentation of skin found in pregnancy and give two examples.**

Melanocyte stimulating hormone (MSH) is elevated from the end of the second month of pregnancy to term. Estrogen and progesterone may have melanocyte stimulating properties. Estrogen and progesterone may also stimulate the hypertrophy of the intermediate lobe of the pituitary, which is where MSH and β-endorphin are formed from the metabolism of pro-opiomelanocortin. Two examples are the linea nigra and the melasma gravidarum.

○ **What are the glands of Montgomery?**

Normal finding of hypertrophic sebaceous glands scattered throughout the areola of a pregnant woman's breast.

○ **What is the average weight gain in pregnancy?**

11 kg (25 lb).

○ **What percentage of maternal weight gain is contributed by the fetus and placenta at term?**

Approximately 30%.

○ **What percentage of maternal weight gain is contributed by blood, amniotic fluid, and extravascular fluid at term?**

Approximately 30%.

○ **What percentage of maternal weight gain is contributed by maternal fat?**

30%.

○ **At term, what is the water content in liters of the fetus, placenta, and amniotic fluid?**

3.5 L.

○ **What is the total amount of extra water that a pregnant woman retains during normal pregnancy?**

6.5 L total—3.5 L for the fetus, placenta, and amniotic fluid and 3.0 L for the increased volume of blood, uterus, and breasts.

○ **Why do water retention, a normal physiological alteration of pregnancy, and edema occur in normal pregnancy?**

Fall in plasma osmolality of 10 mOsm/kg. Prepregnancy plasma osmolality is approximately 290 mOsm/kg. At 4 weeks, it starts to drop and by 8 weeks, it plateaus to approximately 280 mOsm/kg.

○ **Describe the utility of increased body protein during pregnancy?**

One half of the normal increase in body protein during pregnancy (500 g) is contained in the fetus and placenta. The other 500 g of protein is incorporated in contractile proteins in the uterus, glands of the breast, maternal blood proteins, and hemoglobin.

○ **In a healthy pregnant woman, what happens to the fasting plasma glucose level and why?**

It is decreased by 8 to 10 mg/dL in the first trimester with little change after that. This negates fetal demand as the cause, and therefore, it is probably a dilutional effect.

○ **In a healthy pregnant woman, how long does it take to return to fasting glucose levels after a glucose load?**

The levels peak later (55 min when pregnant vs 30 min when not) and remain elevated longer, thereby prolonging the return to fasting level to approximately 2 hours (usually 1 hour in nonpregnant patients).

○ **What is the state of carbohydrate metabolism in normal pregnancy in terms of fasting glucose, postprandial glucose, insulin levels, and insulin resistance?**

Mild fasting hypoglycemia, postprandial hyperglycemia, hyperinsulinemia, and increased insulin resistance.

○ **What are the changes in the pancreas seen in normal pregnancy?**

Beta cell hypertrophy, hyperplasia, and hypersecretion.

○ **In a normal pregnancy, what effect does a glucose stimulus have on glucagon levels?**

Plasma glucagon levels are suppressed.

○ **What is the general trend of serum lipid concentrations in pregnancy?**

Increase continuously throughout gestation. This includes triglycerides, cholesterol, phopholipids, and fatty acids.

○ **At what gestational age does LDL and HDL cholesterol peak in pregnancy?**

36 and 30 weeks respectively.

○ **Are pregnant women more likely to become ketonuric after starvation compared to nonpregnant women?**

Yes. Because there are higher concentrations of lipids and lower concentrations of glucose during fasting. The lipids are preferentially metabolized to ketones. This is known as accelerated starvation.

○ **What is the effect of pregnancy on folate and B_{12} levels?**

Both levels decrease (there is wide variation).

○ **What is the effect of pregnancy on erythropoetin levels?**

There is a steady increase causing increased red cell mass. This is a paradoxical finding because erythropoetin is stimulated by tissue hypoxemia. Hypoxemia is unusual during normal pregnancy because there is more total circulating hemoglobin, better oxygen carrying capacity, and a reduced arteriovenous oxygen difference at the heart (better oxygenated blood is returned to the heart).

○ **What is the general effect of pregnancy on electrolyte concentrations?**

Sodium, potassium, calcium, magnesium, and zinc are all mildly decreased by no greater than approximately 10% of nonpregnant levels.

○ **What is the effect of pregnancy on copper concentrations in serum?**

Increases from approximately 1.0 mg/L to 2.0 mg/L because of increased ceruloplasmin (copper binding protein) levels and fetal demand (fetal liver has 10 times the amount of copper found in an adult liver). Increased estrogen levels have been shown to increase copper and ceruloplasmin.

○ **How do the bicarbonate levels change during pregnancy?**

They decrease by approximately 4 mEq/L to a level of 18 to 22 mEq/L.

○ **Why are bicarbonate levels decreased during pregnancy?**

One postulate explains that the developing fetus must off load its bicarbonate. To allow for this, the mother normally hyperventilates causing a respiratory alkalosis. The pCO_2 of the maternal blood is then lowered. In compensation for this, the maternal kidney excretes bicarbonate, therefore, lowering the level and maintaining serum pH at normal or slightly elevated levels.

○ **Which two serum protein concentrations decrease during pregnancy and why?**

(1) Total protein (70 g/L to 60 g/L—major decrease in the first trimester).

(2) Albumin (45 g/L to 35 g/L—major decrease in the first trimester).

This is probably because of decreased production early in pregnancy, as plasma volume does not start to expand until the end of the first trimester. Further decreases are believed to be dilutional.

○ **What is the normal total body iron content in a nonpregnant woman?**

2 g—approximately one half that of men.

○ **What is the total iron requirement from the beginning to the end of pregnancy?**

Approximately 1 g.

○ **What is the total iron requirement per day necessary in the latter half of pregnancy?**

6 to 7 mg/d.

○ **Describe the utilization of iron in the body during pregnancy?**

The total iron content of a healthy woman is 2 g, however, the iron stores are only approximately 300 mg. The fetus and placenta take 300 mg. Normal excretion consumes 200 mg. The increase in total volume of circulating erythrocytes (450 mL) requires another 500 mg.

○ **Why is supplemental iron necessary in pregnancy?**

The iron stores and the iron absorbed from the diet are not enough to provide for the increase in red cells and as plasma volume increases, anemia will result unless exogenous iron is provided. Supplementation is beneficial but will not completely correct the problem.

○ **Does the reticulocyte count normally change during pregnancy?**

Yes, it increases slightly as there is moderate erythroid hyperplasia in the bone marrow, which is correlated with increased erythropoetin levels. This occurs after 20 weeks.

○ **Describe the changes in serum transferrin levels during pregnancy.**

Transferrin levels increase during pregnancy, as do other carrier proteins. The level may increase by as much as 100% by the end of the second trimester. This is the reason that the total iron binding capacity (TIBC) also increases 25% to 100%. Iron supplementation does not decrease the TIBC to prepregnancy levels.

○ **What is thought to be the etiology of the increase in binding proteins (like transferrin and thyroid binding globulin) during pregnancy?**

Increased levels of circulating estrogens are thought to stimulate the liver to increase binding proteins. Women taking oral contraceptives also have increased levels of binding proteins.

○ **During pregnancy, how much do the total erythrocyte volume (TEV), hemoglobin, hematocrit, and MCV change both with and without iron supplementation?**

Iron Supplementation	No Iron Supplementation
• TEV *increases* by 30%	• TEV *increases* by 15%
• Hemoglobin *decreases* by 2%	• Hemoglobin *decreases* by 10%
• Hematocrit *decreases* by 3%	• Hematocrit *decreases* by 5%
• MCV *increases* to an average of 89.7 μm³	• MCV *does not change* from prepregnancy mean = 84.6 μm³

○ **Does the mean erythrocyte volume (MCV) change during pregnancy?**

Without iron supplementation, the MCV does not change, but with iron supplementation, the MCV increases to an average.

○ **What hemoglobin concentration should be considered abnormal in a pregnant woman?**

Values below 11.0 g/dL are present in only 6% of normal pregnant women taking iron and are considered to be in the range for anemia in the first and third trimesters. A woman should be considered anemic in the second trimester if the hemoglobin value is less than 10.5 g/dL. Value less than these numbers should prompt a workup for anemia.

○ **What is the most helpful parameter to make the diagnosis of iron deficiency anemia in a pregnant woman?**

MCV, as it is one of the only hematologic parameters not changed during pregnancy in women not taking iron and is increased in women taking iron. Microcythemia is only caused by three entities—thalassemia, iron deficiency, and lead poisoning. A progressive decrease in MCV to below 82 μm^3 is usually a sign of iron deficiency as the other causes are rare and easily ruled out.

○ **Describe the normal white blood cell count in pregnancy.**

Normal range is 5,000 to 12,000/mL. During labor and the puerperium, it may increase markedly to 25,000 or more.

○ **Which type of immunity (cell mediated vs humoral) is affected by pregnancy and how?**

Clinical evidence shows that cell-mediated immunity is weakened (Th1 responses) and humoral immunity, that is, immunosuppression is strengthened (Th2 responses). Th1 and Th2 cells are functionally distinct subsets of CD4+ T-lymphocytes or helper cells. The weakened cell mediated immunity is responsible for the decreased production of IL2, gamma interferon, and tumor necrosis factor by the Th1 cells, which are harmful to the maintenance of pregnancy. The strengthened humoral immunity is responsible for the increase in immunosuppressive cytokines IL4 and IL10 produced by the Th2 cells.

○ **What is the physiology of the maternal immune system in pregnancy in general terms?**

Pregnancy represents a 50% allograft from the paternal contribution. As a result there is a general suppression of immune function. Therefore, one might have increased susceptibility to infections, improvement of the humoral-mediated autoimmune diseases, and worsening of other cellular-mediated autoimmune diseases.

○ **Does the platelet count change in normal pregnancy?**

Yes, there is a moderate decrease in the number of platelets per unit volume; however, the normal range remains the same for pregnant women (150,000–450,000/mm^3). The mechanism is not clear. Dilution may contribute, but there is some evidence of increased consumption in pregnancy. Thrombocytopenia is defined as platelets less than 100,000/mm^3.

○ **Is the bleeding time affected by pregnancy?**

No. Bleeding time is not different when compared to nonpregnant women.

○ **By how much does the maternal resting heart rate increase in pregnancy?**

10 to 15 beats per minute.

○ **Describe the change in the position and size of the heart in pregnancy.**

The heart is displaced 15 degrees to the left and upward and is rotated laterally causing a larger silhouette in radiographs. The cardiac volume may increase by 10% between early and late pregnancy.

○ **Can a pericardial effusion be normal in pregnancy?**

Yes, small effusions are considered normal in pregnancy.

○ **Stroke volume increases during pregnancy. Is this a function of an increased inotropic effect?**

No, increased stroke volume in a singleton pregnancy is directly proportional to the increased end-diastolic volume caused by increased blood volume (Starling phenomenon). In multifetal pregnancies, however, there has been an increased inotropic effect demonstrated to further increase stroke volume.

○ **What is the prepregnancy stroke volume compared to the pregnancy stroke volume?**

Normal prepregnancy stroke volume is approximately 60 mL. This increases to approximately 70 mL in pregnancy. *Remember:* stroke volume = cardiac output/heart rate.

○ **What normal changes could you see on an EKG during pregnancy?**

Left axis deviation, absent Q wave in aVf, T wave flattening or inversion in lead III. All of these are caused by the positional shift of the heart. The rhythm may be irregular as atrial and ventricular extrasystoles are common.

○ **What are the normal changes in the auscultative heart examination during pregnancy?**

Exaggerated split S1 with increased loudness of both components, systolic ejection murmurs heard at the left sternal border are present in 90% of patients, soft and transient diastolic murmurs are heard in 20%, continuous murmurs from breast vasculature are heard in 10%. The significance of murmurs in pregnancy must be carefully evaluated and clinically correlated. Harsh systolic murmurs and all diastolic murmurs should be taken seriously and worked up before being attributed to pregnancy.

○ **Why is the erythrocyte sedimentation rate (ESR) not a useful test during pregnancy?**

The ESR is elevated normally during pregnancy for unclear reasons. A plausible explanation is the increased clumping of red cells caused by increased levels of fibrinogen and globulin. The elevation is different between whole blood samples and citrated blood samples. For whole blood (red top tube), the mean is 78 mm/h with a range of 44 to 114 mm/h. For citrated blood (purple top tube), the mean is 56 mm/h with a range of 20 to 98 mm/h.

○ **Plasma volume and blood volume increase in pregnancy. By how much and at what gestational age does the volume increase?**

	% Increase	Gestational Age	Plateau
Plasma volume	40%–60%	12–36 weeks	34–36 weeks
Blood volume (plasma and erythrocytes)	45%	24–28 weeks (peak) starts in first trimester	34–36 weeks

○ **Which three clotting factors decrease during pregnancy?**

- Factor XI.
- Factor XIII.
- Antithrombin III (anti factor Xa).

○ **All vitamins are found in human breast milk except which one?**

Vitamin K. This is why vitamin K is administered to newborns.
Formula is also deficient in vitamin K.

○ **The increase and decrease of which factors cause the increased risk of deep vein thrombosis in pregnancy?**

Patients who are pregnant are known to have an increase in clotting factors VII, VIII, X, and XII as well as an increase in prothrombin and fibrinogen. Also, they are found to have a decrease in the anticoagulant protein S.

○ **What is the normal fibrinogen level in pregnancy?**

A normal fibrinogen (factor I) during pregnancy can reach a level of 600 mg/dL at term. This increases from a prepregnancy value of 300 mg/dL.

○ **How does pregnancy affect cardiac output?**

Cardiac output increases to its maximum in the first trimester and this increase continues to term. The increase is 1.5 L/min more than the nonpregnancy average.

○ **Blood flow to most organ systems increases during pregnancy. Which vital organ system does not receive more flow during pregnancy?**

Cerebral blood flow remains unchanged.

○ **How does pregnancy affect arterial blood pressure?**

There is relatively little change in systolic blood pressure. Diastolic blood pressure decreases from 12 to 26 weeks and increases to reach the nonpregnancy value at 36 weeks. This causes an increase in pulse pressure during the second trimester.

○ **What is the definition of mean arterial blood pressure?**

$$MAP = \frac{SBP + 2(DBP)}{3}$$

○ **How does pregnancy affect systemic vascular resistance (SVR)?**

Both SVR and pulmonary vascular resistance are decreased. *Remember:* $MAP = SVR \times CO$. MAP does not change that much in pregnancy; however, CO is very much increased. SVR must decrease by definition. By midpregnancy, the SVR is approximately 1000 dynes/sec/cm^{-5} compared to the nonpregnancy value of 1500 dynes/sec/cm^{-5}. Be aware that SVR may increase, if the patient is in the supine position because of aortic compression.

○ **Does pulmonary capillary wedge pressure (PCWP) change in late pregnancy?**

No. PCWP and central venous pressure (CVP) are not changed significantly in late pregnancy when compared to 12 weeks postpartum. Normal averages are 6 mm Hg and 4 mm Hg, respectively.

○ **What is the normal glomerular filtration rate (GFR) in pregnancy?**

125 cc/min. The average prepregnancy rate is 90 cc/min.

○ **At what gestational age does the GFR reach the maximum level?**

20 weeks and then persists to term. The etiology is not well specified except that renal blood flow is increased by as much as 50% by the beginning of the second trimester. Near term, there is a 15% decrement in the GFR.

○ **Does urine output change in pregnancy?**

No, urine output changes little despite the increase in GFR, indicating that the increased filtered load of water is reabsorbed efficiently.

○ **By how much does the kidney increase in size during pregnancy?**

The length increases by 1 cm.

○ **Which nutrients are lost in greater amounts in the urine of pregnant women?**

Glucose, amino acids, and water-soluble vitamins.

○ **Describe the changes in blood urea nitrogen (BUN) and creatinine during pregnancy.**

BUN and creatinine decrease in pregnancy by approximately 25% with the nadir at 32 weeks. This is thought to be because of an increased GFR. The normal mean creatinine for a pregnant woman is 0.68 mg/dL. The mean BUN level in pregnancy is 10 mg/dL. Renal insufficiency should be suspected with values of creatinine greater than 0.9 mg/dL and urea greater than 14 mg/dL.

○ **What is the best way to calculate GFR in pregnancy?**

A 24 h urine collection for creatinine clearance is preferred as the formula because body weight is not accurate in pregnancy. In pregnancy, the patient's weight does not reflect kidney size as it does prepregnancy.

○ **What is the daily urine protein loss during normal pregnancy?**

Urinary protein loss changes little as a result of pregnancy. The normal range goes up to 300 mg/24 h. Losses greater than 300 mg/24 h may be a result of urinary tract infection or preeclampsia.

○ **How is the function of the renin-angiotensin system unique in the pregnant state?**

In the nonpregnant state, renin is secreted when blood flow to the kidney is compromised causing the formation of angiotensin I and its conversion to angiotensin II. Angiotensin II is a potent vasoconstrictor causing an increase in blood pressure, which maintains perfusion to the kidney. Angiotensin II also stimulates the release of aldosterone, which allows sodium retention and conservation of volume. Despite the hypervolemic state of pregnancy, the levels of renin and angiotensin II increase during pregnancy to approximately five times normal. The expected vasoconstriction and increase in blood pressure do not occur rendering normal pregnancy as a state of refractoriness to angiotensin II. Moreover, the negative feedback exerted by angiotensin II on renin release is not seen in the pregnant state as renin and angiotensin II levels rise simultaneously.

○ **Postpartum, how long does it take for the physiological hydronephrosis of pregnancy to completely resolve?**

12 to 16 weeks.

○ **How does the bladder and urethra compensate for the pressure exerted by the uterus?**

Bladder pressure doubles from 8 to 20 cm H_2O at term and the urethra lengthens by 5 mm as bladder capacity decreases. Compensation occurs by way of increasing intraurethral pressure from 70 to 93 cm H_2O.

○ **What are the normal pregnancy-induced changes known in pulmonary function tests?**

Tidal volume, inspiratory capacity, minute ventilatory volume, and minute oxygen uptake increase by as much as 40% as pregnancy advances. Respiratory rate changes little but may be slightly increased. In general, all of the residual measures are reduced-including functional residual capacity, residual volume, and expiratory reserve volume. The maximum breathing capacity and forced expiratory volume (FEV_1), and peak expiratory flow rate remain unchanged.

○ **Why are the residual capacities of the lungs decreased in pregnancy?**

The resting level of the diaphragm is 4 cm higher in pregnancy.

○ **How much do oxygen requirements increase in pregnancy?**

30 to 40 mL/min.

○ **What anatomic changes occur in the pregnant lungs to facilitate maximal oxygenation?**

- Diaphragm excursion increases from 4.5 cm (prepregnancy) to 6 cm at term.
- The subcostal angle increases from 68 degrees to 100 degrees.
- The diameter of the thoracic cage increases by 2 cm.
- The pulmonary diffusing capacity or rate at which gases diffuse from the alveoli to the blood is increased.

○ **Does pCO_2 increase or decrease during pregnancy?**

There is normally a dramatic decrease in the pCO_2 from a nonpregnancy range of 35–40 mm Hg to 28–30 mm Hg in pregnancy. This occurs from the increased respiratory drive induced by progesterone on the respiratory center. Medroxyprogesterone has been shown to stimulate the respiratory drive in obese nonpregnant patients who hypoventilate.

○ **Describe the trend of gastric acid production in pregnancy?**

It is reduced into the second trimester (36 mg/45 min) from prepregnancy values (60 mg/45 min) but begins to increase in late pregnancy (100 mg/45 min).

Keep in mind that mucus production increases with a protective effect.

○ **Does peptic ulcer disease (PUD) improve or worsen during pregnancy?**

Because there is a decrease in HCl production, PUD is rarely found in pregnancy. Disease that is already present usually improves during the pregnant state.

○ **What is thought to be the cause of the decreased transit time throughout all parts of the alimentary system in pregnancy?**

Increased progesterone levels cause smooth muscle relaxation. Decreased levels of motilin cause loss of smooth muscle stimulating effects. This is evidenced by decreased esophageal, gastric, and intestinal motility and decreased lower esophageal sphincter tone.

○ **What is epulis of pregnancy?**

A focal, highly vascular swelling of the gums that regresses spontaneously after delivery.

○ **Is gastric emptying time increased or decreased during pregnancy?**

In nonpregnant women 60% of a meal is emptied in 90 min. This time is found to almost double during pregnancy.

○   **Do liver function tests change appreciably in normal pregnancy?**

LFT	Increased	Decreased	No change
AST			+
ALT			+
LDH			+
Bilirubin			+
Alkaline phosphatase	+		
Albumin		+	
PT			+
INR			+
PTT			+

○   **If a healthy pregnant woman were to undergo a liver biopsy, what would you see histologically?**

Normal liver morphology even with electron microscopy.

○   **What is the regulator of gall bladder contraction and why is it compromised in pregnancy?**

Cholecystokinin (CCK) causes gall bladder contraction and pancreatic enzyme release. It is formed in the type I mucosal cell of the duodenum and proximal jejunum. High levels of estrogen and progesterone inhibit CCK action on smooth muscle cells in the gall bladder causing impaired contraction and high residual volume.

○   **Name two GI disorders of pregnancy that present most commonly in the third trimester?**

Acute fatty liver of pregnancy and cholestasis of pregnancy.

○   **Hyperplasia of the pituitary occurs in pregnancy. How large does the pituitary grow?**

The pituitary enlarges by 135% compared to nonpregnant controls. This does not compress the optic chiasm.

○   **Is it possible to maintain a pregnancy after a hypophysectomy?**

Yes, the pituitary gland is not necessary for the maintenance of pregnancy.
Women have undergone hypophysectomy and completed pregnancy with replacement of glucocorticoids, thyroid hormone, and vasopressin.

○   **Which thyroid function tests reflect true thyroid function in pregnancy?**

TSH, free T_3, and free T_4 are the three tests not affected by pregnancy after the first trimester. The other parameters (total T_4, total T_3, and T_3 uptake) are altered because of the increase in thyroid binding globulin that occurs as a result of the high estrogen state.

○ **Name the thyroid hormones that cross the placenta?**

In humans, transfer of thyroxine, triiodothyronine, or reverse triiodothyronine from the maternal to the fetal compartment is minimal, if any. The fetal thyroid function is independent of the maternal thyroid status except in the case of autoimmune thyroid disease when stimulatory or inhibitory IgG crosses the placenta and affects the fetal thyroid. Thyroid-releasing hormone, however, can cross the placenta and may stimulate the fetal pituitary to secrete TSH.

○ **Describe the trend of TSH in pregnancy. Does it cross the placenta?**

TSH decreases in the first trimester then normalizes throughout the rest of the pregnancy. TSH levels are inversely correlated with hCG levels. TSH does not cross the placenta.

○ **What percentage of pregnant women will have "hyperthyroid" levels of TSH during each trimester?**

- 13% of gravidas in the first trimester.
- 4.5% in the second trimester.
- 1.2% in the third trimester.

The undetectable TSH levels occur in the absence of thyroid disease because of the effects of β-hCG.

○ **Why does rising hCG cause a decrease in the TSH level?**

Both contain a homologous alpha subunit. The hCG may act as TSH and stimulate the pituitary to secrete thyroid hormones, which in turn suppress the release of TSH.

○ **Does the basal metabolic rate increase or decrease in pregnancy and by how much?**

Increases. Oxygen consumption increases by 25% as a result of fetal metabolic activity.

○ **At what gestational age does thyroid-binding globulin plateau?**

The peak increase begins early in the first trimester with a plateau at approximately 500 nmol/L at 20 weeks until term.

○ **Describe the trend in the free T$_4$ and free T$_3$ levels in pregnancy.**

- Both levels decrease from 6 weeks to a nadir and plateau at 20 weeks.
- Both remain within the normal nonpregnant reference range.
- Both correspond to decreasing thyroxine binding globulin saturation, which decreases from 40% to 30%.

○ **List the six most important factors responsible for calcium metabolism in pregnancy.**

- Serum calcium levels.
- Magnesium levels.
- Phosphate levels.
- Parathyroid hormone.
- Calcitonin.
- Vitamin D.

○ **Why is pregnancy termed a "hyperparathyroid state"?**

The feto-maternal unit has the primary goal of transporting calcium across the placenta (by active transport) for fetal skeletal development. This consumes most of the maternal calcium. Calcium concentration is maintained within normal range despite the increased and expanding extracellular volume. As calcium needs are very great, parathyroid hormone levels are increased by 30% to 50% to bring calcium from the maternal bone, kidney, and intestine into the serum.

○ **Describe the trend of calcitonin in pregnancy.**

Calcitonin is secreted from the parafollicular cells of the thyroid gland. Calcitonin levels have been shown to increase from 13 to 16 weeks with a peak at 25 weeks (230 pg/mL) then a return to prepregnancy levels at approximately 35 weeks (200 pg/mL). Not only does the level increase but the responsiveness to hypocalcemia also increases in order to protect the maternal skeleton from calcium loss.

○ **Which form of vitamin D is increased in pregnancy and why?**

The activated form 1,25 vitamin D is increased in pregnancy with nonpregnant values doubling to a range of 75 to 100 pg/mL. This is a PTH related mechanism. As PTH increases, the hydroxylation of 25-vitamin D at the 1 position is increased at the level of the kidney. In addition, vitamin D binding protein also increases in pregnancy, which may increase 1,25 vitamin D levels.

○ **Does parathyroid hormone and or calcitonin cross the placenta?**

No, neither hormone crosses the placenta.

○ **Which of the substances produced by the adrenal cortex are decreased in pregnancy?**

The substances produced by the adrenal cortex are sex steroids (testosterone, androstenedione, and dehydroepiandrosterone sulfate), cortisol, and aldosterone. All of these are significantly increased in pregnancy except one. Dehydroepiandrosterone sulfate (DHEAS) remains unaltered or slightly decreased through extensive 16 alpha-hydroxylation.

○ **If testosterone is increased in the maternal serum, why is the female fetus not masculinized?**

Total testosterone is doubled from nonpregnancy levels of 0.5 μg/L to 1.0 μg/L. Free testosterone levels are decreased in pregnancy by approximately one half. Little or no testosterone enters the fetal circulation as testosterone. There is complete conversion of testosterone to 17β-estradiol by the trophoblast. This has been documented in women who have very high testosterone levels because of androgen secreting tumors.

○ **Describe the ACTH response to pregnancy.**

ACTH levels rise in pregnancy after an initial decrease early in pregnancy. The levels rise despite a dramatically increased cortisol level (3 times nonpregnancy values). This is a paradox postulated to be caused by a resetting of the feedback system secondary to tissue refractoriness to cortisol.

○ **A pregnant woman complains that her contact lenses are painful to wear recently. Is this normal?**

Yes, corneal thickness increases in pregnancy and can cause discomfort when wearing lenses fitted before pregnancy.

○ **Is vision affected by pregnancy?**

No, visual acuity remains the same. A transient loss of accommodation has been reported during pregnancy and lactation.

○ **Which hormones, aside from hCG, increase the most in pregnancy?**

Hormone	Increase
Human placental lactogen (HPL)	5,000-fold
Progesterone	1,000-fold
Estradiol	400-fold
Prolactin	10-fold

○ **At what gestational age is the breast ready for lactation?**

Lactation is possible after 16 weeks of gestation.

○ **What mechanism prevents lactation from actually occurring prior to delivery?**

The effect of prolactin is blocked by progesterone.

○ **Describe the lesions of polymorphic eruption of pregnancy?**

Also known as pruritic urticarial papules and plaques of pregnancy, these lesions consist of small erythematous papules located most commonly on the abdomen and spare the palms, soles of the feet, and periumbilical area.

○ **Other than polymorphic eruption of pregnancy, name three other dermatologic lesions that may be specific to pregnancy?**

Three other lesions are pruritic folliculitis (erythematous papules most commonly found on the back and chest), pemphigoid gestationis (also known as herpes gestationis characterized by pruritic bullous disease of the skin), and prurigo of pregnancy (characterized by pruritic, erythematous, nodular lesions and is frequently a diagnosis of exclusion).

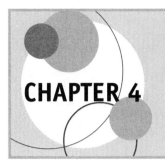

CHAPTER 4

Antepartum Fetal Monitoring and Fetal Surveillance

Michael Lempel, DO

○ **How is the perinatal mortality rate (PMR) defined by the National Center for Health Statistics?**

The number of late fetal deaths (fetal deaths of 28 weeks gestation or more) plus early neonatal deaths (deaths of infants 0 to 7 days of age) per 1000 live births plus late fetal deaths.

○ **What is the definition of the neonatal mortality rate?**

It is defined as the number of neonatal deaths (deaths of infants 0 to 27 days of age) per 1,000 live births.

○ **Before what gestational age do the majority of fetal deaths occur?**

Before 32 weeks.

○ **What information does antepartum fetal assessment provide?**

A reassuring test suggests the fetus is not asphyxiated at the time of the test and no intervention is necessary.

○ **What aspects of the fetal condition might be predicted by antepartum testing?**

Perinatal death, intrauterine growth restriction, nonreassuring fetal status, neonatal asphyxia, postnatal motor and intellectual impairment, premature delivery, congenital abnormalities, and need for specific therapy.

○ **At what gestational age can antepartum testing be initiated to find the fetus at risk?**

26 to 28 weeks for high-risk patients and 32 to 34 weeks for at risk patients.

○ **What are the indications for antepartum fetal monitoring?**

Patients at high risk of uteroplacental insufficiency, fetal compromise suggested by other tests, patients with a previous poor obstetric outcome, and routine antepartum surveillance.

○ **What medical factors place patients at risk for uteroplacental insufficiency?**

Prolonged pregnancy, diabetes mellitus, hypertension, previous stillbirth, severe asthma, suspected IUGR, substance abuse, and advanced maternal age.

○ **How much of time does a near-term fetus spend in a quiet sleep state?**
25%.

○ **How much time is spent in an active sleep state in a near-term fetus?**
60% to 70%.

○ **What does the fetal heart rate exhibit in an active sleep state?**
Increased variability and frequent accelerations with movement.

○ **When can fetal heart tones first be heard via transabdominal Doppler?**
10 to 12 weeks.

○ **When can fetal heart tones first be auscultated via nonelectronic fetoscope?**
18 to 20 weeks.

○ **What is the normal range of the fetal heart rate in the third trimester?**
110 to 160 beats per minute.

○ **What is a prolonged fetal heart rate deceleration?**
A deceleration of the fetal heart rate for longer than 2 minutes, but less than 10 minutes.

○ **What is the definition of fetal bradycardia?**
A deceleration of the fetal heart rate for 10 minutes or longer.

○ **What does the fetal heart rate exhibit during quiet or non-REM sleep?**
Lower heart rate and reduced variability.

○ **How long do periods of quiet sleep and active sleep last in a near-term infant?**
Quiet sleep may last 20 minutes and active sleep approximately 40 minutes.

○ **Approximately, how long are periods of active fetal body movement?**
40 minutes.

○ **How long are periods of quiet fetal movement?**
20 minutes.

○ **At what time of day do fetal movements appear to peak?**
Between 9:00 PM and 1:00 AM.

○ **What maternal physiologic condition is associated with decreased fetal movement?**
Hypoglycemia.

○ **By what gestational age should all pregnant women begin monitoring fetal activity?**

24 weeks or the currently accepted gestational age of viability.

○ **Which technique has been found to be ideal in assessing fetal movement?**

Kick counts.

○ **What is the count-to-ten approach in maternal assessment of fetal movement?**

The patient should count a minimum of 10 movements in a 2-hour period.

○ **What are the fetal and placental factors that influence the maternal assessment of fetal activity?**

Placental location, the length of fetal movements, the amniotic fluid volume, and fetal anomalies.

○ **What placental location is associated with decreased perception of fetal movements?**

Anterior.

○ **What types of anomalies are associated with decreased activity?**

CNS anomalies.

○ **What maternal factors influence the evaluation of fetal movement?**

Maternal activity, obesity, and medications.

○ **Which position do mothers appear to appreciate fetal movements best?**

Left lateral recumbent position.

○ **Which maternal medications depress fetal movement?**

Narcotics and barbiturates.

○ **How should the contraction stress test (CST) be performed?**

The patient is place in the semi-Fowler's position at a 30- to 45-degree angle with a slight left tilt to avoid the supine hypotensive syndrome. Fetal heart rate is recorded and uterine contractions are monitored. Maternal blood pressure is determined every 5 to 10 minutes to detect maternal hypotension. Baseline fetal heart rate and uterine tone are recorded for 10 to 20 minutes. A CST then requires uterine contractions of moderate intensity, either spontaneous or stimulated, lasting approximately 40 to 60 seconds with a frequency of three in ten minutes.

○ **How can uterine activity be stimulated?**

Nipple stimulation or intravenous oxytocin can be started.

○ **How is oxytocin administered for the CST?**

By an infusion pump at 0.5 mU/min. The infusion rate is doubled every 20 minutes until adequate uterine contractions are produced.

○ **What is the advantage of generating uterine contractions with nipple stimulation versus intravenous oxytocin administration?**

The CST can be completed in less time (on average, 30 minutes as opposed to 90 minutes). Also, an intravenous infusion is not required.

○ **How is nipple stimulation achieved for the CST?**

One of two methods may be utilized. The patient may apply a warm moist towel to each breast for 5 minutes. If uterine activity is not adequate, the patient is asked to massage one nipple for 10 minutes. The second method involves using intermittent nipple stimulation. The patient gently strokes the nipple of one breast with the palmer surface of her fingers through her clothes for 2 minutes and then stops for 5 minutes. The cycle is repeated only as needed to achieve adequate uterine activity.

○ **How long should a patient be monitored after the CST has been completed?**

The patient should be observed until uterine activity has returned to baseline.

○ **What are the contraindications to the contraction stress test?**

Patients at high risk for premature labor, such as those with premature rupture of membranes, multiple gestation, and cervical incompetence, and patients in whom uterine contractions should be avoided, such as those with placenta previa, previous classical cesarean section, or previous uterine surgery.

○ **How is a CST interpreted?**

A *negative* CST has no late decelerations appearing anywhere on the tracing with adequate uterine contractions of at least 3 in 10 minutes.

A *positive* CST has late decelerations that are consistent and persistent, present with the majority (>50%) of contractions without excessive uterine activity. If persistent late decelerations are seen before the frequency of contractions is adequate, the test is interpreted as positive.

A CST is called *equivocal* if decelerations are seen with uterine hyperstimulation, isolated late decelerations are seen, or one is unable to achieve adequate contractions (3 contractions in 10 minutes).

○ **What is the incidence of perinatal death within one week of a negative CST?**

0.4/1000.

○ **A CST cannot predict what kind of fetal compromise?**

Acute, such as deaths attributed to cord accidents, malformations, placental abruption, and acute deterioration of glucose control in patients with diabetes mellitus.

○ **What is the likelihood of perinatal death after a positive CST?**

7% to 15%.

○ **What is the greatest limitation to the CST?**

A high incidence of false positives (30%).

○ **What are false-positive CSTs a result of?**

Misinterpretation of the tracing; supine hypotension, which decreases perfusion; uterine hyperstimulation, which is not appreciated using the tocodynamometer; or an improvement in fetal condition after the CST has been performed.

○ **Is a positive CST an indication for an elective cesarean section?**

No. A trial of labor can be attempted if the cervix is favorable for induction so that fetal heart rate monitoring and uterine contractility monitoring can be carefully assessed.

○ **When should a suspicious or equivocal CST be repeated?**

Within 24 hours.

○ **How is a nonstress test (NST) performed?**

The patient is seated in a reclining chair and tilted to the left slightly with a Doppler ultrasound transducer monitoring the fetal heart rate and a tocodynamometer detecting uterine contractions. The patient's blood pressure is recorded before the test begins and repeated at 5- to 10-minute intervals.

○ **How is a reactive nonstress test (NST) defined?**

A reactive NST requires that at least two accelerations of the fetal heart rate of 15 bpm amplitude and 15 seconds duration be observed in 20 minutes of monitoring after 32 weeks or at least two accelerations of the fetal heart rate of 10 bpm amplitude and 10 seconds duration be observed in 20 minutes of monitoring after 28 weeks.

○ **What pathway is required for a healthy fetus to exhibit accelerations greater than the baseline fetal heart rate?**

An intact neurologic coupling between the CNS and the fetal heart.

○ **What fetal condition can disrupt this pathway?**

Fetal hypoxia.

○ **What is the most common cause of absent fetal heart rate accelerations?**

A quiet fetal sleep state.

○ **What are other causes for absence of fetal heart rate accelerations?**

CNS depressants such as narcotics and phenobarbital, β-blockers such as propranolol, and chronic smoking.

○ **If in 20 minutes of monitoring the NST is nonreactive, what is the next step?**

The test can be extended for an additional 20 minutes.

○ **If in 40 minutes of monitoring the NST continues to be nonreactive, what is the next step?**

A CST or biophysical profile should be performed.

○ **When is the NST most predictive?**

If normal or reactive.

○ **What is the perinatal mortality rate associated with a nonreactive NST?**

30 to 40/1000.

○ **What is the false-positive rate associated with a nonreactive NST?**

75% to 90%.

○ **What percentage of NSTs is nonreactive between 24 and 28 weeks' gestation?**

Up to 50%.

○ **What percentage of NSTs remains nonreactive between 28 and 32 weeks?**

15%.

○ **How can vibroacoustic stimulation be utilized during an NST?**

It can be utilized to change fetal state from quiet to active sleep and shorten the length of the NST.

○ **What is the false-negative rate of a reactive NST (i.e., what is the incidence of stillbirth occurring within one week of a reactive NST)?**

1.9/1000.

○ **What is the fetal biophysical profile (BPP)?**

It is the use of real-time ultrasonography to perform an in utero physical examination and evaluate dynamic functions reflecting the integrity of the fetal CNS.

○ **What five parameters are assessed by the fetal biophysical profile?**

NST, fetal breathing movements, fetal body movement, fetal tone, and amniotic fluid volume.

○ **How are the various BPP parameters measured?**

The presence of each parameter is given a score of 2 and the absence or abnormality found is given 0 points.

○ **What must be present in order to receive 2 points for tone on the BPP?**

At least one episode of active extension and return to position of flexion of fetal limbs or spine; or an episode of opening and closing of fetal hand; or upper and lower extremities in positions of full flexion and head flexed on chest.

○ **What must be present in order to receive 2 points for fluid on the BPP?**

A cord and limb-free pocket of amniotic fluid measuring at least 2 × 2 cm; or AFI > 5 cm.

○ **What must be present in order to receive 2 points for movement on the BPP?**

At least three discrete episodes of gross body movements or movements of extremities.

○ **What must be present in order to receive 2 points for breathing on the BPP?**

Fetal breathing movements sustained for at least one episode of 30 seconds duration.

○ **What components make up a modified BPP?**

NST and amniotic fluid volume (AFI).

○ **What is the false-positive rate of a well-performed BPP?**

As low as 20%.

○ **What is the false-negative rate of a BPP?**

0.8 per 1000 tests.

○ **How early can a BPP be used?**

26 to 28 weeks' gestation.

○ **What is the management of BPP scores of 4/10 and less than 4/10?**

Deliver if ≥36 weeks gestation. Repeat BPP if <32 weeks, need to individualize treatment. If less than 4/10 then deliver.

○ **What is the management of a BPP score of 6/10?**

If term then deliver, if preterm then repeat in 24 hours.

○ **If BPP score 2/10, how long can the test be extended?**

120 minutes.

○ **How much time is allotted for the biophysical profile?**

30 minutes.

○ **In the presence of risk factors, how often should the fetal heart rate be auscultated during the active phase of the first stage of labor?**

FHR should be evaluated and recorded at least every 15 minutes after a contraction.

○ **In the presence of risk factors, how often should the fetal heart rate be auscultated during the second stage of labor?**

FHR should be evaluated and recorded at least every 5 minutes.

○ **What does an external fetal heart rate monitor measure?**

Continuous Doppler detects cardiac valve closure.

○ **What is the largest increased risk associated with continuous electronic fetal heart rate monitoring?**

Increased cesarean section rate.

○ **How are early decelerations described?**

Mirror image of the contraction with the nadir of the deceleration matching the peak of the contraction, returning to baseline by the time the contraction has ended.

○ **What is the classic cause of early decelerations?**

Head compression.

○   **How are variable decelerations described?**

V or W-shaped decelerations with an abrupt drop from the baseline and quick return to baseline, variable in degree and timing. The deceleration should decrease from the baseline 15 bpm or more with a duration of 15 seconds or more but less than 2 minutes.

○   **What is the classic cause of variable decelerations?**

Cord compression.

○   **How are late decelerations described?**

Smooth, often shallow decelerations with the nadir of the deceleration after the peak of the contraction. The duration between the onset and the nadir of the deceleration must be greater than or equal to 30 seconds.

○   **What is the classic cause of late decelerations?**

Uteroplacental insufficiency.

○   **What is the positive predictive value of continuous electronic fetal monitoring in detecting a fetus compromised by hypoxia?**

Only 15% to 25%.

○   **When monitoring the fetal heart rate, what is the most sensitive measure of fetal well-being?**

Variability.

○   **What is fetal scalp stimulation?**

Stroking the fetal scalp to stimulate the sympathetic nervous system and monitoring the fetal heart monitor for resultant accelerations.

○   **What does the presence of fetal scalp stimulation represent?**

A nonacidotic fetus.

○   **How is fetal scalp sampling performed?**

With patient in lithotomy or Sims position, direct visualization of the fetal scalp is performed, the scalp is punctured, and fetal capillary blood is obtained.

○   **How is fetal scalp blood pH used to assess fetal well-being?**

7.25 reassuring

7.20 to 7.25 borderline, preacidotic, should be reassessed in 20 to 30 minutes

<7.20 acidosis

<7.00 critical or potentially damaging acidosis

○   **What factors increase the likelihood of variable decelerations?**

Ruptured membranes, oligohydramnios, vasa previa, nuchal cord, short or prolapsed cord.

○ **What are the advantages of an internal scalp electrode monitor?**

Beat-to-beat variability is more apparent, easier to continuously follow fetal heart rate despite movement of fetus or mother, and decreased chance of inadvertently monitoring maternal pulse instead of fetal heart rate.

○ **What are the disadvantages of an internal scalp electrode monitor?**

Necessity of rupture of membranes for placement and a slightly increased risk of fetal infection or scalp hematoma.

○ **In what maternal conditions should application of a fetal scalp electrode be avoided?**

Hepatitis B and HIV infection.

○ **What are potential causes of a sinusoidal fetal heart rate pattern?**

Maternal–fetal hemorrhage, Rh isoimmunization and fetal hypoxia, often resulting from severe chronic fetal anemia, or administration of narcotic drugs to the mother.

○ **What are potential causes of fetal tachycardia?**

Maternal fever, chorioamnionitis, fetal anemia, illicit drug use, congenital heart disease, sympathomimetic drugs (i.e., terbutaline), fetal hypoxia and acidosis.

○ **What are potential causes of fetal bradycardia?**

Acute cord compression or prolapse, rapid descent of the fetal head in labor, uterine hyperstimulation, maternal hypotension, congenital heart block, inadvertent monitoring of maternal pulse, uterine dehiscence, severe fetal hypoxia, placental abruption.

○ **What are potential causes of decreased variability?**

Fetal quiet sleep state cycle, hypoxia, narcotics, CNS anomalies, magnesium sulfate.

○ **What maneuvers should be performed for intra-uterine resuscitation with late decelerations?**

Administer oxygen via facemask.
Turn patient to side to minimize supine hypotension and improve uterine blood flow.
Correct hypotension, if present.
Stop oxytocin infusion.
Consider terbutaline, especially in presence of uterine hyperstimulation.
Validate fetal well-being with scalp stimulation or scalp sampling.
Administer intravenous colloids to increase maternal cardiac output.

○ **What is the mechanism of supine hypotension?**

Uterine compression of the vena cava leads to decreased return of blood to the heart, decreasing maternal cardiac output, causing maternal hypotension and decreased uterine blood flow.

○ **What does this fetal heat rate monitoring tracing represent? [Fig. 4–1]**

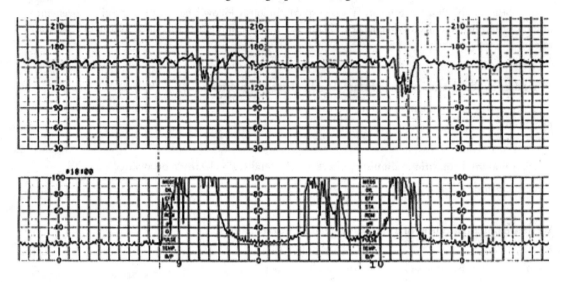

Variable deceleration.

○ **What does this fetal heat rate monitoring tracing represent? [Fig. 4–2]**

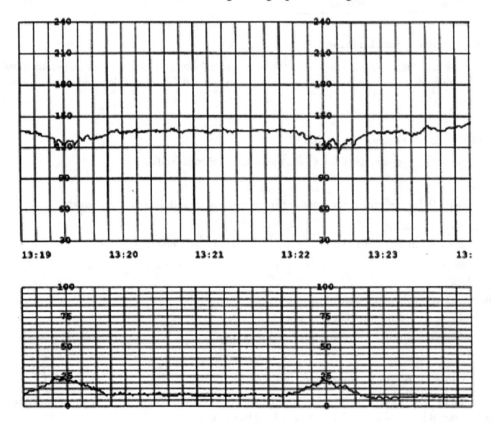

Early deceleration.

○   **What does this fetal heat rate monitoring tracing represent? [Fig. 4–3]**

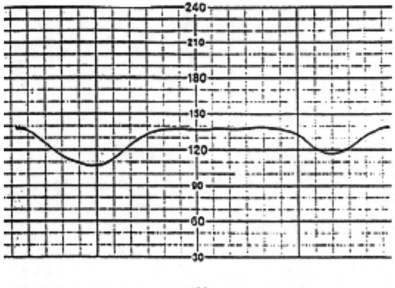

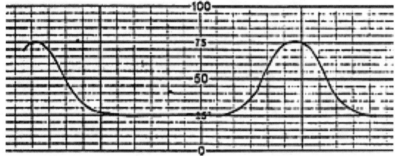

Late deceleration.

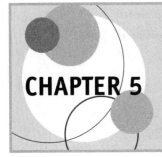

CHAPTER 5 Labor and Delivery

Frank J. Craparo, MD

○ **What is the definition of labor?**

Labor is defined as the initiation of regular and rhythmic contractions that results in serial dilatation and effacement of the cervix.

○ **How many stages of labor exist?**

Labor is traditionally divided into three stages, and some consider there to be a fourth stage.

○ **What is the definition of the first stage of labor?**

The first stage of labor is defined as the onset of regular contractions that results in cervical change. This stage ends when the cervix is fully dilated.

○ **What is the definition of the second stage of labor?**

The second stage of labor is defined from the time of full dilatation of the cervix until delivery of the infant.

○ **What is the definition of the third stage of labor?**

The third stage of labor begins with the delivery of the infant and ends with the delivery of the placenta.

○ **Is there a fourth stage of labor?**

Some consider the 1- to 2-hour time period after delivery of the placenta to be the fourth stage. This is not part of the traditional description of labor.

○ **What is a common complication of this "fourth stage"?**

This is a time when postpartum hemorrhage is most likely to occur.

○ **What is the latent phase of labor?**

The latent phase of labor is the initiation of contractions with slow cervical change, which continues until accelerated cervical change occurs.

○ **Is there a time difference in the latent phase for nulliparous versus multiparous patients?**

In the nulliparous patient, the average latent phase is 6.4 hours. In the multiparous patient, the average is 4.8 hours.

○ **What is the definition of the active phase of labor?**

The active phase of labor is defined as when the expected phase of maximal slope has been accomplished. The majority of patients (90%) are in this phase when they are approximately 5 cm dilated.

○ **What is the average cervical change during the active phase for a nulliparous patient?**

The expected cervical dilatation in the nulliparous patient is greater than or equal to 1.2 cm/h.

○ **What is the average cervical change for a multiparous patient?**

The expected cervical change in a multiparous patient in the active phase of labor is 1.5 cm/h.

○ **What is the average length of time pushing for a multiparous patient?**

The multiparous patient usually pushes for no more than 1 hour. However, this may be extended to 2 hours if there is regional anesthesia.

○ **What is the average length of time pushing for a nulliparous patient?**

The average time may last up to 2 hours in the nulliparous patient or extended to 3 hours if the patient has had regional anesthesia.

○ **What is the definition of precipitous labor?**

Traditionally, this is defined as labor resulting in delivery in less than 3 hours. In a nulliparous patient, labor is also considered precipitous if the cervical dilatation is greater than 5 cm/h.

○ **What is "failure to progress"?**

"Failure to progress" is defined as labor not resulting in cervical dilatation or descent of the fetus.

○ **What is cephalopelvic disproportion?**

Cephalopelvic disproportion is the difference in the dimensions of the fetal head and the maternal pelvis resulting in obstruction of labor.

○ **What is protracted labor?**

Protracted labor can be the result of protracted dilatation or protracted descent. Protracted dilatation is progress less than 1.2 cm/h in a nulliparous patient and less than 1.5 cm/h in a multipara patient. Protracted descent is defined as descent less than 1 cm/h in a nullipara patient or less than 2 cm in the multiparous patient.

○ **What is the Bishop score?**

The Bishop score is a description of the cervix to help evaluate "ripeness."

○ **How is the Bishop score defined?**

There are five parts to the Bishop score including dilatation, effacement, station, consistency, and the position of the cervix in the pelvis.

○ **What is considered a favorable Bishop score?**

Greater than or equal to nine.

○ **What is considered an unfavorable Bishop score?**

Four or less is considered unfavorable.

○ **How are dilatation and effacement defined?**

Dilatation is defined in centimeters. Effacement is defined in percentage and refers to the thinning of the cervix.

○ **How frequently is the fetus vertex at term?**

95% of all patients at term present as vertex.

○ **What do the cardinal mechanisms of labor refer to?**

They refer to the changes in the position of the fetal head as it passes though the birth canal.

○ **Why does the fetal head need to change position at this time?**

These changes are needed secondary to the asymmetric shape of the fetal head and maternal bony pelvis.

○ **How are these changes accomplished?**

The changes occur as the result of the propulsive forces of uterine activity during labor.

○ **How many changes occur during the cardinal movements?**

Seven.

○ **Name the cardinal movements of labor.**

Engagement, descent, flexion, internal rotation, extension, external rotation, and expulsion.

○ **How is engagement defined?**

Engagement occurs when the descent of the biparietal diameter (BPD) is below the level of the pelvic inlet.

○ **What is the average distance between the pelvic inlet and the ischial spines?**

The average distance is 5 cm.

○ **When does the greatest rate of descent occur?**

It most often occurs during the deceleration phase of the first stage of labor and during the second stage of labor.

O   **How does flexion usually occur?**

Flexion usually occurs as a passive motion.

O   **Approximately what percentage of pregnant patients have factors that can be identified prenatally that place the patient at increased risk?**

Approximately 20% of patients have identifiable risk factors.

O   **Of the patients identified with risk factors, how many of these will result in a poor outcome?**

20% of patients identified with risk factors may account for greater than 50% of poor outcomes.

O   **What percentage of patients are identified with risk factors when they present in labor?**

An additional 5% to 10% will be identified at this time.

O   **How many of these will result in poor outcomes?**

These patients account for approximately 20% to 25% of poor outcomes.

O   **What percentage of patients with poor outcomes have no identifiable risk factors?**

20%.

O   **What are the goals of assisted spontaneous deliveries?**

Assisted spontaneous deliveries should result in decreased maternal trauma and decreased fetal injury.

O   **What are the "proposed advantages" of routine episiotomy?**

The "proposed advantages" include easier repair of a surgical incision, reduction in the second stage of labor, and reduction of trauma to the pelvic floor musculature.

O   **What are the "proposed disadvantages" to episiotomy?**

The "proposed disadvantages" include increased blood loss, increased maternal pain, and unnecessary surgical incision.

O   **What are the four types of the pelvic shapes?**

Gynecoid, anthropoid, android, and platypelloid.

O   **What are Leopold maneuvers?**

Palpation of the uterus to determine fetal lie and position.

O   **What is the definition of prolonged latent phase?**

The latent phase is defined as prolonged if this period lasts greater than 20 hours in a nulliparous patient or greater than 14 hours in a multiparous patient.

○ **What is the most common treatment for prolonged latent phase of labor?**

Maternal rest.

○ **What percentage of patients will proceed to active labor following maternal rest?**

Approximately 85% will proceed to active labor and approximately 10% will stop having contractions.

○ **How is dysfunctional labor defined?**

Dysfunctional labor is defined when the active phase of dilatation is in the less than fifth percentile.

○ **What is the less than fifth percentile for nulliparous patients?**

Less than 1.2 cm/h.

○ **What is the less than fifth percentile for multiparous patients?**

Less than 1.5 cm/h.

○ **What is the definition of the secondary arrest of labor?**

It is defined as lack of cervical change for 2 hours following normal dilatation.

○ **What are the most common units used to describe uterine activity?**

Montevideo units—a uterine activity unit.

○ **How are these units defined?**

Montevideo units refer to the strength of contractions in millimeters of mercury multiplied by the frequency per 10 minutes. The uterine activity unit is defined as 1 mm Hg/min.

○ **When is oxytocin indicated?**

When uterine activity is less than 50 mm Hg every 3 minutes or less than 200 Montevideo units.

○ **What is the duration (half-life) of intravenous oxytocin?**

The half-life is 3 to 4 minutes.

○ **Name a maternal systemic effect of oxytocin.**

Antidiuresis.

○ **An anthropoid pelvis is often associated with what presentation?**

Occipitoposterior.

○ **An android pelvis is often associated with:**

Deep transverse arrests.

○ **A transverse presentation is frequently seen with which pelvis type.**

Platypelloid.

○ **What percentage of women has a gynecoid pelvis?**

Approximately 50%, making this the most common pelvis type.

○ **The critical distance of the anterior–posterior diameter of the pelvis is?**

10 cm.

○ **The uterus receives what percentage of cardiac output at term?**

Approximately 10%.

○ **What is the average blood flow to the uterus at term?**

Approximately 600 mL/min.

○ **Name the principal prostaglandins produced by the amnion and the decidua?**

The principal prostaglandin of the amnion is PGE2. The principal prostaglandin produced by the decidua is PGF2alpha.

○ **When the fetal vertex enters the pelvis, what is the most common position?**

Left occiput transverse.

○ **In what percentage of pregnancies is there a nuchal cord?**

10% to 25%.

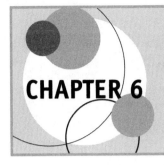

CHAPTER 6

Operative Obstetrics

Richard Latta M.D.

○ **What type of needle tip should be used to close the fascia of a Pfannenstiel skin incision?**

Taper needles. Cutting needles or reverse cutting needles increase the risk of pull through. Blunt needles are used for friable tissues.

○ **What tissues are disrupted in a first-degree laceration?**

This is defined as superficial laceration of the vaginal mucosa or perinatal body not requiring suturing.

○ **What tissues are involved in a second-degree laceration or episiotomy?**

This involves the vaginal mucosa, perineal skin, and deeper subcutaneous tissue and requires suturing.

○ **Define a fourth-degree laceration.**

This involves extension of an episiotomy or laceration into the rectal mucosa.

○ **True or False: Episiotomy increases the risk of disruption of the rectal sphincter.**

True.

○ **Myonecrosis of the deep fascia is most often associated with infection by which organism?**

Clostridium perfringens.

○ **What type of locking devices are shown with the forceps in the above figure?**

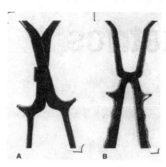

(1) Keiland forceps with a sliding lock.

(2) Simpson forceps with a fixed English lock.

○ **Modern forceps were developed by this family in England (that maintained forceps as their family secret until the late 18th century).**

The Chamberlen family.

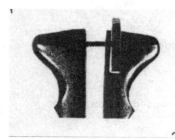

○ **The type of lock seen above is found on what type of forceps?**

Elliot

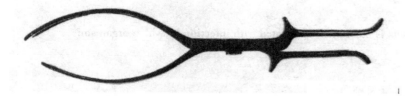

○ **What type of forceps is shown above?**

Keiland forceps.

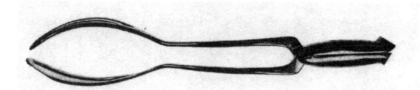

○   **The forceps demonstrated above is used for delivery in what situation?**
Breech.

○   **What is the name of the forceps from the last question?**
Piper forceps.

○   **How would you describe a delivery from a +2 station with a 35-degree rotation?**
Low forceps, nonrotational delivery.

○   **How would you describe a forceps delivery with a sagittal suture in the AP diameter with the fetal scalp visible at the introitus?**
Outlet forceps.

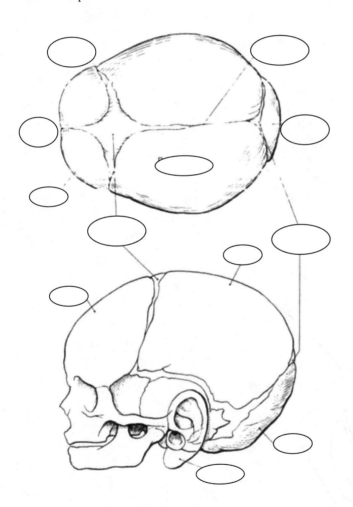

O   **Label the structures on the associated figure.**

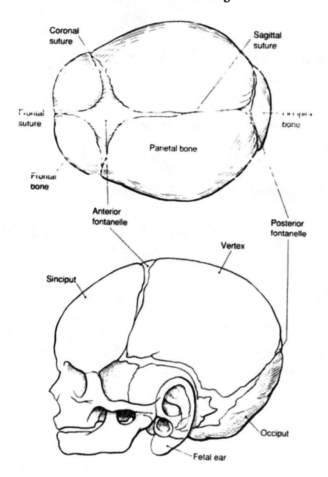

Coronal suture

Sagittal suture

Frontal suture

Parietal bone

Frontal bone

Anterior fontanelle

Posterior fontanelle

Vertex

Sinciput

Occiput

Fetal ear

=

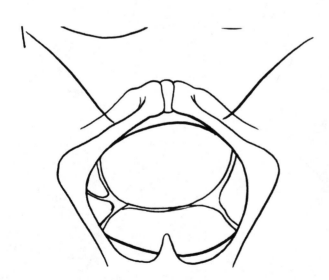

○ **Describe the presentation of the fetus in figure above.**

Left occiput transverse with anterior asynclitism.

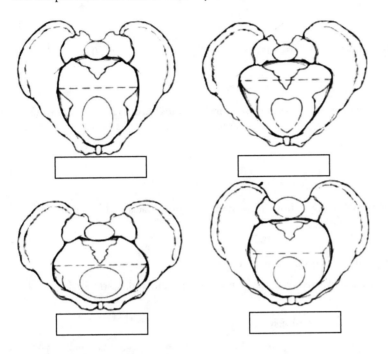

○ **Label the pelvis types noted above.**

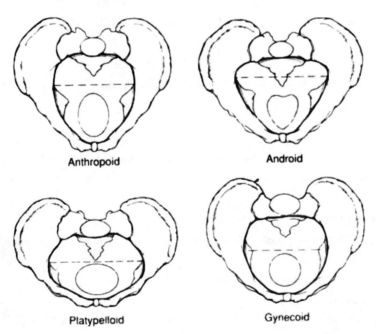

Anthropoid   Android

Platypelloid   Gynecoid

○ **What are the common contraindications to cervical cerclage?**

Active bleeding, premature labor, ruptured membranes, chorioamnionitis, hydramnios, or confident diagnosis of a lethal fetal anomaly.

○ **What are the common intrapartum complications associated with cervical cerclage placement?**

Cervical lacerations occurring in 3% to 13% of patients and cervical stenosis secondary to scarring in approximately 5% of patients.

○ **What type of cervical cerclage is currently the most common?**

McDonald.

○ **What cervical cerclage involves the dissection of the anterior cervicovaginal mucosa just distal to the bladder refection?**

Shirodkar.

○ **Define cervical incompetence.**

A repetitive, acute, painless, second trimester evacuation of the uterus without associated bleeding or contractions.

○ **How does the stroma of the cervix differ from the uterine corpus?**

There is a relative lack of smooth muscle compared to the amount of collagenous and elastic tissue.

○ **Specify at least one indication for cervical cone biopsy during pregnancy.**

Suspected microinvasion on colposcopy or colposcopy directed biopsy or persistent cytologic evidence of invasive disease not explained by colposcopy or cervical biopsy or Adenocarcinoma in situ.

○ **What is the current maternal mortality associated with legal abortion in the United States?**

Less than 1 in 100,000.

○ **Osmotic dilators used for dilating the cervix prior to abortion include laminaria tents. What are laminaria tents derived from?**

Dried seaweed of the *Japonicum species.*

○ **What four complications almost equally contribute to the mortality related to legal abortion?**

Embolism, infection, hemorrhage, and anesthesia.

○ **What is the reported incidence of uterine perforation at abortion?**

0.2 per 100; however, the real incidence may be higher because of asymptomatic and unsuspected perforations.

○ **What are the two most common causes of postabortal hemorrhage?**

Uterine hypotonus and retained products of conception.

○ **What is the treatment of postabortal bleeding, if uterine atony is suspected to be the cause?**

General uterine massage and parenteral uterotonics (oxytocin, methylergonovine, 15-Methylprostaglandin F2 alpha).

○ **What combination of medications is approved for use of "medical abortion" in the United States?**

A combination of mifepristone (RU-486) and misoprostol.

○ **The majority of midtrimester abortions are performed in the United States by what technique?**

Dilation and evacuation.

○ **What is the safest method for termination of pregnancy in terms of mortality and morbidity between 13 and 16 weeks gestation?**

Dilation and evacuation.

○ **Of the procedures curettage, D&E, instillation procedures, and hysterotomy, what procedure is associated with the highest case-fatality rate?**

Hysterotomy.

○ **At what gestational age should elective repeat cesarean delivery be performed?**

ACOG recommends elective delivery at or beyond 39 weeks with the following criteria met: (1) normal menstrual cycles; (2) no recent oral contraceptive use; (3) one of the following: fetal heart tones auscultated by 10 menstrual weeks, positive pregnancy test by 4 menstrual weeks, ultrasound confirming menstrual dates prior to 20 weeks gestation.

○ **What is the most frequent indication for primary cesarean delivery in the United States?**

Labor dystocia.

○ **What are the three common uterine incisions used to perform a cesarean delivery?**

Low transverse, low vertical, and classical.

○ **What is the most common abdominal operation performed in the United States?**

Cesarean section.

○ **List the ACOG indications for operative vaginal (there are four indications):**

Prolonged second stage for a nulliparous woman: lack of continuing progress for 3 hours with regional anesthesia or 2 hours without regional anesthesi

Prolonged second state for a multiparous woman: lack of continuing progress for 2 hours with regional anesthesia or 1 hour without regional anesthesia.

Suspicion of immediate or potential fetal compromise. Shortening of the second stage for maternal benefit.

○ **True or False: In 1988, ACOG redefined the classification of station and types of forceps deliveries. The revised classification uses the level of the leading bony point of the fetal head in centimeters at or below the level of the maternal ischial spines to define station (0–5 cm), instead of the previously used method of describing the birth canal in terms of thirds (0−3+).**

True.

○   **The definition of midforceps.**

Station is above +2 cm but head is engaged.

○   **True or False: According to the ACOG practice bulletin, vacuum extractors are designed to limit the amount of traction on the fetal skull because detachment can occur. Nevertheless, traction achieved with vacuum extraction is substantial (up to 50 lb) and can result in significant fetal injury, if misused.**

True.

○   **The two FDA recommendations for use of the vacuum device are:**

Rocking movements or torque should not be applied to the device; only steady traction in the line of the birth canal should be used, and clinicians caring for the neonate should be alerted that a vacuum device has been used so that they can adequately monitor the neonate for the signs and symptoms of device-related injuries.

○   **According to the ACOG practice bulletin, the lowest rate of neonatal intracranial hemorrhage is associated with: Vacuum delivery alone, cesarean section with labor, cesarean section without labor, forceps delivery alone.**

Cesarean section without labor.

○   **According to the ACOG practice bulletin, the lowest rate of neonatal death is associated with: Vacuum delivery alone, cesarean section with labor, cesarean section without labor, forceps delivery alone.**

Vacuum delivery alone.

○   **True or False: The vacuum extractor is associated with an increased incidence of complications including neonatal cephalohematomata, facial nerve palsy, retinal hemorrhages, and jaundice when compared with forceps delivery.**

False; neonatal cephalohematomata, retinal hemorrhages, and jaundice are greater with the vacuum extractor but facial nerve palsy is increased with forceps delivery.

○   **True or False: Assuming that there is adequate operator experience, both forceps and vacuum extractors are acceptable and safe instruments for operative vaginal delivery.**

True.

○   **The definition of nonrotational low forceps requires (two-part answer):**

Leading point of fetal skull is at station ≥+2 cm and rotation is 45 degrees or less.

○   **The single greatest risk factor for third- or fourth-degree lacerations.**

The performance of a median episiotomy.

○   **True or False: Episiotomy has been identified as an independent risk factor for dyspareunia or delayed return to sexual activity when compared with equally severe perineal trauma in women who did not have an episiotomy.**

False.

○ True or False: Restricted use of episiotomy is preferable to routine use of episiotomy.

True.

○ True or False: Mediolateral episiotomy is associated with higher rates of injury to the anal sphincter and rectum than is median episiotomy.

False.

○ True or False: Currently the major known benefit of routine episiotomy helps to prevent pelvic floor damage leading to incontinence.

False.

○ True or False: To avoid anal sphincter or rectal injury, mediolateral episiotomy is superior to median episiotomy.

True.

○ True or False: According to the ACOG practice bulletin, the fetal benefits of episiotomy include cranial protection, especially for premature infants, reduced perinatal asphyxia, less fetal distress, and better Apgar scores.

False, none of the above are benefits of episiotomy.

○ True or False: Operative vaginal delivery is contraindicated, if the fetus is known to have osteogenesis imperfecta.

True.

○ True or False: Operative vaginal delivery is contraindicated if the fetus is known to occiput posterior.

False.

○ True or False: Operative vaginal delivery is contraindicated if the fetus is known to have alloimmune thromobocytopenia.

True.

○ True or False: Operative vaginal delivery is contraindicated if the fetus is known to have von Willebrand disease

True.

○ Comparing fetuses delivered by cesarean section during labor vs fetuses delivered by cesarean section after attempted vacuum or forceps. The relative risk of intracranial hemorrhage is __ times greater.

Three times greater

○ **True or False: The American and Gynecologist practice bulletin would consider patients with two previous low transverse cesareans and no prior vaginal deliveries to be a candidate for vaginal birth after cesarean section College of Obstetricians.**

False.

○ **The rate of uterine rupture for a classical uterine incision is approximately:**

4% to 9 %.

○ **The rate of uterine rupture for a T-shaped uterine incision is approximately:**

4% to 9 %.

○ **The rate of uterine rupture for a low vertical uterine incision is approximately:**

1% to 7 %.

○ **The rate of uterine rupture for a low transverse uterine incision is approximately:**

0.2% to 1.5 %.

○ **True or false: Patients with pregnancies complicated by known HIV infection should be counseled that vertical transmission to the fetus is approximately 2% with zidovudine and scheduled cesarean delivery.**

True.

○ **True or false: Patients with pregnancies complicated by known HIV infection should be counseled that vertical transmission to the fetus is approximately 2% among women with viral loads less than 1000 copies/mL, even without systematic use of scheduled cesarean delivery.**

True.

○ **Placenta accreta has increased ___ fold in the last 10 years.**

10-fold

○ **Risk factors for placenta accreta include:**

(1) prior cesarean section

(2) placenta previa

(3) prior myomectomy

(4) Asherman's syndrome

(5) submucous leiomyomata

(6) maternal age greater than 35

○ **What is the term used for the tendency of suture material to return to its original shape after deformation, for example, tying?**

Memory.

○ **What is the term used for a suture's tendency to return to original form after stretching?**
Elasticity.

○ **What are the three surgical needle types that are currently available?**
Swaged, controlled release ("pop-off"), and open.

○ **Of the forceps (pickups): dressing, tissue, or Russian, which may be used to grab the needle?**
None. Although occasional use of the forceps to grab a needle is of little consequence, none of these should be used for grasping the needle.

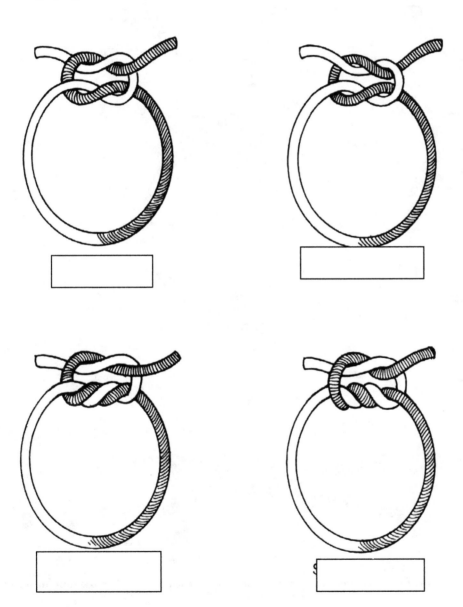

○   **Label the types of knots pictured above.**

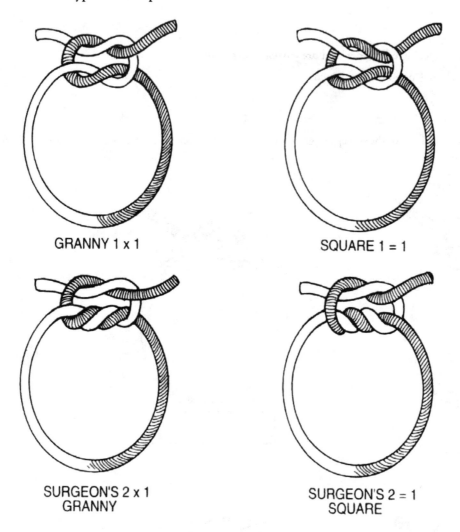

GRANNY 1 x 1   SQUARE 1 = 1

SURGEON'S 2 x 1   SURGEON'S 2 = 1
GRANNY   SQUARE

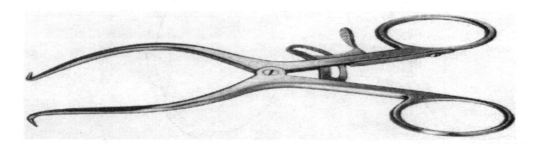

○   **What is the name of this self-retaining perineal retractor that may be used to provide retraction for repair of vaginal tears?**

Gelpi.

○ **What is the National Research Council's classification of surgical wounds for a cesarean section in labor?**

Contaminated.

○ **What is the name of the maneuver used to control the fetal breech head where the obstetrician applies the index finger and middle finger of one hand over the maxilla, with two fingers of the other hand hooked over the fetal neck and grasping the fetal shoulders?**

Mauriceau-Semllie-Viet maneuver.

○ **The Pinard maneuver is sometimes used in the case of a frank breech. Describe the maneuver.**

The obstetrician's fingers are kept parallel to the femur. Pressure is placed in the popliteal fossa, resulting in flexion of the fetal knee.

○ **Entrapment of the fetal head is potentially life-threatening to a breech delivery. Describe a surgical correction of this problem.**

Duhrssen's incision. The technique involves two or three incisions in the cervix at the two-, six-, and ten-o'clock positions.

○ **Of frank breech, complete breech, or footling breech, which presentation has the highest frequency of umbilical cord prolapse?**

Footling breech; 15% to 18%.

○ **True or False: Congenital anomalies are two to three times greater with a fetus in the breech presentation compared to the cephalic presentation.**

True.

○ **In approximately what percentage of twin deliveries are both twins cephalic/cephalic?**

40%.

○ **What is the approximate incidence of shoulder dystocia?**

0.2% to 0.5% of all deliveries; although there is a wide variation in the definition and methods of reporting.

○ **List at least three interpartum risk factors for shoulder dystocia.**

(1) First stage labor abnormalities, including protraction disorders or arrest disorders.

(2) Prolonged second stage of labor.

(3) Oxytocin augmentation of labor.

(4) Midforceps and midvacuum delivery.

○ **What is the incidence of shoulder dystocia in a patient with diabetes mellitus and a fetus greater than 4500 g birthweight?**

50%.

○ **Name at least three antepartum risk factors for shoulder dystocia.**

    (1) Fetal macrosomia

    (2) Maternal obesity

    (3) Diabetes mellitus

    (4) Postterm pregnancy

    (5) Male gender

    (6) Advanced maternal age

    (7) Excessive weight gain

    (8) Prior shoulder dystocia

    (9) Platypoid pelvis or contracted pelvis

    (10) Prior macrosomic infant

○ **What is the first necessity in the management of shoulder dystocia?**

Additional help is summoned, including anesthesia and pediatrics.

○ **What is the name of the maneuver in which the legs are sharply flexed upon the abdomen in an attempt to relieve shoulder dystocia?**

McRobert's maneuver.

○ **What is the most common risk factor for the development of puerperal hematomas?**

Episiotomy, predominantly left medial lateral.

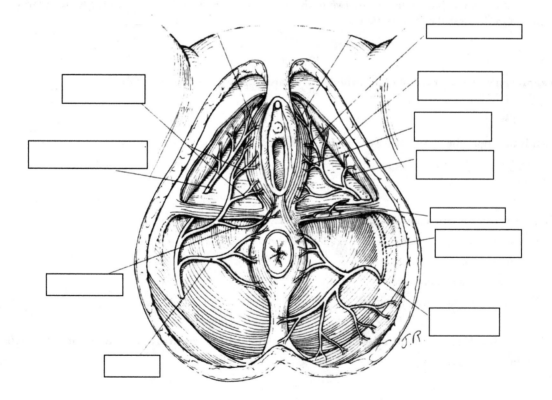

O **Label the structures of the pelvis.**

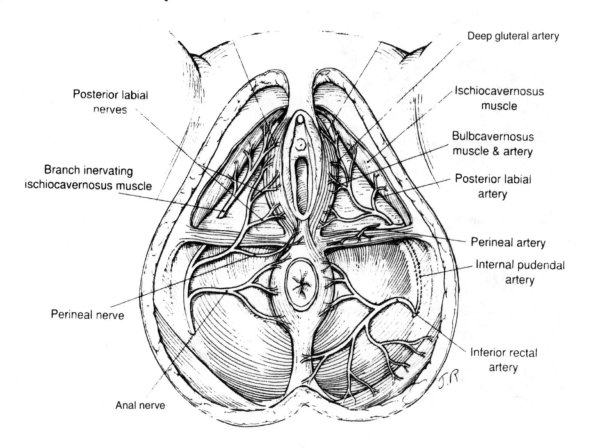

Deep gluteral artery

Posterior labial nerves

Ischiocavernosus muscle

Bulbcavernosus muscle & artery

Posterior labial artery

Branch inervating ischiocavernosus muscle

Perineal artery

Internal pudendal artery

Perineal nerve

Inferior rectal artery

Anal nerve

O **What are the blood vessels most commonly injured during vulvar hematomas?**

Branches of the pudendal artery: inferior rectal, transverse perinatal, and posterior labial arteries.

O **What percentage of women undergoing cesarean section for placenta previa in the presence of one or more prior scars subsequently require cesarean hysterectomy for placenta accreta?**

25%.

O **What is the most frequent cause of serious postpartum hemorrhage?**

Uterine atony.

O **In the management of postpartum uterine atony, fundal compression has not stopped the bleeding. At what dose would you request oxytocin to be begun?**

Oxytocin, 40 U/L, with rapid infusion.

O **What are the common contraindications and relative contraindications to routine newborn circumcision?**

Low birth weight—less than 2500 g, bleeding abnormalities, family history of bleeding disorder not ruled out in the infant, infection, unstable infant, hypospadias and other genitourinary abnormalities, abnormal body temperature, and abnormal feeding.

○ **What infection is much less common in circumcised boys than in uncircumcised boys?**

Urinary tract infections are reduced by 10 to 39 times with circumcision.

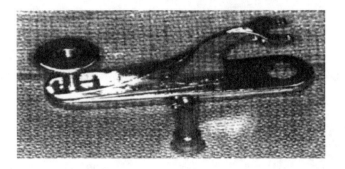

○ **What is the name of this device used for circumcision?**

Gomco.

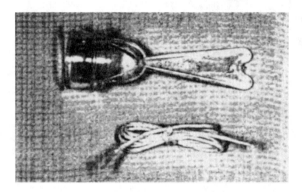

○ **What is the name of this device used for circumcision?**

Plastibell

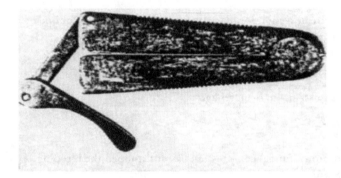

○ **What is the name of this device used for circumcision?**

Mogan.

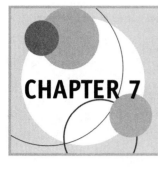

CHAPTER 7 Multiple Gestations

Roberto Prieto-Harris, MD

○ **What percentage of all pregnancies is twins and higher order multiple gestations?**

With the increased use of fertility treatments, multiple gestations represent approximately 3% of all pregnancies.

○ **What is the overall frequency of twins and vanishing twin?**

Improved ultrasound techniques have facilitated sonographic studies of early gestation, which show that the first trimester incidence of twins is much greater than the incidence of twins at birth. Multiple gestations are now estimated to occur in 12% of all spontaneous conceptions but only 14% of them survive at term.

○ **What is superfecundation?**

Refers to the fertilization of two ova within a short period of time but not at the same coitus and not necessarily by the sperm from the same male.

○ **What is the difference between chimera and mosaicism?**

Chimera: Individual whose cells originated from more than one fertilized ovum.

Mosaicism: Two or more cell lines from different chromosomal composition arise from the same zygote as a consequence of nondisjunction.

○ **What are the different etiologies of multiple fetuses?**

Twin fetuses can arise from the fertilization of two separate ova (dizygotic or fraternal) or from a single fertilized ovum that subsequently divides into two similar structures (monozygotic or identical). Slightly more than 30% are monozygotic twins; nearly 70% are dizygotic.

Characteristics of Monozygotic and Dizygotic twins

Zygocity	Etiology	Affected by Ethnicity?	Frequency	Rate
Monozygotic (identical)	Arise from single fertilized ovum	Not affected by ethnic background	One set per 250 live births	Constant
Dizygotic twins (fraternal)	Fertilization of two separate ova	Yes, the highest rate of twinning occurs in African Americans, followed by Caucasians and lowest in Asians	Approximately 1 in 83 conceptions	Depends on race, hereditary factors, ART, age, and parity

○ **What percentage of multiple fetus pregnancies or multiple infant births from ART represent triplets or higher order gestations?**

4% to 5% of all live births resulting from ART are triplets or higher order gestations.

○ **Do female descendants of twins have higher twining rate among their offspring?**

Yes. Women who are dizygotic twins or who are siblings of dizygotic twins have higher rates. The father's genetic contribution plays little or no part.

○ **Is the incidence of twinning affected by age?**

Yes, the incidence of twinning increases with maternal age.

○ **The incidence of twins peak at what age?**

35 to 40 years.

○ **What is the incidence of multiple pregnancies with the use of clomiphene citrate?**

The rate of twinning is approximately 8% with less than 1% triplets or higher order gestations.

○ **What is the incidence of multiple pregnancies with the use of gonadotropin therapy?**

The multiple gestation rates are approximately 20–25% with approximately 1% to 2% triplets or higher order gestations.

○ **How does the timing of division of the fertilized ovum affect monozygotic twins?**

Division within the first 72 hours after fertilization results in a diamniotic, dichorionic twin pregnancy. Division between 4 and 8 days after fertilization results in a diamniotic, monochorionic gestation. Division between 8 and 13 days after fertilization results in a monoamniotic, monochorionic gestation. Division after 13 days leads to conjoined twins.

○ **What type of monozygotic twins is more common?**

Monochorionic-diamniotic.

○ **How does examination of the placenta aid in the determination of zygosity?**

In cases of like-sex twins evaluation of the relationship of the amnion(s) and chorion(s) will aid in determining the zygosity. Twins of the opposite sex are dizygotic.

○ **Other than gender, what is the most predictive way to diagnose mono vs dichorionic gestations via ultrasound?**

The membrane character and thickness are different for mono- vs dichorionic gestations. In dichorionic gestations, the membrane is >2 mm (Figure 7.2) thick with 3 to 4 layers identified and a "twin peak" sign seen on ultrasound (Figure 7.1) where the chorion attaches to the amnion. In monochorionic gestations, the membrane is thin and "hair-like" with only two layers and a "T" sign is noted on ultrasound where the chorion and amnion attach.

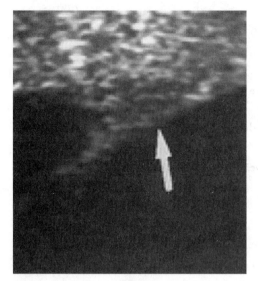

Figure 7.1 *Twin Peak Sign*

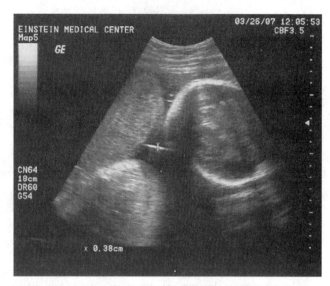

Figure 7.2 *Dichorionic gestation. Membrane thickness >2mm*

○ **Which type of twin placenta is at highest risk for vascular communications?**

Monochorionic placentas are at highest risk for vascular communications.

○ **What maternal changes are more frequently observed with multiple gestations?**

(1) Anemia often develops secondary to a greater demand of iron from the fetuses

(2) Respiratory tidal volume is increased, but women pregnant with twins often feel "breathless," possibly secondary to a higher progesterone levels.

(3) Marked uterine distension and increased pressure on adjacent viscera.

(4) Theca-lutein cysts form more frequently during multiple gestations as a result of higher levels of chorionic gonadotrophin.

(5) Urinary tract infection is at least twice as common.

○ **What complications of multiple gestations affect pregnancy outcome?**

(1) Increased incidence of spontaneous abortion.

(2) Increased incidence of malformations.

(3) Intrauterine growth restriction.

(4) Increased incidence of preterm birth.

(5) Placenta previa is more frequently encountered because of large size of placenta or placentas.

(6) Gestational hypertension. The risk is increased three to five times more in multiple gestations than in single pregnancies.

(7) Gestational diabetes.

(8) Acute fatty liver.

(9) PUPPS.

(10) Pulmonary embolus.

(11) Uterine atony.

(12) Abruption.

(13) Malpresentation.

○ **What physiologic effects occur in twins affected with twin–twin transfusion syndrome?**

The donor twin is underperfused, anemic, growth restricted, microcardiac, hypotensive, and develops oligohydramnios. The recipient twin is overperfused, polycythemic, hypertensive, and develops polyhydramnios.

○ **What is the prognosis of twin–twin transfusion syndrome?**

The earlier in gestation that twin–twin transfusion syndrome develops, the worse the prognosis. If diagnosed before approximately 28 weeks, mortality is in the range of 60% to 80%.

○ **What antenatal factors predict a poor outcome in pregnancies with twin–twin transfusion syndrome?**

Factors such as early gestation at the time of diagnosis, severe polyhydramnios requiring multiple therapeutic amniocenteses, hydrops, or absent- or reversed end diastolic flow.

○ **What is the most common cause of neonatal morbidity and mortality in twins?**

Preterm delivery is the most common cause of neonatal morbidity and mortality in twins.

○ **What percentage of twins are born preterm (before 37 weeks gestation)?**

Almost 50% of twin gestations are born preterm.

○ **What is the mean duration of gestation in twins and triplets?**

Twins, on an average, deliver around 35 weeks and triplets around 33 weeks.

○ **How much greater is the perinatal death rate for twins compared to singletons?**

The perinatal death rate is three times greater for twins compared to singletons.

○ **How much greater is the perinatal death rate for monozygotic twins compared to dizygotic twins?**

The perinatal death rate is 2.5 times greater for monozygotic twins compared to dizygotic twins.

○ **What percentage of twins are affected by intrauterine growth restriction?**

Up to two-thirds of twins can be affected by intrauterine growth restriction.

○ **What criteria are used to diagnose intrauterine growth restriction in twins?**

Intrauterine growth restriction is diagnosed when the estimated fetal weight falls below 10% for a singleton gestation or when there is discordance of greater than 20% between the twins.

○ **What antenatal monitoring should be done once intrauterine growth restriction has been diagnosed?**

Once intrauterine growth restriction has been diagnosed, the pregnancy should be followed closely with serial ultrasounds every 2 to 3 weeks, antenatal testing (nonstress test twice/week) and early delivery should be considered.

○ **Has bed rest been shown to reduce the risk of preterm delivery in twins?**

Numerous studies have failed to show that bed rest reduces the incidence of preterm delivery, lengthens gestation, or improves neonatal morbidity.

○ **Should maternal dietary intake change in multifetal pregnancies?**

Maternal dietary intake should increase by approximately 300 kcal more than that for singleton gestations.

○ **What is the recommended weight gain for women carrying twins?**

The Institute of Medicine recommends a 35 to 45 pound total weight gain at term.

○ **What percentage of twin–twin contamination occurs when CVS is performed on a twin gestation?**

Twin–twin contamination occurs in approximately 5% of cases.

○ **What is the most common clinical presentation for a vanishing twin?**

First trimester bleeding.

○ **What is the pregnancy loss rate in multifetal reduction?**

Pregnancy loss rates range from 5% to 25% depending on the starting number of gestations.

○ **What gestational age is multifetal reduction performed?**

Multifetal reduction is performed around 10 to12 weeks of gestational age.

○ **What is the positive predictive value of routine cervical exams or sonographic cervical measurements in predicting preterm delivery?**

These systems have been associated with a positive predictive value of 75%, which is associated with a fourfold increased relative risk of preterm delivery.

○ **If one twin dies, what complications can occur to the surviving twin?**

Recent evidence suggests that death or morbidity in the surviving twin results from acute hypotension and partial exsanguanation into the dying twin. The surviving twin can develop renal cortical necrosis and multicystic encephalomalacia.

○ **Do twins develop pulmonary maturity at the same rate as singletons?**

Twins appear to develop pulmonary maturity 3 to 4 weeks earlier than singletons.

○ **What are the two most common presentations of twins at the time of delivery?**

The most common presentation of twins at the time of delivery is vertex–vertex (∼40%) followed by vertex–breech (∼25%).

○ **How should vertex–vertex twins be delivered?**

Vaginal delivery is recommended.

○ **How should vertex–nonvertex twins be delivered?**

The delivery of vertex–nonvertex twins is controversial. Some data suggest that the Apgar scores are lower and perinatal complications are increased by vaginally delivering the second nonvertex twin.

○ **What are the vaginal delivery options for the vertex–breech delivery?**

Delivery options for second twin in a vertex–breech delivery include external cephalic version of the second breech twin or internal podalic version and breech extraction.

○ **How should a nonvertex-presenting twin be delivered?**

In general, cesarean delivery is the method of choice when the first twin is nonvertex.

○ **What is the minimum estimated fetal weight of a nonvertex second twin that you would consider attempting a vaginal delivery?**

>1500 g.

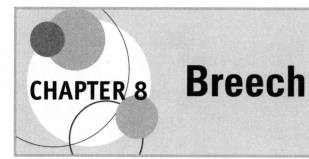

CHAPTER 8 Breech

Rachel Cohen, DO, and Julio Mateus, MD

○ **What is the percentage of infants who are breech after 37 weeks, at 29 to 32 weeks, and at 21 to 24 weeks?**

5% to 7%

14%

33%

○ **What are the types of breech presentation?**

Frank breech—flexed thighs and extended knees (50%–75%).

Complete breech—flexed thighs and knees (5%–10%).

Footling breech—one or both legs extended below the buttocks (20%–24%).

(Figures reproduced, with permission from Cunningham FG et al. *Williams Obstetrics*, 22nd ed. New York: McGraw-Hill, 2005, pp. 566–567.)

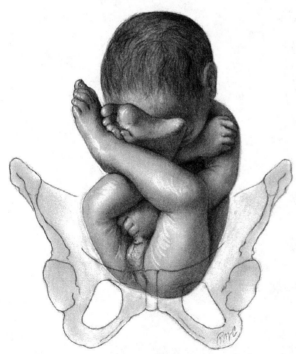

Frank breech

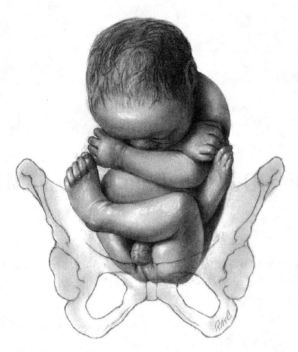

Complete breech

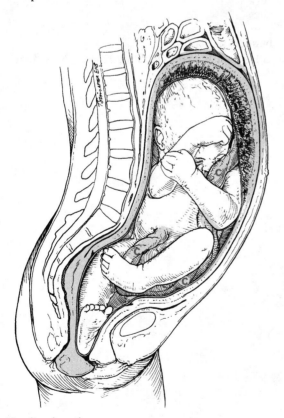

Footling breech

○ **Does perinatal mortality increase in breech presentation?**

Yes, perinatal mortality is increased two- to fourfold regardless of the mode of delivery.

○ **What are the risk factors for breech presentation?**

1. Altered intrauterine contour or volume:
   - Uterine anomalies (bicornuate, septate uterus)
   - Space occupying lesions (uterine myomas)
   - Placental abnormalities (placenta previa, cornual placenta)
   - Multiple gestations
   - Polyhydramnios or oligohydramnios
2. Altered fetal shape or mobility:
   - Fetal anomalies (anencephaly, hydrocephaly, sacrococcygeal teratoma)
   - Impaired fetal growth
   - Short umbilical cord
   - Fetal death
   - Neurologic impairment

○ **What are the three ways to deliver a breech through the vagina?**

Spontaneous—the infant is delivered entirely spontaneously without traction or manipulation.

Assisted breech extraction—the infant is delivered spontaneously to the umbilicus with the rest of the body being extracted.

Total breech extraction—entire body of the infant is extracted.

○ **What is the best indicator of pelvic adequacy for a breech delivery?**

Satisfactory progression of labor.

○ **What percentage of breech presentations undergo cesarean section in the United States?**

90%.

○ **Who are the candidates for external cephalic version (ECV)?**

Women with breech presentation, reassuring fetal heart tracing, and no contraindications for vaginal delivery at 36 weeks and beyond.

○ **What is the most consistent factor associated with the success of ECV?**

Parity.

○ **What other factor is associated with the success of ECV?**

Gestational age—the more remote from term, the higher success rate of the version.

○ **What factors are associated with unsuccessful attempts at version?**

Diminished amniotic fluid, obesity, anterior placenta, cervical dilation, descent of breech into the pelvis, and positioning of the fetal spine.

○   **What are the absolute contraindications for ECV?**

Multiple gestations with a breech presenting fetus, contraindications to vaginal delivery (e.g., genital herpes simplex virus infection, placenta previa), and nonreassuring fetal status.

○   **What are the relative contraindications for ECV?**

Polyhydramnios or oligohydramnios, fetal growth restriction, malformation, and fetal anomaly.

○   **What steps are taken to complete a version?**

   1. Ultrasound to confirm position and vertical pocket of at least 2 cm of amniotic fluid
   2. Reactive nonstress test (NST).
   3. Terbutaline 0.25 mg subcutaneously (not required).
   4. Attempted "forward roll" of fetus 20 minutes after terbutaline.
      (Reproduced, with permission, from Cunningham FG et al. *Williams Obstetrics*, 22nd ed. New York: McGraw-Hill, 2005, p. 583.)

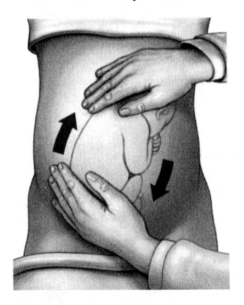 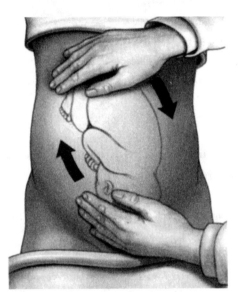

○   **For what reasons is the version attempt abandoned?**

Excessive discomfort, persistent abnormal fetal heart rate after multiple failed attempts.

○   **Is D-immune globulin given to D-negative unsensitized women after version?**

Yes.

○   **Is regional anesthesia recommended for ECV?**

There is not enough consistent evidence favoring the use of regional anesthesia during ECV attempts.

○   **What test is performed after the version?**

NST.

○ **What are the complications of a version?**

Placental abruption, uterine rupture, fetal distress, fetomaternal hemorrhage, brachial plexus injury, fetal death (no reported fetal deaths from external version since 1980), and preterm labor.

○ **What is the overall success rate of external cephalic version?**

58%.

○ **What is the average cesarean delivery rate among those undergoing an attempted version?**

37% (compared to 83% of controls).

○ **What percentage of infants with breech presentation will have congenital anomalies?**

6% to 18% (whereas vertex presentation is 2%–3%).

○ **In what circumstances can total breech extraction be performed?**

Total breech extraction should be used only for a noncephalic second twin.

○ **What are the injury rate and mortality rate of total breech extraction for the singleton breech?**

Injury rate is 25% and mortality rate is around 10%.

○ **What are the steps in the delivery of a frank breech?**

Episiotomy generally required, delivery of posterior hip spontaneously, delivery of anterior hip, delivery of legs, fetal bony pelvis is grasped with both hands using a towel (with fingers resting on superior iliac crest and thumbs on the sacrum), apply gentle downward traction until scapulas are visible; once one axilla is visible the anterior shoulder and arm should be delivered, rotate trunk to deliver other shoulder and arm, the fetal head is then delivered by maintaining flexion with suprapubic pressure provided by an assistant with simultaneous pressure on the maxilla by the operator.

○ **Who needs to be present during an assisted vaginal breech delivery?**

An obstetrician with an assistant, an anesthesiologist, and a pediatrician.

○ **What is the name given to the maneuver where the index and middle finger are placed over the maxilla to flex the head?**

Mauriceau-Smellie-Veit maneuver.

○ **Which forceps can be used if the Mauriceau maneuver cannot be easily accomplished?**

Piper forceps.

○ **What problem associated with the fetal head can occur during a vaginal breech delivery?**

Head entrapment (88/1,000); head circumference is greater than abdominal or thoracic circumference at about 36 weeks.

○ **What two maneuvers can be performed to deliver an infant with head entrapment?**

1. *Duhressen incisions:* If the cervix cannot be slipped over the trapped head, incisions in the cervix at 2-, 6-, and 10-o'clock positions can be made.

2. *Abdominal rescue*

○ **What are the most frequent complications of Duhressen incisions?**

Maternal hemorrhage and extension into the lower uterine segment.

○ **What percentage of fetuses have hyperextended heads during breech labor?**

3% to 5%.

○ **Hyperextension of the head is associated with what injury?**

Spinal cord (21% risk).

○ **When is the Prague maneuver used?**

Prague maneuver consists of two fingers of one hand grasping the shoulders of the back-down fetus while the other hand draws the feet up of the abdomen and is used when the fetal trunk fails to rotate anteriorly.

○ **Which maneuver is used to deliver a foot into the vagina (or during cesarean section) in the case of a frank breech presentation?**

Pinard maneuver.

○ **Why are membranes kept intact as long as possible in breech deliveries?**

Decreases risk of cord prolapse and intact membranes may assist in the dilation of the cervix owing to the pressure.

○ **Which breech presentation has the lowest rate of cord prolapse and the highest?**

Lowest incidence in frank breech (0.5%).
Highest incidence in footling (10%).

○ **What is a nuchal arm?**

When one or both fetal arms are found around the infant's neck.

○ **How does one deliver an infant with a nuchal arm?**

Place two fingers over the humerus and sweep arm over infant's chest; the humerus should be splinted with the operator's fingers to help prevent fracture.

Or, the fetus may be rotated through half a circle so that the elbow is drawn toward the infant's face facilitating delivery of the arm. Lastly, the arm can be forcibly extracted by hooking a finger over it. (High risk of fracture of humerus or clavicle.)

○ **What maternal complications can occur as a result of a vaginal breech delivery?**

Increased risk of infection (because of intrauterine maneuvers).
Laceration of cervix.
Deep perineal tears/extension of episiotomy.

○ **What fetal complications can occur as a result of a breech delivery?**

Fracture of humerus and clavicle

Perineal tears (because of spiral electrode use)

Hematoma of sternocleidomastoid muscles

Separation of epiphyses of scapula, humerus or femur

Skull fractures

Paralysis of the arm

Testicular injury

Increased risk of sudden infant death syndrome

○ **Under what two conditions may term singleton breech delivery be considered?**

(1) Patients presenting with advanced labor, likely to have an imminent delivery of a fetus in breech presentation.

(2) Patients whose second twin is in a nonvertex presentation.

○ **What is the recommended mode of delivery for persistent breech presentation?**

Planned cesarean delivery.

○ **Are perinatal mortality, neonatal mortality, and serious neonatal morbidity significantly lower in a planned cesarean group compared with planned vaginal breech birth group?**

Yes 1.6% vs 5.0%, according to the Term Breech Trial Collaborative Group study published in 2000 in the *Lancet*.

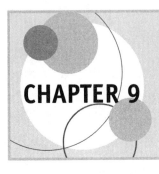

CHAPTER 9

Postdates Pregnancy and Fetal Demise

Stephen J. Smith, MD

○ **Define postterm pregnancy.**

A pregnancy that has extended to or surpassed 42 weeks of gestation or 294 days from the first day of the last menstrual period.

○ **Name the most common cause of postterm pregnancy.**

Error in dating the pregnancy accurately.

○ **What is Naegele's rule?**

A method used to calculate the estimated date of confinement. Using the date of the first day of the last menstrual period as the starting point, subtract 3 months and then add 7 days.

○ **During which trimester is pregnancy dating most accurate?**

First trimester.

○ **What is the margin of error for an ultrasound evaluation of pregnancy dating in the third trimester?**

The margin of error can be as great as plus or minus 3 weeks.

○ **What is the incidence of postterm pregnancy?**

Approximately 10% (range 3%–4%).

○ **List the risk factors for postterm pregnancy.**

Primiparity
  Prior postterm pregnancy
  Fetal anencephaly
  Placental sulfatase deficiency
  Fetal gender: male

○   **List the fetal risks associated with postterm pregnancy.**

Increased perinatal mortality
> Uteroplacental insufficiency leading to oligohydramnios and IUGR
> Meconium aspiration
> Intrauterine infection
> Macrosomia
> Dysmaturity syndrome
> Increased risk of death within 1 year of life

○   **What is the cause of dysmaturity syndrome?**

Dysmaturity syndrome results from chronic intrauterine growth restriction caused by uteroplacental insufficiency.

○   **What is the incidence of dysmaturity syndrome in postterm pregnancy?**

Approximately 20%.

○   **Describe the appearance of the infant with dysmaturity syndrome.**

Dry, parchment-like skin with desquamation.
> Wasted, malnourished appearance with long, thin arms.
> Meconium staining in some cases.
> Long nails.
> Sparse or absent lanugo.
> Increased alertness with "wide-eyed" look.

○   **What intrapartum and neonatal complications are observed in the infant with dysmaturity syndrome?**

Intrapartum: Umbilical cord compression from oligohydramnios
Meconium aspiration
Nonreassuring fetal heart tracing
Neonatal: Hypoglycemia
Seizures
Respiratory insufficiency

○   **List the maternal complications associated with postterm pregnancy?**

Labor dystocia
> Perineal injury
> Cesarean section
> These complications result from the higher risk of macrosomia

○ **What maternal complications are seen with higher frequency following cesarean section vs vaginal delivery?**

Endometritis
Hemorrhage
Thromboembolism

○ **Why does the American College of Obstetricians and Gynecologists (ACOG) recommend the initiation of antepartum fetal surveillance between 41 and 42 weeks gestation?**

The perinatal mortality rate doubles at 42 weeks compared to 40 weeks. Fetal surveillance may decrease perinatal mortality.

○ **What form of antenatal surveillance may be used to assess the postterm fetus?**

Options include
nonstress test;
biophysical profile;
modified biophysical profile;
contraction stress test.
No single method has been shown to be superior, but an assessment of amniotic fluid volume should be incorporated into the surveillance scheme.

○ **What are the criteria for oligohydramnios requiring delivery in the postterm pregnancy?**

Amniotic fluid index $\leq$ 5 cm or largest vertical pocket of amniotic fluid $\leq$ 2 × 2 cm.

○ **What is the most reasonable management plan for the patient with an inducible cervix at 42 weeks gestation?**

Induction and delivery.

○ **In the patient with an uninducible cervix, what are the potential benefits to labor induction at 41 to 42 weeks gestation vs continued expectant management?**

Lower perinatal mortality rate
Reduced risk of meconium-stained fluid
Higher patient satisfaction

○ **True or False: Induction of the patient with an uninducible cervix at 41 to 42 weeks gestation increases the risk of cesarean section.**

False.

○ **What is the modified biophysical profile?**

Nonstress test plus amniotic fluid volume estimation.

○ **The intrapartum fetal heart rate tracing of a patient at 42 weeks gestation is shown below. What intrapartum complication does this tracing suggest?**

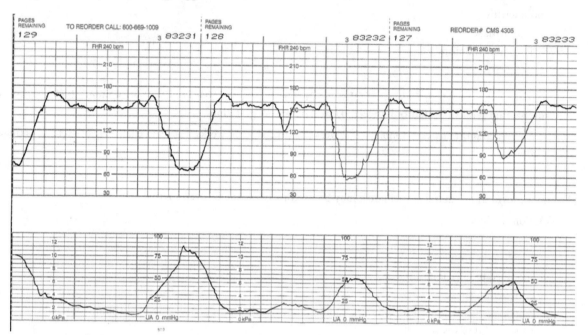

Severe variable decelerations indicative of oligohydramnios and umbilical cord compression.

○ **The nonstress test shown below was performed on a patient at 41 weeks gestation. The amniotic fluid index was 10 cm. Her cervix is uninducible. What are the options for management?**

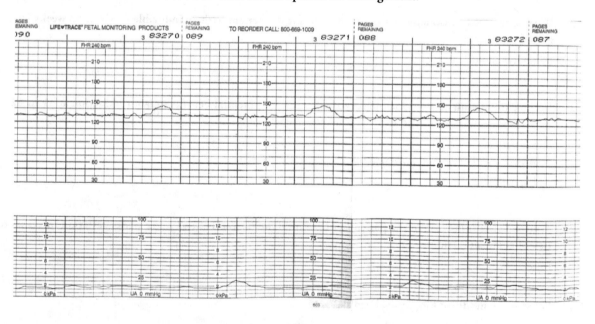

This is a reactive nonstress test in a patient with normal amniotic fluid volume. Reasonable options include continued expectant management or induction of labor.

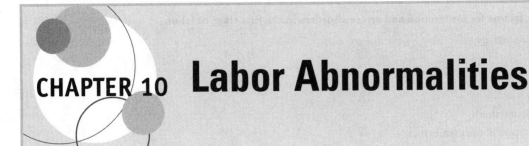

CHAPTER 10 Labor Abnormalities

Stephen J. Smith, MD

○ **What is the definition of labor?**

The presence of uterine contractions of sufficient intensity, frequency, and duration to cause effacement and dilation of the cervix.

○ **What is the definition of labor dystocia?**

Abnormal labor resulting from abnormalities in "power, passenger, or passage."

○ **In the United States, the most common indication for primary C-section is:**

Dystocia.

○ **Many repeat cesarean sections are performed after primary cesarean sections for dystocia. Taking this fact into account, what percentage of all cesarean sections performed in the United States is attributable to the diagnosis of dystocia?**

60%.

○ **Latent phase is considered prolonged if:**

It exceeds 20 hours in nulliparas or 14 hours in multiparas.

○ **The latent phase is completed when the cervix is:**

A minimum of 4 cm dilated.

○ **Management of choice for prolonged latent phase is:**

Therapeutic rest induced with morphine.

○ **What percentage of patients treated with therapeutic rest for prolonged latent phase will progress to active phase?**

85%.

○ **List the risk factors for protraction and arrest disorders in the first stage of labor.**

Advanced maternal age

Diabetes

Hypertension

Oligohydramnios

Previous perinatal death

Premature rupture of the membranes

Chorioamnionitis

Macrosomia

Epidural anesthesia

Pelvic contractures

Nonreassuring fetal heart rate pattern

○ **List the risk factors for dystocia in the second stage of labor.**

Occiput posterior presentation

Prolonged first stage of labor

Nulliparity

Short maternal stature

Macrosomia

High station at complete cervical dilation

○ **Is amniotomy beneficial for the patient with prolonged latent phase?**

Amniotomy can shorten the latent phase of labor if used with active management of labor protocols. One meta-analysis found that is shortened the first stage by up to 39 minutes.

○ **Describe the effect of amniotomy (performed during the active phase) on labor duration, maternal fever, cesarean section, and nonreassuring fetal heart rate patterns.**

Labor duration: Reduction by 1 to 2 hours.

Maternal fever: Increased incidence.

Cesarean section: No effect.

Nonreassuring fetal heart rate patterns: No effect.

○ **Complete the table, indicating the criteria for second stage arrest in nulliparas and multiparas.**

	No Regional Anesthesia	**Regional Anesthesia**
Nullipara	_____ h	_____ h
Multipara	_____ h	_____ h

	No Regional Anesthesia	Regional Anesthesia
Nullipara	2 h	3 h
Multipara	1 h	2 h

○ **Traditionally, what two criteria must be met to diagnose an arrest disorder in the first stage of labor**

(1) Latent phase complete. (2) Uterine contraction pattern exceeding 200 Montevideo units for 2 hours without cervical change (the 2-hour rule) calculated using an intrauterine pressure catheter.

○ **True or False: In making the diagnosis of active phase arrest, 4 hours of sustained uterine contractions without cervical change may be more appropriate than the traditional "2-hour rule."**

True.

○ **Treatment of active phase arrest includes:**

Amniotomy and/or oxytocin augmentation.

○ **Minimally effective uterine activity is defined as:**

Three contractions per 10 minutes of at least 25 mm Hg above baseline or a contraction pattern exceeding 200 Montevideo units per 10 minute window without cervical change.

○ **Hyperstimulation is defined as:**

Persistent pattern of more than five contractions in 10 minutes, contractions lasting 2 minutes or more, or contractions of normal duration occurring within 1 minute of each other.

○ **Mean plasma half-life of oxytocin is:**

3 to 5 minutes.

○ **The interval to reach a steady state concentration of oxytocin in plasma is between:**

20 to 40 minutes.

○ **True or False: X-ray pelvimetry is generally considered of a little value in the treatment of active phase arrest.**

True.

○ **Maximal dose of oxytocin is generally considered to be:**

30 to 40 mU/min.

○   **In patients with documented disorders of labor, what percentage responds to oxytocin infusion resulting in a vaginal delivery?**

80%.

○   **Calculate the Montevideo units for the 10-minute window in this illustration (round to the nearest 50). Assume an internal pressure transducer is being used.**

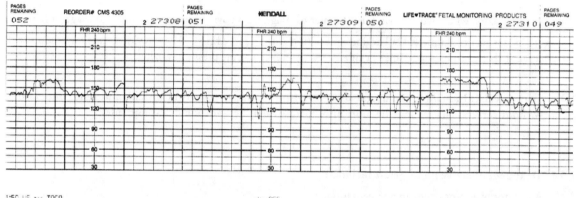

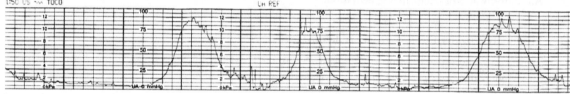

250

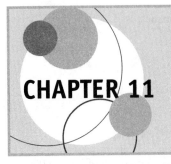

CHAPTER 11 The Puerperium

Maria A. Giraldo-Isaza

○ **Define the puerperium.**

The period that extends from just after birth to 6 weeks postpartum.

○ **How many weeks does it take for the uterus to regain its nonpregnant size?**

The uterus regains its nonpregnant size approximately 4 weeks after delivery.

○ **What is the process called by which the uterus shrinks to its nonpregnant size?**

Involution.

○ **What is the term used to describe the arrest of the normal process of uterine involution?**

Subinvolution. Subinvolution is recognized on examination by the presence of a uterus that is larger and softer than normal for the particular postpartum time. It is usually associated with irregular or excessive uterine bleeding.

○ **What are the two most common causes of subinvolution?**

Retained placental fragments and uterine infection.

○ **What is the definition of puerperal fever?**

Temperature greater than or equal to 100.4°F on any two of the first ten postpartum days, exclusive of the first 24 hours.

○ **What is the most significant risk factor for the development of postpartum uterine infection?**

Mode of delivery.

○ **What are the risk factors for postpartum uterine infection?**

Mode of delivery, prolonged rupture of membranes, multiple cervical examinations, prolonged labor, internal fetal monitoring, intra-amniotic infection, lower socioeconomic class, vaginal colonization with Group B *Streptococcus, Chlamydia, Mycoplasma, Ureaplasma,* or *Gardnerella.*

○   **True or False: Postpartum uterine infection is usually caused by a single organism.**

False.

○   **What organism most commonly causes late onset postpartum metritis?**

Chlamydia.

○   **What are the clinical signs of postpartum uterine infection?**

Fever, abdominal tenderness, tachycardia, foul-smelling lochia, elevated white blood count of 15,000 to 30,000.

○   **What is the incidence of bacteremia associated with postcesarean uterine infection?**

10% to 20%.

○   **List the organisms most commonly causing postpartum uterine infection.**

Aerobes

    Enterococcus

    Staphylococcus aureus

    Group A, B, D streptococci

    Gram-negative bacteria—*E. coli, Klebsiella, Proteus*

Anaerobes

    Peptococcus species

    Peptostreptococcus species

    Bacteroides species

    Clostridium species

    Fusobacterium species

Other

    Mycoplasma

    Gonorrhea

    Chlamydia trachomatis

○   **What are the risk factors for postcesarean section wound infection?**

Obesity, diabetes, corticosteroid therapy, immunosuppression, anemia, wound hematoma, uterine infection.

○   **What is the treatment for wound infection?**

Antibiotics and surgical drainage.

○   **What is necrotizing fasciitis?**

A rare complication of wound infection involving the deep soft tissues, including muscle and fascia.

○   **What are the risk factors for necrotizing fasciitis?**

Diabetes, obesity, intravenous drug use, age greater than 50, hypertension, malnutrition, malignancy, cirrhosis, and peripheral vascular disease.

○ **True or False: Wound infection resulting in necrotizing fasciitis is usually monobacterial.**

False (Usually polymicrobial caused by anaerobes and aerobes. If monobacterial, usually group A beta-hemolytic *Streptococcus*).

○ **Name common extra-pelvic causes of puerperal fever?**

Atelectasis, pneumonia, pyelonephritis, breast engorgement, thrombophlebitis.

○ **In a woman with postcesarean wound infection, what is the most common presenting symptom, and how many days after cesarean section does the symptom usually occur?**

Fever on postoperative day 4.

○ **List complications of postpartum uterine infection that result in persistent fever.**

Wound infection, peritonitis, pelvic abscess, parametrial phlegmon, pelvic hematoma, septic pelvic thrombophlebitis, and antibiotic-resistant bacteria.

○ **How long after delivery does ovarian abscess complicating postpartum uterine infection usually present?**

1 to 2 weeks.

○ **True or False: Ovarian abscess complicating postpartum uterine infection is usually bilateral.**

False.

○ **What is the parametrial phlegmon?**

An area of induration in the broad ligament resulting from parametrial cellulitis and postpartum metritis.

○ **What is the approximate incidence of wound infection following cesarean section?**

3% to 15%.

○ **True or False: Enigmatic fever is associated with postpartum septic thrombophlebitis.**

True.

○ **What is the one constant clinical characteristic of enigmatic fever?**

Hectic fever spikes following initial response to antimicrobial treatment of postpartum pelvic infection.

○ **What are the clinical features of ovarian vein thrombosis?**

Lower abdominal or flank pain on postpartum day 2 to 3, possible fever, possible palpable tender adnexal mass.

○ **True or False: Pulmonary embolism is commonly associated with septic thrombophlebitis.**

False.

○ **What is the incidence of episiotomy infection or breakdown after vaginal delivery?**

Less than 1%.

○ **What is the primary cause of episiotomy breakdown?**

Infection.

○ **What are the three most common symptoms of episiotomy infection?**

Pain, purulent discharge, fever.

○ **How is episiotomy infection treated?**

Open and drain wound, broad-spectrum antibiotics.

○ **True or False: Vulvar hematomas most commonly result from injury to the branches of a descending uterine artery.**

False (Pudendal artery).

○ **What is the most common presenting symptom of vulvar hematoma?**

Pain.

○ **True or False: Surgical drainage is the best treatment for a 3 cm nonexpanding hematoma in a patient experiencing a mild degree of pain.**

False (Expectant management is appropriate).

○ **What is the definition of secondary postpartum hemorrhage?**

Postpartum hemorrhage occurring after 24 hours and before 6 to 12 weeks after delivery.

○ **What are the three main causes of secondary postpartum hemorrhage?**

Abnormal involution of the placenta site, retained placenta, and uterine infection.

○ **True or False: Breast feeding is contraindicated in women with HIV infection because of the risk of transmission.**

True. The frequency of breast milk transmission is estimated to be 15% to 20%.

○ **True or False: Breast feeding is absolutely contraindicated in hepatitis B.**

False. Breastfeeding is not contraindicated if hepatitis B immune globulin and vaccine are given to the infants of seropositive mothers.

○ **True or False: Breast feeding is contraindicated in the mother with active herpes simplex virus.**

False. Breastfeeding is appropriate if there are no breast lesions and the mother is meticulous about hand washing before handling the infant and breast feeding.

○ **True or False: For late postpartum hemorrhage, uterine curettage is the initial treatment of choice.**

False. Curettage is reserved for failed medical management.

○ **How many days or weeks postpartum is mastitis most commonly seen?**

Four to five weeks.

○ **True or False: Mastitis is usually bilateral.**

False.

○ **What are the clinical signs and symptoms of mastitis?**

Marked breast engorgement, fever, chills, hard reddened painful area of breast.

○ **What is the approximate incidence of abscess complicating mastitis?**

10%.

○ **What is the most common organism causing mastitis?**

Staphylococcus aureus.

○ **What is the source of the organism causing mastitis?**

The infant's nasopharynx.

○ **True or False: A woman with mastitis should immediately discontinue breast feeding.**

False (Discontinuation has been associated with an increased risk of abscess formation).

○ **List the symptoms experienced by women with postpartum blues.**

Insomnia, weepiness, depression, anxiety, poor concentration, irritability, and moodiness.

○ **True or False: Approximately 50% of childbearing women experience postpartum blues.**

True.

○ **List some factors that most likely contribute to the development of postpartum blues.**

The discomforts of the puerperium.
A new mother's anxieties over her capabilities for caring for her infant.
Fatigue from loss of sleep.
Fears that she has become less attractive.
The emotional letdown following the anticipation and excitement of delivery.

○ **True or False: Postpartum depression usually does not recur.**

False (Up to a 70% recurrence risk).

○ **True or False: Adolescent women have an increased risk for postpartum depression.**

True.

○   **What are the risk factors for postpartum psychosis?**

History of psychotic illness, primiparity, and family history of psychiatric illness.

○   **How long should antibiotics be given for the condition shown?**

Antibiotics should be given for 10 to 14 days for mastitis.

○   **What is the predominant immunoglobulin found in breast milk?**

Secretory IgA.

○   **True or False: Bromocriptine is indicated for lactation inhibition.**

False. Bromocriptine is not recommended for this indication as it has been shown to have significant side effects like stroke, MI, seizures, and psychiatric disorders.

○   **What is the treatment for breast engorgement?**

Ice packs, well fitting brassiere, and oral analgesics for 12 to 24 hours.

○   **What is the most common neuropathy associated with deliveries?**

Lateral femoral cutaneous.

○   **True or False: Elective cesarean section delivery should be considered after pelvic joint separation in prior delivery.**

True. Recurrence is more than 50% in subsequent pregnancy.

○   **What is the most important criteria for the diagnosis of postpartum metritis?**

Fever.

○   **What is the gold standard treatment for pelvic infection following C-section?**

Clindamycin 900 mg + gentamicin 1.5 mg/kg IV q8h.

○   **True or False: Antepartum treatment of asymptomatic women with vaginal infection has been shown to prevent postpartum endometritis.**

False.

○   **What is the layer that is separated in a wound dehiscence?**

Fascia.

○   **What is the treatment for wound dehiscence?**

Secondary closure of incision in OR.

○   **What is diagnostic test for septic thrombophlebitis?**

CT or MRI pelvis.

○   **How is postpartum hemorrhage classified?**

Primary hemorrhage occurs within the first 24 h postpartum, while secondary hemorrhage occurs between 24 h and 6–12 week postpartum.

○   **What is the main etiology of primary postpartum hemorrhage?**

Uterine atony.

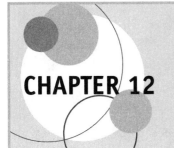

CHAPTER 12 Obstetric Complications

Amy Mackey, MD

○ **Beta-sympathomimetics may cause which electrolyte abnormalities?**

Hypokalemia, hypocalcemia.

○ **What is antidote for magnesium sulfate toxicity?**

1 g calcium gluconate IV push.

○ **Name the contraindication to terbutaline.**

Maternal cardiac disease (structural, ischemic, dysrhythmic), hypertensive disease, antepartum hemorrhage, uncontrolled diabetes mellitus, and uncontrolled maternal hyperthyroidism.

○ **What is the incidence of preterm birth in the US?**

11.8%.

○ **What endogenous substances have been linked to preterm labor?**

Bacterial endotoxins (lipopolysaccharides), platelet activating factor, interleukins 1 and 6, and tumor necrosis factor.

○ **What substance is released when the amnion begins to separate from the decidua?**

Fetal fibronectin.

○ **What is the significance for testing cervical secretions for fetal fibronectin?**

Negative predictive value 95% of not delivering within 14 days when test negative.
Positive predictive value 40% of delivery when test positive in symptomatic women.

○ **Low lying placenta with a marginal insertion, soft abdomen, a minimal amount of bleeding and acutely distressed fetus suggests:**

Vasa previa.

○ **What percentage of vasa previa is detected by antepartum ultrasound?**

<10%.

○ **What is the signature hepatic lesion of preeclampsia?**

Periportal necrosis.

○ **When do convulsions occur during eclampsia?**

50% before the onset of labor, and the other 50% equally divided between intrapartum and postpartum.

○ **What are the benefits of antepartum corticosteroids in premature babies?**

- Increased lung compliance, increased surfactant production, and decreased respiratory distress syndrome
- Decreased intraventricular hemorrhage
- Decreased necrotizing enterocolitis
- Decreased neonatal mortality

○ **What are the NIH recommendations for steroid use in preterm premature rupture of membranes?**

Recommended for less than 30 to 32 weeks in the absence of chorioamnionitis.

○ **Of all IUGR babies, how many show symmetric growth lag?**

20%.

○ **Of all IUGR babies, how many are affected by a chromosomal abnormality, congenital malformation, or genetic syndrome?**

10%.

○ **What metabolic problems are commonly found in IUGR neonates?**

Hypocalcemia, hypoglycemia, hyponatremia, hypothermia, and polycythemia.

○ **At what gestational age does maternal IgG begin to crossover the placenta and provide protection for the fetus?**

16 weeks. By 26 weeks, fetal and maternal IgG serum levels are similar.

○ **How is *Toxoplasma gondii* infection diagnosed in the fetus?**

Cord blood fetal anti-Toxoplasma IgM or amniotic fluid PCR.

○ **What percentage of adults in the US has antibodies (and thus immunity) to *Toxoplasma*?**

40% to 50%, and the prevalence is the highest in lower socioeconomic populations.

○ **What percentage of childbearing age women shows immunity to varicella zoster (chicken pox)?**

95%.

○ **What life threatening complications can affect a patient with adult onset varicella infection?**

Encephalitis and pneumonia.

○ **What is the role of varicella zoster immune globulin (VZIG) and varicella vaccine in pregnancy?**

VZIG is administered within 96 hours of significant exposure, and is 60% to 80% effective in preventing infection. Varicella vaccine is an attenuated live virus, and should NOT be given during pregnancy. Acyclovir can also be effective in preventing varicella when given prophylactically (800 mg po 5 times per day for 5–7days).

○ **What is the fetal effect of maternal parvovirus B-19 infection in pregnancy?**

Most fetuses are unaffected. An increased risk of miscarriage is seen with early exposure, and rarely, a syndrome of nonimmune hydrops can be seen. Parvo B-19 is thought to cause anemia by reducing supply rather than increasing destruction of erythrocytes. Treatment is intrauterine blood transfusion.

○ **What is missing on microscopic examination of the placenta when placenta accreta, increta, and percreta?**

Nitabuch's layer, a line of separation between myometrium and invading trophoblasts.

○ **Name risk factors for placental abruption.**

Smoking, trauma, cocaine, hypertension, preterm premature rupture of membranes, retroplacental fibroids, multiple gestation, inherited thrombophilia, and possibly advanced age/parity.

○ **The recurrence rate of placental abruption is:**

5% to 17%.

○ **What complications can be anticipated in the use of a cell-saver autotransfusion for uterine or adnexal surgery in the pregnant patient?**

Potential amniotic fluid contamination (minimal after processing) and Rh incompatibility between maternal and fetal blood.

○ **Virtually all postpartum patients with septic shock have a source of infection requiring surgical drainage. What microorganisms are associated with each clinical picture?**

Endomyometritis: Prevotella (was Bacteroides) biviens and/or *Gardnerella* (60%), aerobic gram-negative bacilli (*E. coli, Klebsiella pneumoniae, Proteus*), group B *Streptococcus*

Late onset endomyometritis: *Chlamydia, Mycoplasma*

Pelvic abscess: *Prevotella, Bacteroides*

Necrotizing fasciitis:

Group A *Streptococcus* + *Staphylococcus*

Mixed aerobe + anaerobes including *Clostridia*

Group B *Streptococcus* + anaerobes

○ **Postpartum patient presenting with mild fever, hip tenderness, paravaginal tenderness. Delivery record shows an uncomplicated vaginal delivery with a pudendal block for anesthesia. What is going on?**

Retroperitoneal mixed aerobe and anaerobic abscess following needle track along trochanter and/or psoas muscle. Start antibiotics and confirm with CT.

○ **What is the average gestational age for delivery in cases of multiple gestations beyond 24 weeks?**

Twins: 36 to 37 weeks

Triplets: 33 to 34 weeks

Quadruplets: 30 to 31 weeks

Three or more fetuses reduced to twins: 35 to 36 weeks

○ **At what gestational age is it generally not recommended to use a vacuum to assist delivery?**

34 weeks or less.

○ **What is the risk of using a vacuum below this age limit?**

Intraventricular hemorrhage.

○ **What is the risk of placenta accreta in women who have a placenta previa?**

After first C/S: 3%

After second C/S: 11%

After third C/S: 40%

After fourth C/S: 61%

○ **What is the maternal mortality rate associated with placenta accreta?**

7%.

○ **What is the difference between placenta accreta, increta, and percreta?**

Accreta—placental villi are attached to the myometrium with absent Nitabuch layer.

Increta—invasion of placental villi into the myometrium.

Percreta—invasion penetrates through the full thickness of the myometrium.

○ **What is the technique for replacement of the uterus in an inverted uterus when replacement is refractory to manual replacement?**

Huntington's technique: Perform a laparotomy with a tenaculum placed on the uterus to sequentially replace the fundus. If the cervical band is too tight, use the Haultain technique. This is incising the ring posteriorly (to avoid the bladder) and correcting the inversion.

○ **Most fetal survivors of a perimortem C/S are delivered within what time frame?**

5 minutes of cardiac arrest.

○ **What are the two leading causes of anesthesia related maternal morbidity and mortality?**

Failed intubation and pulmonary aspiration.

○ **What is the recurrence risk of shoulder dystocia?**

1% to 16.7%.

○ **What is the advantage of placing heroin addicted pregnant women on methadone during pregnancy?**

1. It avoids the risks of STDs such as HIV and Hepatitis from IV drug use.
2. It decreases the risk of intrauterine demise from cyclical withdrawal.

○ **What is the incidence of conjoined twins? When does the embryonic division occur in conjoined twins?**

1/50,000 births
Days 13 to 15 after fertilization

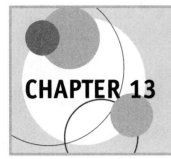

CHAPTER 13

Hypertension and Pregnancy

Shai Pri-Paz, MD

○ **What is the incidence of hypertensive disease in pregnancy?**

12% to 22%.

○ **What is gestational hypertension?**

A systolic blood pressure level of 140 mm Hg or higher or a diastolic blood pressure level of 90 mm Hg or higher that occurs after 20 weeks of gestation in a woman with previously normal blood pressure, and blood pressure returns to normal within 12 weeks postpartum. The elevated blood pressure should be documented on two separate occasions at least six hours apart, but no more than seven days apart.

○ **What is preeclampsia?**

Hypertension (as defined before) with proteinuria (urinary excretion of 300 mg protein or higher in a 24 hour urine specimen or persistent 1+ or more on dipstick in random urine samples).

○ **What is eclampsia?**

Presence of new onset grand mal seizures (that cannot be attributed to other causes) in a woman with preeclampsia.

○ **What is superimposed preeclampsia?**

New onset proteinuria in a woman with hypertension before 20 weeks of gestation, a sudden increase in proteinuria if already present in early gestation, a sudden increase in hypertension, or the development of HELLP syndrome.

○ **What are the criteria for diagnosis of severe preeclampsia?**

One or more of the following: systolic blood pressure of 160 mm Hg or higher or diastolic 110 mm Hg or higher on two occasions at least 6 hours apart while the patient is on bed rest; proteinuria of 5000 mg or higher in a 24 hour urine specimen or 3+ or greater on two random urine samples collected at least 4 hours apart; oliguria of less than 500 mL in 24 hours; cerebral or visual disturbances; pulmonary edema or cyanosis; epigastric or right upper quadrant pain; impaired liver function; thrombocytopenia; fetal growth restriction.

○ **What is the diastolic blood pressure?**

The pressure when the sound disappears (Korotkoff phase V).

○ **What is an appropriate size cuff?**

Length 1.5 times upper arm circumference or a cuff with a bladder that encircles 80% or more of the arm.

○ **How should the blood pressure be measured?**

In an upright position (or left lateral recumbent position with the patient's arm at the level of the heart) after a 10 minute or longer rest period. Tobacco or caffeine should not be used for 30 minutes prior to the measurement.

○ **What is the incidence of preeclampsia?**

5% to 8%.

○ **What are some risk factors for preeclampsia?**

First pregnancy, multifetal gestations, preeclampsia in a previous pregnancy, chronic hypertension, pregestational diabetes, vascular and connective tissue disease, nephropathy, antiphospholipid antibody syndrome, obesity, age 35 years or older, African American race.

○ **What is the pathophysiology of preeclampsia?**

Vascular endothelial damage with vasospasm, transudation of plasma, and ischemic and thrombotic sequelae.

○ **Name a few suggested etiologies for the development of preeclampsia.**

Abnormal (incomplete) trophoblastic invasion of uterine vessels, immunological intolerance of fetoplacental tissue, maladaption to inflammatory or cardiovascular changes of pregnancy, dietary deficiencies, and genetic influence.

○ **What term is used to describe the arterial changes noted in preeclampsia?**

Atherosis.

○ **How does the prostacycline:thromboxane A2 ratio change in preeclampsia?**

It decreases and thus there is increased sensitivity to infused angiotensin 2, which results in vasoconstriction.

○ **How does the blood volume differ with the different conditions?**

In average size women, there is an expected increase in the blood volume at the end of normal pregnancy from 3500 to 5000 mL. With gestational hypertension, a normal blood volume is expected. Different degrees of hemoconcentration are expected with preeclampsia depending on the severity, and absence of much or all of the anticipated volume excess is expected with eclampsia.

○ **What is the characteristic hepatic lesion?**

Periportal hemorrhage in the liver periphery.

○ **What changes can be associated with preeclampsia?**

Vascular	Hypertension
	Hemoconcentration
	Intense vasospasm
Hematologic	Thrombocytopenia
	Hemolysis
Hepatic	Elevated AST and ALT
	Hyperbilirubinemia
	Hepatic hemorrhage
Neurologic	Temporary blindness
	Headache
	Blurred vision
	Scotomata
	Hyperreflexia
	Eclampsia
Renal	Oliguria
	ATN
	Absence of decrease in serum creatinine
Fetal	IUGR
	Oligohydramnios
	Placental abruption
	Non-reassuring fetal status

○ **Name a few imitators of severe preeclampsia/HELLP syndrome. –**

Acute fatty liver of pregnancy, thrombotic thrombocytopenic purpura, hemolytic uremic syndrome, and acute exacerbation of systemic lupus erythematosus.

○ **What may a high fever associated with preeclampsia indicate?**

A central nervous system hemorrhage.

○ **What is the recommended screening test for preeclampsia?**

A variety of tests have been studied, such as uric acid, fibronectin, PAI-1 levels and ratio, and homocysteine level, but no test is currently recommended.

○ **Can preeclampsia be prevented?**

No treatment is currently recommended to prevent preeclampsia, but a study regarding treatment with vitamin C and vitamin E showed promising findings that should be confirmed in a larger study. The Cochrane review does report small to moderate benefits when using antiplatelet agents for prevention of preeclampsia (15% reduction in the risk of preeclampsia associated with the use of antiplatelet agents).

The Cochrane review reports that calcium supplementation appears to almost halve the risk of preeclampsia, and to reduce the rare occurrence of the composite outcome without any other clear benefits or harms.

○ **Name a few treatments that may prevent preeclampsia?**

Calcium supplementation, fish oil, low-dose aspirin, and antioxidants.

○ **How should preeclampsia be treated?**

Maternal and fetal risks have to be balanced while deciding when to deliver the pregnancy and is the definitive treatment.

For mild disease with a preterm fetus, continued observation may be appropriate. It may include weekly NST and or BPP (or twice weekly for suspected IUGR or oligohydramnios), and US for growth scan and amniotic fluid assessment every 3 weeks. Maternal evaluation should include platelet count, liver enzymes, renal function, and 24 hour urine collection for protein weekly.

If continued observation is chosen for a severe disease (remote from term), it may include daily evaluation of fetal and maternal status including laboratory evaluation, depending on the severity and the progression.

○ **When should antihypertensive treatment be given during expectant management of preeclampsia?**

When systolic blood pressure is above 150 to 160 mm Hg or diastolic blood pressure above 100 to 110 mm Hg; since at these levels, there is a higher risk of maternal complications, such as cerebral hemorrhage. The only proven effect of treatment of mild preeclampsia is a reduced incidence of severe preeclampsia.

○ **What is the initial treatment of severe preeclampsia prior to 34 weeks?**

Hospitalization, during which the maternal and the fetal status are evaluated: blood pressure monitoring; strict documentation of intake and output; 24 hour urine collection; and laboratory studies such as CBC, basic metabolic panel, liver function tests and possibly LDH, uric acid, albumin, and coagulation studies. The fetal status is evaluated by NST, AFI, fetal growth, and possible umbilical artery Doppler velocimetry. Corticosteroids should be administered and magnesium should be given for seizure prophylaxis.

○ **What about women who develop preeclampsia before 23 to 25 weeks?**

They should be delivered, with no role for expectant management.

○ **Who is a candidate for expectant management?**

Asymptomatic women with laboratory abnormalities that resolve within 24 to 48 hours; severe preeclampsia because of severe proteinuria alone; severe preeclampsia based solely on fetal growth restrictions; severe preeclampsia based solely on blood pressure criteria.

○ **What are contraindications to expectant management (in which the pregnancy is not even prolonged enough to receive the second dose of steroids)?**

Maternal shock, non-reassuring fetal testing, severe blood pressure unresponsive to medications, persistent headache, visual disturbances or epigastric/RUQ pain, eclampsia, pulmonary edema, renal failure, some laboratory abnormalities, such as coagulopathy, placental abruption, gestational age more than 34 weeks, maternal request, and HELLP syndrome.

○ **Is there a role for outpatient management of preeclampsia?**

Hospitalization is often initially recommended for new onset preeclampsia. Ambulatory management is possible for selected women such as those with mild gestational hypertension or preeclampsia remote from term. If severe preeclampsia or worsening of preeclampsia is diagnosed, hospitalization is indicated and, therefore, it is indicated for women who have difficulty with compliance.

○ **What is the medical management during labor and delivery?**

The treatment is aimed at preventing seizures or eclampsia and controlling hypertension. Magnesium sulfate is effective in severe preeclampsia/GHTN and eclampsia, but there are different opinions regarding its use in women with mild disease. Antihypertensive treatment is generally recommended for diastolic blood pressure of 105 to 110 mm Hg or higher or systolic blood pressure more than 160 mm Hg.

○ **Why is the use of magnesium sulfate in mild disease controversial?**

The risk of seizures in this group is considered low and is balanced against the toxicity of magnesium. A report from Parkland in 2006 demonstrated an increase in the incidence of eclampsia following their decision not to treat mild gestational hypertension with magnesium.

○ **Name the two most common antihypertensive medications used for acute therapy?**

Labetalol (20 mg IV followed by 40, 80, and 80 as needed with 10 minutes interval) or hydralazine (5 to 10 mg IV every 15 to 20 minutes).

○ **What is the optimal mode of delivery?**

Mild preeclampsia—vaginal delivery. For severe preeclampsia, it should be individualized. (Some recommend a scheduled cesarean delivery for pregnancies at less than 30 weeks with a low Bishop score.)

○ **What is the preferred anesthesia?**

For preeclampsia and eclampsia, the preferred method is regional anesthesia. This anesthesia is contraindicated in the presence of coagulopathy or severe thrombocytopenia (platelet count less than $50,000/mm^3$).

○ **When does the blood pressure usually normalize?**

Within the first week postpartum for gestational hypertension, and 2 weeks for preeclampsia.

○ **Describe the classic eclamptic seizure.**

Generalized tonic clonic. Usually begins with facial twitching, followed after a few seconds by a phase of generalized muscular contraction for 15 to 20 seconds. During the clonic phase, which may last approximately a minute, all the muscles contract and relax alternately, usually starting at the jaws and the eyelids. The movements then gradually subside, becoming smaller and less frequent until the woman eventually lies motionless.

○ **How should eclampsia be managed?**

Medical stabilization is necessary in order to prevent maternal injury. The first step will include supportive care, maintaining an open airway, and maternal oxygenation (supply oxygen at 8–10 L/min). Magnesium sulfate (IV or IM) should be used to control convulsions and prevent recurrence. Antihypertensive medications should be used for diastolic blood pressure of 105 to 110 mm Hg or higher. Delivery should be done in a timely fashion.

○ **What is the regimen of intravenous magnesium?**

Loading dose of 4 to 6 g for 15 to 20 minutes, followed by maintenance of 2 g/h. The magnesium level is measured every 4 to 6 h to adjust the level to 4.8 to 8.4 mg/dL.

○ **When should magnesium sulfate be discontinued?**

Usually 24 hours after delivery or after the onset of convulsions. A randomized controlled trial published in 2006 (Ehrenberg and Mercer, 2006) concluded that for mild preeclampsia, discontinuation of magnesium 12 hours after delivery was associated with infrequent disease progression and a clinical course similar to that with 24-hour therapy.

○ **How is magnesium cleared?**

Renal excretion.

○ **What is the main side effect of magnesium?**

Flushing.

○ **At what level do the patellar reflexes disappear?**

9.6 to 12 mg/dL.

○ **How should magnesium toxicity be treated?**

Calcium gluconate 1 g IV for 5 to 10 minutes.

○ **May magnesium be used in association with calcium channel blockers, such as nifedipine?**

The simultaneous use of these drugs may, on very rare occasions, result in profound neuromuscular blockade, including cardiac depression and muscle weakness. (Reversal can be achieved with 10% solution calcium gluconate.)

○ **Does magnesium affect the fetal heart rate pattern?**

It may decrease the variability.

○ **How should you treat a recurrent eclamptic seizure in spite of magnesium treatment (approximately 10% of cases)?**

An additional 2 g dose of magnesium should be given IV and may be repeated once in some women.

○ **When should sodium amobarbital be used?**

250 mg intravenously over 3 to 5 minutes may be used to treat recurrent convulsions in spite of adequate magnesium therapy.

○ **What percentage of eclamptic seizures develops before overt proteinuria is identified?**

10% to 14%.

○ **Can eclampsia occur without hypertension?**

In 16% of the eclamptic cases, hypertension is absent. (It is severe in 20% to 54% and mild in 30% to 60%).

○ **When does eclampsia develop?**

More than 90% develop at or beyond 28 week, 38% to 53% develop antepartum, 18% to 36% intrapartum, and 11% to 44% postpartum.

○ **Which condition may be associated with eclampsia prior to 20 weeks?**

Molar pregnancy.

○ **Name the common symptoms, which may precede eclampsia.**

Persistent occipital or frontal headaches, blurred vision, photophobia, epigastric pain, right upper quadrant pain.

○ **When is cerebral imaging indicated?**

For patients with focal neurological deficits or prolonged coma, and for patients with atypical features of eclampsia, such as onset before 20 weeks, late postpartum eclampsia, or eclampsia refractory to adequate therapy with magnesium sulfate.

○ **What conditions are in the differential diagnosis of eclampsia?**

Hypertensive encephalopathy, seizure disorder, brain tumors, hypoglycemia, thrombophilia, thrombotic thrombocytopenic purpura, vasculitis, encephalitis, meningitis, and ruptured cerebral aneurysm.

○ **What percentage of eclamptic seizures occurs in late postpartum eclampsia (beyond 48 hours postpartum but less than 4 weeks)?**

25% (attributed to improved prenatal care).

○ **Is fetal bradycardia following a seizure an indication for a stat cesarean?**

No. Fetal bradycardia is common after a seizure because of maternal hypoxemia and lactic acidemia. This usually resolves after 3 to 5 minutes of intrauterine resuscitation. If persistent for more than 10 minutes, then an imminent delivery must be considered, as it may indicate other complications such as placental abruption.

○ **What patterns of fetal heart rate may be noted during and after a seizure?**

Bradycardia, transient late decelerations, decreased beat-to-beat variability.

○ **Name the maternal complications that may follow a seizure. –**

Pulmonary edema, aspiration pneumonitis, cerebral hemorrhage resulting in hemiplegia or sudden death, blindness, psychosis, placental abruption, DIC, acute renal failure, and cardiopulmonary arrest.

○ **What is the rate of preeclampsia in a subsequent pregnancy after eclampsia in the index pregnancy?**

25%.

○ **What is the rate of recurrent eclampsia?**

2%.

O   **What does HELLP stand for?**

Hemolysis, elevated liver enzymes and low platelets.

O   **What are the diagnostic criteria of HELLP syndrome?**

Criterion	Laboratory Findings	Associated Clinical Findings (nondiagnostic)
Hemolysis—microangiopathic hemolytic anemia	Abnormal peripheral smear— schistocytes, burr cells. Elevated indirect bilirubin in the serum Low serum haptoglobin levels Elevated LDH (isoforms 1 and 2) Significant drop in hemoglobin level	Malaise
Elevated liver function tests	Elevated AST and ALT (usually more than two times the upper limit of normal) Abnormal bilirubin levels	Right upper quadrant or epigastric pain Nausea Vomiting
Low platelet count	Less than 100,000/mm^3	Mucosal bleeding Hematuria Petechial hemorrhages Ecchymosis

O   **Is HELLP syndrome always associated with hypertension?**

No. Hypertension may be absent in 12% to 18%. It may be only mild in 15% to 50%.

O   **Is HELLP syndrome always associated with proteinuria?**

No. It may be absent in up to 14%.

O   **What is the differential diagnosis for a patient with HELLP syndrome?**

Acute fatty liver of pregnancy, thrombotic thrombocytopenic purpura, hemolytic uremic syndrome, immune thrombocytopenic purpura, systemic lupus erythematosus, antiphospholipid syndrome, cholecystitis, viral hepatitis, pancreatitis, upper respiratory infection, disseminated herpes simplex, and hemorrhagic or septic shock.

O   **What maternal morbidities are associated with HELLP syndrome?**

Pulmonary edema, acute renal failure, DIC, placental abruption, liver hemorrhage or failure, ARDS, sepsis, stroke, and death (1%).

O   **What is the reported perinatal mortality rate?**

7.4% to 20.4%, mainly because of severe prematurity.

○   **What is the rate of prematurity in HELLP syndrome?**

70%.

○   **How is a suspected case of HELLP syndrome managed?**

Immediate hospitalization and observation. Diagnostic measures include blood tests such as complete blood count, a peripheral smear, coagulation studies, AST, ALT, creatinine, glucose, bilirubin, and LDH. Therapeutic measures are those for severe preeclampsia including magnesium for seizure prophylaxis and antihypertensives to keep blood pressure below 160/105 mm Hg.

○   **What is the definitive treatment of HELLP syndrome?**

Delivery. While there is consensus regarding prompt delivery beyond 34 weeks (and prior to 24 weeks), some may advocate expectant management in selected stable patients prior to 34 weeks (i.e., in the absence of multiorgan dysfunction, DIC, liver infarction or hemorrhage, renal failure, placental abruption or non-reassuring fetal condition). This management might include delivery in 24 to 48 hours thus allowing completion of steroid course or may include prolonging the pregnancy even further, until other indications for delivery occur. Expectant management for more than 48 hours was found to be associated with significant rate of fetal death, and no improvement in overall perinatal outcome, compared to those who were delivered within 48 hours.

○   **What is the role of steroids in the treatment of HELLP syndrome?**

As with severe preeclampsia, steroids prior to 34 weeks improve perinatal outcome, and may also be associated with transient improvement of the thrombocytopenia. There are two possible regimens: 12 mg of betamethasone IM every 24 hours for two doses or 6 mg of dexamethasone IM every 12 hours for a total of 4 doses.

Other regimens of steroids including high dose, treatment after 34 weeks or postpartum are experimental. There is insufficient evidence to determine whether adjunctive steroid use in HELLP syndrome decreases maternal and perinatal mortality.

○   **Which methods for pain control are contraindicated in HEELP syndrome?**

Pudendal block is contraindicated because of the risk of bleeding and hematoma formation. Epidural anesthesia is contraindicated, especially, when thrombocytopenia is less than $75,000/mm^3$.

○   **What are the indications for platelet transfusion?**

A level less than $20,000/mm^3$ or the presence of significant bleeding. Some recommend transfusion of six units of platelets prior to surgery, if the level is less than $40,000/mm^3$.

○   **What is the recommended postpartum treatment?**

Supportive therapy with continuation of magnesium sulfate prophylaxis for 24 to 48 hours and the use of antihypertensives to keep blood pressure below 155/105 mm Hg.

○   **What is the rate of preeclampsia in subsequent pregnancies?**

Approximately 20%.

○   **What is the rate of recurrent HELLP syndrome?**

2% to 19%.

○   **How is chronic hypertension defined?**

Hypertension (systolic pressure of 140 mm Hg or above, diastolic pressure of 90 mm Hg or above) present before the 20th week of pregnancy (not attributable to gestational trophoblastic disease), or hypertension present before pregnancy, or hypertension that persists longer than 12 weeks post delivery.

○   **How is chronic hypertension classified according to the Joint National Committee (2003)?**

Prehypertension (systolic 120 to 139 or diastolic 80 to 90), stage 1 hypertension (140 to 159 or 90 to 99), and stage 2 hypertension (160 or above or 100 or above).

○   **What are some benefits associated with antihypertensive treatment in nonpregnant women?**

Decreased mortality, stroke, and major cardiac events.

○   **Describe some lifestyle modifications recommended for managing hypertension.**

Weight reduction, physical activity, dietary sodium reduction, smoking cessation, and moderation of alcohol consumption.

○   **What is the most common cause of chronic hypertension in pregnant women?**

Essential or familial hypertension (more than 90%).

○   **Which pregnancy complications are associated with chronic hypertension?**

Premature birth, IUGR, small for gestational age, fetal demise, placental abruption (1% to 2% and up to 8.4% with severe chronic hypertension), cesarean delivery, superimposed preeclampsia, perinatal mortality.

○   **Name a few risk factors for the development of superimposed preeclampsia.**

Severe hypertension in early pregnancy, hypertension for at least 4 years, preeclampsia during a prior pregnancy, and abnormal uterine artery Doppler velocimetry (increased impedance at 16 to 20 weeks).

○   **When does the physiologic decrease in blood pressure reach its lowest level?**

At 16 to 18 weeks of gestation.

○   **Which clinical tests are useful in the initial evaluation of a pregnant woman with hypertension?**

It is recommended especially with long standing hypertension, to have electrocardiography, echocardiography, ophthalmologic examination, and renal ultrasonography. Baseline laboratory evaluations include serum creatinine, blood urea nitrogen and 24-hour urine evaluation for total protein and creatinine clearance. Uric acid of at least 5.5 mg/dL could indicate an increased likelihood of having superimposed preeclampsia.

Some would also recommend urinalysis, urine culture, glucose, and electrolytes in an attempt to rule out etiologies, such as renal disease or chronic pyelonephritis or to identify comorbidities, such as diabetes.

○   **Who should be treated for chronic hypertension during pregnancy?**

Even though antihypertensive treatment would be the standard with sustained diastolic blood pressure of 90 mm Hg or systolic of 140 mm Hg in nonpregnant women, the management during pregnancy is debated. Women with mild hypertension generally do not require antihypertensive medications. It is reasonable to either stop or reduce medication in women who are already taking antihypertensive therapy, but therapy could be increased or reinstituted for women with blood pressures exceeding 150 to 160 mm Hg systolic or 100 to 110 mm Hg diastolic. In women with severe hypertension (systolic of 180 mm Hg or more or diastolic of 110 mm Hg or more) antihypertensive therapy should be initiated or continued for maternal indications.

End organ dysfunction diastolic blood pressure of 90 mm Hg or higher may be considered an indication for treatment.

○ **Which medications are contraindicated during pregnancy?**

Angiotensin converting enzyme inhibitors because of teratogenic risk (underdeveloped calvarial bone, renal failure, oligohydramnios, anuria, renal agenesis, pulmonary hypoplasia, IUGR, fetal death, neonatal renal failure, and neonatal death). Angiotensin II receptor blockers are also contraindicated. The beta blocker atenolol may be associated with growth restriction and is not recommended in pregnancy. The use of diuretics, which may affect volume expansion, is not contraindicated unless uteroplacental perfusion is already reduced such as with IUGR and preeclampsia. Nitroprusside is contraindicated in the later stages of pregnancy because of possible fetal cyanide poisoning.

○ **Which medications should not be used postpartum if the patient is breast-feeding?**

ACE inhibitors and angiotensin receptor antagonists should be avoided in the first few weeks. Diuretics should be avoided as they can reduce the milk volume.

○ **Name a few acceptable medications for treatment of chronic hypertension during pregnancy.**

Methyldopa, labetalol, and nifedipine.

○ **What is the recommended fetal surveillance for pregnancies complicated by chronic hypertension?**

It should be individualized. Some investigators recommend baseline US at 18 to 20 weeks, then repeat at 28 to 32 weeks and then monthly for fetal growth. NST or BPP is recommended in case of IUGR or superimposed preeclampsia.

CHAPTER 14

Medical and Surgical Complications in Pregnancy

Shai Pri-Paz, MD

INFECTIONS

○ **What is the incubation period of herpes?**

2 to 12 days.

○ **What are the three stages of HSV infection?**

Primary: infection in a patient without preexisting antibodies to HSV 1/2.

Recurrent: reactivation with homologous antibodies present.

Nonprimary first episode: infection with one type of HSV in presence of antibodies to the other type of HSV.

○ **What is the incidence of new herpes infection among susceptible pregnant women?**

Approximately 2%.

○ **What is the reason for most neonatal HSV infections?**

Delivery through an infected birth canal usually in asymptomatic mothers.

○ **What is the classification of neonatal disease?**

1. Localized disease of the skin, eye, and mouth—the most common (45%). No mortality.
2. CNS disease with or without skin, eye, and mouth disease (30%)—4% mortality.
3. Disseminated disease (25%)—30% mortality.

○ **What is the maternal fetal vertical transmission rate?**

Primary, 30% to 60%; nonprimary first episode, 33%; recurrent, 0% to 3%.

○ **What is the risk of transmission for women with a history of recurrent disease and no visible lesions at delivery?**

2:10,000.

○   **What are possible effects of maternal infection during pregnancy?**

A primary infection during the first trimester is associated with anomalies such as microcephaly, microphthalmia, intracranial calcifications, skin lesions, and chorioretinitis. There might also be increased rate of miscarriages, but recent studies do not support such a risk. A primary infection after the first trimester increases the risk of preterm delivery and the risk of transmission to the newborn.

○   **What are the treatment options for herpes**

	Class	First Clinical Episode	Suppressive Therapy	Recurrent Episodes
Acyclovir	B	200 mg orally five times a day or 400 mg orally three times a day for 7–10 days	400 mg orally twice a day or three times daily from 36 weeks until delivery	400 mg orally three times a day for 5 days or 800 mg orally twice a day for 5 days or 800 mg orally three times a day for 2 days
Valacyclovir	B	1 g orally twice a day for 7–10 days	500 mg orally daily or twice a day or 1 g orally daily (when 10 or more episodes per year) from 36 weeks until delivery	500 mg orally twice a day for 3 days or 1 g orally once a day for 5 days
Famciclovir	B	250 mg orally three times a day for 7–10 days	250 mg orally twice a day	125 mg orally twice a day for 5 days or 1 g orally twice daily for a day

○   **Who should receive prophylactic therapy for herpes and when?**

Women at or beyond 36 weeks with a first episode of HSV occurring during the current pregnancy benefit the most, including a significant reduction in clinical recurrences at delivery and a reduction in cesarean rates for clinical herpes recurrences (but not in total number of cesarean deliveries). Treatment should also be offered to women at or beyond 36 weeks with active recurrent genital herpes.

○   **Is routine screening for genital herpes recommended during pregnancy?**

No.

○   **In which situations should cesarean delivery be considered?**

In women with active genital lesions or symptoms such as vulvar pain or burning at delivery, which may indicate an impending outbreak. Cesarean delivery is not recommended for women with a history of HSV infection but no active genital disease during labor.

○   **Is cesarean delivery recommended for women with recurrent herpes simplex virus lesions on the back, thigh, or buttock?**

No. These lesions may be covered with an occlusive dressing.

○ **Is there a duration after which cesarean delivery is not indicated for women with active HSV infection and ruptured membranes?**

No.

○ **Are invasive procedures contraindicated in women with HSV?**

Procedures should be delayed in cases of primary infections. With recurrent infections, procedures may be done except for transcervical procedures.

○ **May fetal scalp electrodes be used in women with a history of herpes?**

Yes, if indicated in women with a history of recurrent HSV and no active lesions. The risk of neonatal infection is increased sixfold. Local neonatal infection may occur as vesicular or vesiculopustular lesions and should be treated with systemic antiviral therapy.

○ **What is the most common congenital infection?**

Cytomegalovirus (CMV).

○ **How can vertical transmission of CMV occur?**

Transplacental infection, exposure to contaminated genital tract secretions at parturition or breastfeeding.

○ **When is the risk of transmission of CMV the highest?**

Primary maternal infection has a risk of transmission of 30% to 40%, while a recurrent infection has a risk of 0.15% to 2%. The overall risk of infection is greatest in the third trimester (but is more severe after infection in the first trimester).

○ **What is the sensitivity of CMV IgM serologic assays?**

50% to 90%.

○ **Name a few adverse effects of fetal infection with parvovirus B19.**

Spontaneous abortion, hydrops fetalis, and stillbirth.

○ **When does hydrops develop because of parvovirus B19?**

Usually within 8 weeks from maternal infection.

○ **What are some characteristics of congenital varicella syndrome?**

Skin scarring, limb hypoplasia, chorioretinitis, and microcephaly. The risk is limited to exposure during the first 20 weeks of pregnancy.

○ **What is the most dangerous time for VZV infection with regards to neonatal death?**

When the maternal infection develops from 5 days before delivery up to 48 hours postpartum (these infants should receive VZIG).

○ **What is the treatment for maternal varicella?**

Oral acyclovir. Intravenous route should be used for infections complicated by pneumonia.

○ **How should a susceptible woman exposed to varicella be managed?**

VZIG, as soon as possible no later than 72 hours after exposure.

○ **What is the rate of vertical transmission of toxoplasmosis?**

10% to 15% in the first trimester, 25% in the second trimester, and 60% in the third trimester (but the earlier the fetus is infected, the more severe the disease).

○ **What is the treatment for maternal toxoplasmosis infection?**

Spiramycin. If fetal infection is established, pyrimethamine, sulfadiazine, and folinic acid are added.

○ **What will be considered a positive skin test for tuberculosis in a person with HIV?**

5 mm or greater. This applies also to those with abnormal chest radiography or those with a recent contact with an active case.

○ **When is 10 mm or more considered positive for tuberculosis infection?**

High-risk patients: foreign-born individuals, IV drug user who are HIV negative, low income populations, and those with medical conditions that increase the risk for tuberculosis.

○ **How should a pregnant woman with a positive skin test for tuberculosis be evaluated and treated?**

A chest radiograph. If it is negative, then no treatment is necessary until after delivery, when isoniazid is given for 1 year.

○ **When will skin test positive women be treated during pregnancy?**

Known recent conversion, exposure to active infection, and HIV positive.

○ **What is the initial treatment of a pregnant patient with symptomatic tuberculosis?**

Isoniazid, rifampin, and ethambutol for 9 months or a four-drug regimen with pyrazinamide for 6 months.

○ **Which HIV infected pregnant women should be offered antiretroviral treatment?**

All of them, regardless of T cell count or HIV level.

○ **How should HIV RNA levels be monitored?**

4 weeks after initiation of a change in treatment, then monthly until undetectable, then every 3 months and finally near term.

○ **What is the regimen of zidovudine antepartum?**

100 mg orally five times daily, or 200 mg three times daily, or 300 mg twice daily.

○ **When should intravenous zidovudine be started prior to elective cesarean delivery?**

3 hours prior to surgery.

○ **What is the maternal treatment if the HIV RNA level is more than 1000 copies/mL?**

Combination antiretroviral therapy.

○ **What is the recommended mode of delivery?**

Scheduled cesarean delivery as early as 38 weeks is recommended for HIV-infected women with more than 1000 copies/mL of HIV RNA. Cesarean delivery is unlikely to offer additional benefit when the HIV RNA levels are below 1000 copies/mL since the rate of transmission is very low.

○ **Does vaginal disinfection decrease the risk of transmission from mother to infant?**

Currently there is no evidence of such an effect.

DIABETES

○ **When should the 50 g 1 h oral glucose tolerance test (GTT) be administered?**

24 to 28 weeks.

○ **Should this screening test be done in a fasting state?**

No.

○ **What is the sensitivity of different threshold values?**

80% at 140 mg/dL and 90% for 130 mg/dL.

○ **What is the diagnostic test for gestational diabetes mellitus?**

Women who screen positive to the 50 g oral glucose tolerance test should undergo the 100 g 3 h oral GTT.

○ **How should the 3-hour GTT be performed?**

In the morning, after an overnight fast. No smoking should be allowed before the test and the women should remain seated during the test. A positive diagnosis requires two or more abnormal values.

○ **What is the rate of recurrence of gestational diabetes in a subsequent pregnancy?**

33% to 50%.

○ **What is the effect of primary dietary therapy for gestational diabetes on fetal growth and neonatal outcomes?**

There is no significant effect on birth weight greater than 4000 grams or cesarean deliveries.

○ **When should medical intervention be considered for gestational diabetes mellitus?**

1-hour postprandial values exceeding 130 to 140 mg/dL, or 2-hour postprandial values exceeding 120 mg/dL, or fasting glucose exceeding 95 mg/dL.

○   **What is the prevalence of pregestational diabetes in the United States?**

1% of all pregnancies.

○   **Is insulin resistance increased or decreased during pregnancy?**

Insulin sensitivity is enhanced late in the first trimester by higher levels of estrogen; but later in pregnancy, the insulin resistance increases and is the greatest in the third trimester.

○   **Which hormones contribute to the increase in insulin resistance?**

Placental hormones including human placental lactogen (HPL), progesterone, prolactin, placental growth hormone, and cortisol. TNF alpha and leptin also contribute.

○   **What are the average insulin requirements?**

First trimester, 0.7 to 0.8 U/kg/d; second trimester, 0.8 to 1 U/kg/d; third trimester, 0.9 to 1.2 U/kg/d.

○   **What are the goal values of therapy?**

As same as gestational diabetes: fasting glucose level of 95 mg/dL or less, premeal value of 100 mg/dL or less, 1 hour postprandial 140 mg/dL or less, 2 hours postprandial 120 mg/dL or less.

○   **What is the desired level of hemoglobin A_{1c}?**

6% or less.

○   **What does HbA_{1c} reflect?**

It reflects the glycemic control over the past 2 to 3 months. An HbA_{1c} level of 8% indicates a mean glucose level of 180 mg/dL, with each 1% higher or lower equal to a change of 30 mg/dL.

○   **When should regular insulin be given?**

30 minutes before eating.

○   **How does pregnancy affect diabetic retinopathy?**

May cause acute progression of retinopathy.

○   **What are the laboratory findings associated with diabetic ketoacidosis?**

Low arterial pH (less than 7.3), a low serum bicarbonate level (less than 15 mEq/L), an elevated anion gap, and positive serum ketones.

○   **What does the treatment of diabetic ketoacidosis include?**

Laboratory assessment, IV insulin, fluids, repletion of glucose, potassium, and bicarbonate as needed.

○   **What is the loading dose of insulin?**

0.2 to 0.4 U/kg, followed by maintenance of 2 to 10 U/h.

○ **Does glyburide cross the placenta?**

No.

○ **What are some pharmacokinetics regarding glyburide?**

Onset is 4 hours and duration is 10 hours.

○ **When should antenatal testing be initiated?**

At 32 to 34 weeks, or even earlier in more complicated pregnancies. Testing should be done twice weekly. Doppler velocimetry of the umbilical artery may be useful in cases with vascular complications and poor fetal growth.

○ **When should cesarean delivery be considered in a gestational diabetes patient?**

When EFW is greater than 4500 g.

THYROID DISEASE IN PREGNANCY

○ **Which of the thyroid function test results increase during pregnancy?**

Thyroid binding globulin (TBG), total thyroxine (TT4), and total triiodothyronine (TT3).

○ **When does the fetal thyroid begin concentrating iodine?**

10 to 12 weeks.

○ **Which hormone is the least likely to cross the placenta?**

TSH.

○ **What is the most common etiology of hyperthyroidism in pregnancy?**

Grave disease.

○ **Name a few symptoms and signs more specific to Grave disease.**

Ophthalmopathy (including lid lag and lid retraction) and dermopathy (including localized or pretibial myxedema).

○ **Name other signs and symptoms of hyperthyroidism.**

Tremors, nervousness, tachycardia, frequent stools, sweating, heat intolerance, weight loss (in spite of good appetite), goiter, insomnia, palpitations, and hypertension.

○ **Which maternal complications may result from inadequately treated thyrotoxicosis?**

Preterm delivery, severe preeclampsia, and heart failure.

○ **Which fetal complications may result from inadequately treated thyrotoxicosis?**

LBW, fetal loss.

○   **What effect may maternal Grave disease have in the neonate?**

The neonate may have immune-mediated hypothyroidism or hyperthyroidism because of thyroid stimulating hormone binding inhibitory immunoglobulin (TBII) or thyroid stimulating immunoglobulins (TSI), respectively.

○   **Name a few signs and symptoms of hypothyroidism.**

Fatigue, constipation, intolerance to cold, muscle cramps, hair loss, dry skin, prolonged relaxation phase of deep tendon reflexes, carpal tunnel syndrome, weight gain (even in spite of decreased appetite), intellectual slowness, voice changes, and insomnia. Untreated cases may progress to myxedema coma.

○   **Which neonatal risk is associated with iodine deficient hypothyroidism?**

Congenital cretinism.

○   **What is the most common etiology of hypothyroidism in developed countries?**

Hashimoto disease.

○   **Which antibodies are associated with Hashimoto disease?**

Thyroid antimicrosomal and antithyroglobulin antibodies.

○   **What should be measured initially in a pregnant patient with a suspected thyroid disease?**

TSH and FT4 or FTI.

○   **Which medications can be used to treat hyperthyroidism?**

PTU and methimazole.

○   **Once treatment has started, how often should TSH and FT4 or FTI be checked?**

Every 2 to 4 weeks.

○   **What potential adverse effect is believed to be associated with methimazole?**

Fetal aplasia cutis.

○   **What other side effects are related to treatment with thioamides?**

Agranulocytosis (usually with fever and sore throat), thrombocytopenia, hepatitis and vasculitis. Minor side effects may include rash, nausea, arthritis, anorexia, fever, and loss of taste or smell.

○   **Which treatment for hyperthyroidism is contraindicated in pregnancy?**

Iodine 131 (should avoid pregnancy for 4 months after procedure).

○   **How often should levothyroxine be adjusted?**

Every 4 weeks.

○ **How does thyroid storm present clinically?**

Fever, tachycardia, changed mental status, diarrhea, vomiting, and cardiac arrhythmia. Untreated storm may result in shock, stupor, and coma.

○ **How should thyroid storm be treated?**

PTU (600–800 mg orally immediately, followed by 150–200 mg orally every 4–6 hours), saturated solution of potassium iodide or sodium iodide or Lugol solution, dexamethasone (2 mg IV every 6 hours for four doses) and propranolol (20–80 mg orally every 4–6 hours). In cases of severe agitation, phenobarbital may be used.

○ **Does pregnancy affect the outcome of thyroid cancer?**

No.

○ **What is the incidence of postpartum thyroiditis?**

5%, with 70% risk of recurrence.

○ **Are thyroid function tests indicated in an asymptomatic pregnant woman with a slightly enlarged thyroid gland?**

No.

○ **Is routine screening for hypothyroidism indicated?**

No. There is an observational study that showed significant difference in mean IQ scores between children of untreated hypothyroid women and controls, but there are insufficient data to warrant routine screening at this time.

URINARY SYSTEM

○ **What is the most common bacterial infection during pregnancy?**

Urinary tract infection.

○ **What is the prevalence of asymptomatic bacteriuria in pregnancy?**

2% to 7%.

○ **When does bacteriuria usually present?**

At the first prenatal visit.

○ **What are the consequences of not treating asymptomatic bacteriuria?**

25% will develop an acute symptomatic infection. Some studies show an association with low birth weight and prematurity. Antibiotic treatment is effective in reducing the risk of low birth weight and the risk of pyelonephritis in pregnancy.

○ **What is the suppression regimen for persistent or frequent bacteriuria recurrences?**

Nitrofurantoin 100 mg at bedtime for the remainder of the pregnancy.

○ **What is the probable cause of infection in a woman with frequency, urgency, dysuria, and pyuria, but with a negative urine culture and a mucopurulent cervicitis?**

Chlamydia trachomatis.

○ **In which side is pyelonephritis more common?**

Right side.

○ **What are the most common organisms causing pyelonephritis?**

E. coli is isolated in 75% to 80% of infections, *Klebsiella pneumoniae* in 10%, and *Enterobacter* or *Proteus* in 10%.

○ **How often is bacteremia present in women with acute pyelonephritis?**

15% to 20%.

○ **How can pyelonephritis affect different organs?**

20% develop renal dysfunction; 1% to 2% develop respiratory insufficiency, which may be severe enough to cause ARDS; 33% develop acute anemia because of hemolysis. Women may also experience contractions.

○ **Describe the treatment of acute pyelonephritis during pregnancy.**

Hospitalization, hydration, IV antimicrobial therapy (ampicillin plus gentamicin or cefazolin or ceftriaxone), discharge when afebrile for 24 hours, continuation of antimicrobial therapy for 7 to 10 days and a repeat urine culture 1 to 2 weeks after antimicrobial therapy completed.

○ **What is the next step if a woman does not improve clinically within 48 to 72 hours?**

Urinary tract imaging should be performed to rule out an obstruction.

○ **Which stones are most common during pregnancy?**

Calcium oxalate.

○ **Which stones are associated with *Proteus Klebsiella?***

Struvite stones.

○ **How does acute glomerulonephritis affect pregnancy?**

Increased rate of fetal loss and perinatal mortality. Increased rate of prematurity and growth restriction. Increased incidence of hypertension and worsening of proteinuria.

○ **What are the two most important factors in predicting pregnancy outcome in women with chronic renal disease?**

Degree of hypertension and renal insufficiency.

○ **Which pregnancy complications are associated with chronic renal disease?**

Hypertension, anemia, preeclampsia, preterm delivery, and fetal growth restriction.

○ **When should dialysis be initiated?**

When serum creatinine levels are 5 to 7 mg/dL.

○ **What is the most common reason of acute renal failure in pregnancy?**

Severe preeclampsia—eclampsia.

HEMOGLOBINOPATHIES

○ **Adult hemoglobins consist of four polypeptide chains, two of which are alpha. Match the hemoglobin with the adequate polypeptide.**

A. Hemoglobin A   1. Delta subunits
B. Hemoglobin F   2. Gamma subunits
C. Hemoglobin A_2 3. Beta subunits

A-3, B-2, C-1.

○ **What is the prevalence of sickle cell trait in people of African origin?**

1:12.

○ **How are hemoglobinopathies diagnosed?**

CBC and hemoglobin electrophoresis.

○ **What is acute chest syndrome?**

Noninfectious pulmonary infiltrate with fever that leads to hypoxemia and acidosis.

○ **What are the different types of alpha thalassemia?**

Deletion of one alpha globin gene—alpha thalassemia-2 trait.
Deletion of two alpha globin genes—alpha thalassemia-1 trait with mild asymptomatic microcytic anemia.
Deletion of three alpha globin genes—Hb H disease with mild to moderate hemolytic anemia.
Deletion of four alpha globin genes—alpha thalassemia major (Hb Bart's) with absence of alpha globin and hydrops fetalis, intrauterine death, and preeclampsia.

○ **What are the characteristics of beta thalassemia major (Cooley anemia)?**

Severe anemia with resultant extramedullary erythropoiesis, delayed sexual development, and poor growth.

○ **Which ethnic groups are at a higher risk for being carriers of hemoglobinopathies?**

African, Southeast Asian, and Mediterranean.

○ **Elevated Hb F and elevated Hb A$_2$ (more than 3.5%) are associated with which condition?**

Beta thalassemia.

○ **How can alpha thalassemia trait be diagnosed?**

Only by molecular genetic testing. (It should be done in cases of low MCV without iron deficiency anemia and without beta thalassemia trait.)

○ **Name pregnancy complications associated with sickle cell disease.**

Preterm labor, premature rupture of membranes, antepartum hospitalization, and postpartum infection. Fetal complications include IUGR, LBW, and prematurity.

○ **What is the recommended folic acid supplementation for patients with sickle cell disease?**

4 mg per day.

○ **What is the goal of a blood transfusion in the patient with sickle cell disease?**

To lower the percentage of Hb S to approximately 40% while simultaneously raising the total hemoglobin level to 10 g/dLmg/dL.

ANTIPHOSPHOLIPID SYNDROME

○ **What is the correlation between lupus anticoagulant and anticardiolipin antibodies?**

Approximately 80% of patients with lupus anticoagulant have anticardiolipin antibodies, and 20% of patients positive for anticardiolipin antibodies have lupus anticoagulant.

○ **What is lupus anticoagulant associated with?**

Thrombosis. In spite of that APTT may be prolonged because of interference with the assembly of the prothrombin complex.

○ **What is the most common complication of antiphospholipid syndrome?**

Thrombosis, mainly venous.

○ **What is the risk of pregnancy-related thrombosis in women with antiphospholipid syndrome?**

5% to 12% during pregnancy or the puerperium.

○ **Which obstetric complications are associated with antiphospholipid syndrome?**

Fetal loss, recurrent early pregnancy loss, preeclampsia (not term), IUGR, and preterm deliveries.

○ **What are the laboratory criteria for the diagnosis of antiphospholipid syndrome?**

Presence or absence of lupus anticoagulant (by two sensitive phospholipid dependent clotting assays) and/or medium to high titers of anticardiolipin antibodies of IgG or IgM isotype. Positive results must be repeated at least six weeks apart.

○ **What are the clinical obstetric criteria for the diagnosis of antiphospholipid syndrome?**

Three or more consecutive spontaneous abortions before the 10th week of gestation, one or more unexplained fetal deaths of morphologically normal fetuses at or beyond the 10th week of gestation, severe preeclampsia or placental insufficiency necessitating birth of morphologically normal neonates before the 34th week of gestation.

○ **What are the clinical nonobstetric criteria for the diagnosis of antiphospholipid syndrome?**

Unexplained venous thrombosis, unexplained arterial thrombosis or small vessel thrombosis in any tissue or organ without significant evidence of inflammation of the vessel.

○ **How is antiphospholipid syndrome diagnosed?**

If at least one of the clinical criteria and one of the laboratory criteria are met.

○ **Who should be tested for antiphospholipid syndrome?**

Patients with clinical disorders that are clearly related to antiphospholipid syndrome, i.e., those clinical criteria that are part of the diagnosis.

○ **How should pregnant women with antiphospholipid syndrome but without history of thrombotic events be treated?**

Prophylactic doses of heparin and low dose aspirin during pregnancy and postpartum period (6–8 weeks). Combined unfractionated heparin and aspirin may reduce pregnancy loss by 54%.

○ **How should pregnant women with antiphospholipid syndrome and previous history of thrombosis be treated?**

Full anticoagulation throughout pregnancy and postpartum period (6–8 weeks).

○ **What is the recommended antepartum testing for women with antiphospholipid syndrome?**

Serial US to rule out IUGR and antepartum testing starting at 32 weeks.

THROMBOPHILIA

○ **Which clotting factors rise during pregnancy?**

Factors I, VII, VIII, IX, and X.

○ **Which clotting factors diminish during pregnancy?**

Protein S and fibrinolytic activity.

○ **What is the leading cause of maternal death in the USA?**

Pulmonary embolism.

○ **What are the most common inherited thrombophilias during pregnancy?**

Factor V Leiden, prothrombin G20210A mutation, and MTHFR mutation.

○ **Which thrombophilia is the most common acquired during pregnancy?**

Antiphospholipid antibody syndrome.

○ **Is testing for thrombophilia recommended in cases of severe preeclampsia?**

No.

○ **What is the prevalence of different thrombophilias in women with normal pregnancy outcomes?**

Factor V Leiden mutation—2% to 10%, MTHFR mutation—8% to 16%, prothrombin gene mutation—2% to 6%, protein C and S deficiencies—0.2% to 1%, and anticardiolipin antibodies—1% to 7%.

○ **Should women with placental abruption be screened for thrombophilia?**

No. There is a prospective observational study with more than 5000 asymptomatic pregnant women that showed no association between placental abruption and factor V Leiden mutation.

○ **Which thrombophilias are associated with first trimester loss?**

Factor V Leiden, prothrombin gene mutation, and activated protein C resistance.

○ **Which thrombophilias are associated with late nonrecurring fetal loss?**

Factor V Leiden, prothrombin gene mutation, and protein S deficiency.

○ **Who should be screened for thrombophilia?**

Some authors recommend screening women who have had adverse pregnancy outcomes such as fetal death, severe preeclampsia, IUGR, placental abruption, and recurrent miscarriages since the rate of recurrence with thrombophilia is 66% to 83%.

○ **What is the recommended treatment for women with true antiphospholipid antibody syndrome?**

Low dose aspirin with subcutaneous heparin added once fetal cardiac activity is documented.

○ **Which thrombophilia carries the highest risk of pregnancy-related thromboembolism?**

Antithrombin deficiency (up to 40% with a history of venous thromboembolism).

VENOUS THROMBOEMBOLISM

○ **Is pregnancy alone a risk factor for venous thromboembolism?**

Yes. Pregnancy alone increases the risk by five times.

○ **Which women are at particular risk?**

Women with a known thrombophilia, a history of previous venous thromboembolism or a pregnancy complication requiring prolonged bed rest.

○ **When is prophylaxis recommended during pregnancy?**

History of a previous DVT during pregnancy, artificial heart valve, known thrombophilia, and a prior DVT.

○ **What is the risk of recurrence after a DVT during pregnancy?**

5.6%.

○ **Is subcutaneous unfractionated heparin routinely indicated for patients with cesarean deliveries?**

No. The use of pneumatic compression devices is recommended.

○ **Is prophylactic heparin prescribed for prolonged bed rest?**

Not recommended. Graduated compression stockings may be used. Early ambulation should also be considered.

○ **What is the preferred prophylaxis in a pregnant patient with mechanical heart valves?**

Warfarin. Some recommend subcutaneous unfractionated heparin or low molecular weight heparin during the first and third trimesters. Another approach includes conversion to subcutaneous unfractionated heparin three times daily or low molecular weight heparin twice daily.

○ **What anomalies are associated with warfarin use during pregnancy?**

Nasal hypoplasia, stippled epiphyses, and CNS abnormalities.

○ **When should anticoagulant therapy be stopped prior to induction?**

24 hours before.

○ **How can the anticoagulant effect be reversed?**

Protamine sulfate for unfractionated heparin and fresh frozen plasma for low molecular weight heparin.

○ **When can the anticoagulation therapy be resumed postpartum?**

When the assessment of postpartum bleeding is acceptable. Usually 4 to 8 hours after uncomplicated vaginal delivery and 24 hours after cesarean delivery.

○ **What is the obstetric prophylactic dosage for thromboembolism?**

Subcutaneous unfractionated heparin 5000 units every 12 hours or LMWH 40 mg daily at a fixed dose throughout pregnancy.

○ **What is the therapeutic treatment of thromboembolism?**

Subcutaneous unfractionated heparin may be increased up to 10,000 units two to three times per day with a goal of APTT of 1.5 to 2 times normal. Low molecular weight heparin may be given at 30 to 80 mg every 12 hours.

○ **What is the recommended duration of anticoagulation therapy after venous thromboembolism in pregnancy?**

At least 6 months for the first episode. Postpartum treatment should last 6 weeks to 3 months.

○ **What are the possible treatment options for venous thromboembolism in pregnancy?**

Intravenous unfractionated heparin, subcutaneous unfractionated heparin, or low molecular weight heparin.

○   **What is the preferred treatment of venous thromboembolism in pregnancy?**

Low molecular weight heparin.

○   **What is the target value of APTT in treating venous thromboembolism during pregnancy?**

1.5 to 2 times the upper limit of normal.

SLE

○   **How is worsening lupus activity differentiated from preeclampsia?**

Decreased complement levels or increased anti-DNA titers are useful in identifying worsening lupus activity. Lupus nephritis is associated with proteinuria and/or active urine sediment while preeclampsia is associated with proteinuria alone. Elevated serum levels of liver enzymes and uric acid and decreased urinary excretion of calcium are more suggestive of preeclampsia.

○   **When is the prognosis for the mother and child best?**

When the disease has been quiescent for at least six months prior to pregnancy and the renal disease is stable (normal or near normal).

○   **What is the incidence of preeclampsia in women with SLE?**

13%. Up to 66% in the presence of renal disease.

○   **Which factors increase the risk of fetal loss?**

Hypertension, active lupus, lupus nephritis, hypocomplementemia, elevated levels of anti-DNA antibodies, antiphospholipid antibodies, or thrombocytopenia. Fetal loss usually occurs after 10 weeks gestation.

○   **What is the most serious complication associated with neonatal lupus?**

Complete heart block in the neonate.

○   **What is the recurrence risk of congenital heart block?**

15%.

○   **What is the recommended laboratory work up in the first visit during pregnancy?**

Renal function, CBC, anti-Ro/SSA and anti-La/SSB, lupus anticoagulant and anticardiolipin antibodies, anti double stranded DNA, and complement levels (CH50, C3, and C4).

○   **How should women with lupus and antiphospholipid antibodies, but without clinical features of antiphospholipid syndrome (APLS), be treated?**

Low dose aspirin with or without low dose heparin.

○   **What testing is recommended in the presence of anti-Ro or anti-La?**

Fetal cardiac echo to detect fetal heart block.

○   **Which tests may be recommended at the end of each trimester?**

Renal function (GFR and protein/creatinine ratio), anticardiolipin antibodies, complement level, and anti-dsDNA antibodies. CBC may be repeated monthly.

○   **Which medications should be avoided in treating SLE during pregnancy?**

Mycophenolate mofetil, cyclophosphamide, and methotrexate.

○   **Which drugs have a small risk of fetal harm?**

NSAIDs, glucocorticoids, and azathioprine.

○   **Which congenital malformation is associated with glucocorticoids?**

Cleft palate.

○   **Which medications used to treat SLE are safe during pregnancy?**

NSAIDs in late first and in second trimester and antimalarial drugs.

RHEUMATOLOGIC DISORDERS

○   **How does pregnancy affect rheumatoid arthritis?**

Most women improve during pregnancy.

○   **What effect does pregnancy have on scleroderma associated dysphagia and reflux esophagitis?**

Aggravation.

○   **What is the preferred method of analgesia in labor for women with scleroderma?**

Epidural analgesia. (There is limited ability to open the mouth wide).

○   **Which vasculitis syndrome is associated with hepatitis B antigenemia?**

Polyarteritis nodosa.

○   **What percentage of adults with dermatomyositis has an associated malignant tumor?**

15%.

○   **Which disorder is associated with increased frequency of dissecting and ruptured aneurysms during pregnancy?**

Marfan syndrome.

○   **What complications are associated with Ehlers-Danlos syndrome?**

Preterm rupture of membranes, prematurity, and antepartum and postpartum hemorrhage.

DERMATOLOGY

○ **What is the most common pruritic pregnancy specific dermatosis?**

Pruritic urticarial papules and plaques of pregnancy (PUPPP). This is also known as polymorphic eruption of pregnancy (PEP).

○ **Where do the lesions of PUPPP usually develop first?**

On the abdomen, usually around striae. The lesions are then likely to spread to the buttocks, thighs, and extremities.

○ **How is PUPPP treated?**

Oral antihistamines, skin emollients, topical corticosteroid creams or ointments, and occasionally oral corticosteroids.

○ **How is herpes gestationis (pemphigoid gestationis) treated?**

Topical corticosteroids and oral antihistamines, followed as needed by orally administered prednisone (0.5–1 mg/kg daily).

○ **What is the effect of pregnancy on psoriasis?**

Improvement in up to 50% and worsening in up to 20%.

INTENSIVE CARE

○ **What is the most common cause of respiratory failure in pregnancy?**

Adult respiratory distress syndrome (ARDS).

○ **What are the most common causes of ARDS?**

Sepsis and diffuse infectious pneumonia.

○ **What are the major causes of pulmonary edema during pregnancy?**

Preeclampsia or eclampsia, tocolysis, and cardiac disease.

○ **Name a few frequent causes of obstetrical sepsis.**

Pyelonephritis, chorioamnionitis, and puerperal pelvic infection.

○ **What are the goals of ventilation?**

Obtain arterial oxygen pressure of 60 mm Hg or 90% saturation at inspired oxygen content of less than 50% along with positive end expiratory pressures less than 15 mm Hg.

○ **What are the preferred vasopressors during pregnancy?**

Ephedrine or dopamine.

○ **What is the most common cause of serious life threatening or fatal blunt trauma during pregnancy?**

Motor vehicle accidents.

○ **How frequent is traumatic placental abruption?**

Some degree of abruption complicates 1% to 6% of "minor" injuries and up to 50% of "major" injuries.

○ **How common is uterine rupture because of blunt trauma?**

Less than 1%.

○ **What is the most common cause of fetal maternal hemorrhage associated with blunt trauma?**

Placental tear or "fracture" caused by stretching of the placenta.

○ **What is the incidence of maternal visceral injury with penetrating trauma?**

15% to 40%.

○ **How long after the beginning of CPR should a cesarean delivery be performed?**

Within 4 minutes, if the fetus is viable.

○ **What is the minimum recommended time of posttrauma monitoring?**

At least 4 hours, if there are no other maternal conditions requiring attention.

○ **Name indications for continued monitoring.**

Uterine contractions, nonreassuring fetal heart tracing, vaginal bleeding, significant uterine tenderness or irritability, serious maternal injury or rupture of amniotic membranes.

○ **What is the mean estimated blood volume of injected fetal blood during fetal maternal hemorrhage because of trauma?**

Less than 15 mL (less than 30 mL in more than 90% of cases).

○ **How soon should D immune globulin be administered after trauma?**

Within the first 72 hours.

○ **Should a seat belt be used during pregnancy?**

Yes. The lap belt portion should be placed under the pregnant woman's abdomen, over both anterior superior iliac spines and the pubic symphysis. The shoulder harness should be positioned between the breasts.

ASTHMA

○ **What is the prevalence of asthma in pregnancy?**

4% to 8%.

○ **How often do symptoms occur in mild intermittent asthma?**

Twice per week or less. Nocturnal symptoms may occur twice per month or less.

○ **What severity of asthma correlates with daily symptoms?**

Moderate persistent asthma.

○ **What is the peak expiratory flow rate (PEFR) or forced expiratory volume after 1 second (FEV_1) in severe asthma?**

60% predicted or less, and variability more than 30%.

○ **What is the effect of pregnancy on asthma?**

23% improve and 30% become worse during pregnancy.

○ **How can pregnant patients with asthma be monitored?**

By PEFR and FEV_1.

○ **What is the typical PEFR in pregnancy?**

380 to 550 L/min.

○ **How can asthma affect maternal and perinatal outcome?**

Increased rates of preterm delivery (mainly with severe asthma or with using oral corticosteroids), preeclampsia, cesarean deliveries, gestational diabetes, and SGA.

○ **What is the step care therapeutic approach?**

Using the least amount of drug intervention necessary to control a patient's severity of asthma.

○ **When is a burst of oral corticosteroids indicated?**

Exacerbations not responding to initial beta 2 agonists regardless of asthma severity.

○ **Describe a short course of oral corticosteroids.**

Oral prednisone 40 to 60 mg per day for one week followed by tapering over 7 to 14 days.

○ **What is the preferred treatment for mild intermittent asthma?**

Albuterol as needed.

○ **Which medication increases the risk of pulmonary edema?**

Beta 2 agonist (fourfold increase).

○ **What is the preferred treatment for all levels of persistent asthma during pregnancy?**

Inhaled corticosteroids.

○ **Which inhaled corticosteroid is preferred?**

Budesonide (class B).

○ **What are the indications for theophylline?**

Alternative chronic treatment for mild persistent asthma and an alternative adjunctive treatment for moderate and severe persistent asthma.

○ **What is the recommended concentration of theophylline?**

5 to 12 μg/mL.

○ **Which malformation has been associated with oral corticosteroid use during the first trimester?**

Isolated cleft lip with or without cleft palate.

○ **What is the most effective treatment for allergic rhinitis?**

Intranasal corticosteroids.

○ **Should serial ultrasound examinations be done?**

It should be considered for women with suboptimally controlled asthma with moderate to severe asthma (starting at 32 weeks).

NEUROLOGY

○ **Autonomic dysreflexia during labor is potentially life-threatening condition in which patients?**

Spinal cord injury above T7.

○ **Which anti-epileptics have been associated with birth defects?**

Virtually all.

○ **What problems are associated with valproate and valproic acid in early pregnancy?**

1% to 2% incidence of neural tube defects. Facial anomalies.

○ **What problems have been associated with trimethadione in early pregnancy?**

V shaped eyebrows, low set folded ears, abnormal palate and teeth, severe developmental delay.

○ **What problems have been associated with isotretinoin in early pregnancy?**

Defects of CNS, cardio aortic, ear and clefting defects. Brachial and aortic arch anomalies.

○ **How does pregnancy affect migraine headaches?**

The majority reports improvement of headache during pregnancy.

○   **How is migraine treated during pregnancy?**

Acetaminophen is the initial treatment. Additional medications may include metoclopramide, codeine, caffeine, and butalbital. Opioids should not be used on a chronic basis. Ergot alkaloids are contraindicated, since they may induce hypertonic uterine contractions.

○   **What is the gold standard for diagnosis of cerebral venous thrombosis?**

Magnetic resonance venogram.

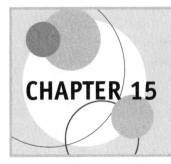

CHAPTER 15

Gastrointestinal Disorders in Pregnancy

Hipolito Custodio III, MD

○ **What are the excess energy requirements during pregnancy (kcal/day)?**

Pregnancy increases energy requirements by 300 kcal/day during the second and the third trimesters. Lactation increases energy requirements by 500 kcal/day.

○ **What dietary micronutrients are needed in much greater amounts during pregnancy?**

Nutrient	Recommended Daily Intake	Add This in Pregnancy/Lactation
Riboflavin	0.6 mg/1000 kcal	0.3–0.5 mg
Niacin	6.6 mg niacin equivalents/1000 kcal	2–5 niacin equivalents
Pyridoxine	1.6–2.0 mg	1 mg
Folic acid	3 μg/kg	400 μg
Vitamin B$_{12}$	2 μg	0.2–0.6 μg
Ascorbic Acid	60 mg	10 mg (pregnancy), 35 mg (lactation)
Iron	15 mg	15 mg
Zinc	0.6 mg/1000 kcal	0.3–0.5 mg

○ **What are the benefits of multiple-micronutrient supplementation during pregnancy?**

Multiple-micronutrient supplementation is associated with a significant decrease in the number of low-birth-weight and small-for-gestational-age babies, as well as of maternal anemia, when compared to supplementation with two or less micronutrients. There were, however, no additional benefits obtained when compared with the WHO-recommended iron-folate supplementation.

○ **What are the most common GI symptoms associated with pregnancy?**

Gingivitis 40% to 100%, Reflux 30% to 50%, Constipation 11%, Hemorrhoids 30% to 40%, Nausea and vomiting 70% to 85%.

The following GI symptoms are also significantly more common among pregnant women: xerostomia, heartburn, eructation, improved appetite, early satiety, epigastric pain, nocturnal pain, and black stools.

○ **What gastrointestinal motility disturbances may occur during pregnancy?**

(1) Abnormal esophageal motility with increased nonpropulsive motor activity and decreased contraction wave amplitude and velocity.

(2) Decreased lower esophageal sphincter pressure.

(3) Decreased LES sensitivity to pharmacologic and physiologic stimulation.

(4) Decreased secretion of acid and pepsin by the stomach.

(5) Prolonged transit through the stomach and small bowel.

(6) Prolonged intervals between interdigestive small bowel myoelectric complexes.

(7) Increased villus height, gut hypertrophy, increased activity of brush border enzymes in the small intestine.

(8) Slower colonic transit.

(9) Enhanced colonic absorption of sodium and water.

(10) Slower gallbladder emptying.

○ **What is the differential diagnosis of nausea and vomiting in pregnancy?**

(1) Gastrointestinal causes: gastroenteritis, gastroparesis, achalasia, biliary tract disease, hepatitis, small bowel obstruction, peptic ulcer disease, pancreatitis, and appendicitis.

(2) Genitourinary causes: pyelonephritis, uremia, ovarian torsion, nephrolithiasis, degenerating fibroids.

(3) Metabolic disease: DKA, porphyria, Addison disease/crisis, hyperthyroidism.

(4) Neurologic disorders: pseudotumor cerebri, vestibular lesions, migraines, CNS tumor.

(5) Pregnancy related conditions: fatty liver of pregnancy and preeclampsia.

(6) Miscellaneous: drug toxicity/intolerance and psychological.

○ **Which hormones influence nausea and vomiting in pregnancy?**

Peak levels of human chorionic gonadotropin correlate temporally with the peak symptoms of nausea and vomiting. The extent of their emetogenic stimulus may be increased in conditions where there is an increased placental mass, such as in multiple gestation or molar pregnancy. Estrogen levels are also correlated with the frequency of nausea and vomiting. Estrogens in OCPs show a dose–response relationship for nausea and vomiting, and women thus sensitized have an increased likelihood of exhibiting nausea and vomiting in pregnancy. Cigarette smokers are less likely to have nausea and vomiting in pregnancy, which may be caused by the associated lower levels of both hCG and estradiol, compared with nonsmokers.

○ **What features are associated with a higher risk of nausea and vomiting of early pregnancy?**

Primigravid status, younger age, nonsmokers, obesity, less than 12 years of education, previous nausea with oral contraceptive use, and corpus luteum primarily on the right ovary.

○ **What physical findings suggest that nausea and vomiting in a pregnant woman may be because of an independent disease process?**

Abdominal pain or tenderness that is worse than the mild epigastric discomfort that occurs after retching, fever, headache, goiter, or an abnormal neurologic examination. A caveat: severe nausea and vomiting may rarely cause a neurologic abnormality, such as thiamine-deficiency encephalopathy or central pontine myelinolysis.

○ **What are the adverse effects of severe nausea and vomiting on the mother and her fetus?**

Significant morbidity to the mother might include Wernicke encephalopathy, splenic avulsion, esophageal rupture, pneumothorax, and acute tubular necrosis. A higher incidence of low birth weight (LBW) is associated with hyperemesis gravidarum, but not with mild to moderate vomiting. Both maternal and fetal deaths are very rare.

○ **What features distinguish hyperemesis gravidarum from the more common nausea and vomiting that occurs during early pregnancy?**

The following criteria are often used to diagnose hyperemesis gravidarum: persistent vomiting not related to other causes, acute starvation with large ketonuria, loss of at least 5% the prepregnancy weight, and electrolyte abnormalities. Hyperemesis is also associated with abnormal liver function tests. Serum bilirubin can be increased up to five times the upper normal limit. Transaminases and alkaline phosphatase can show mild to moderate increases. Serum amylase may be increased; however, the origin of this is mainly the salivary glands.

○ **What are the risk factors for hyperemesis gravidarum?**

The risk factors associated with hyperemesis gravidarum are obesity, multiple gestation, molar pregnancy, and a family history or history of hyperemesis gravidarum in a previous pregnancy. A population-based study from Canada identified several other factors associated with hyperemesis gravidarum severe enough to warrant hospitalization: hyperthyroid disorders, psychiatric illness, previous molar pregnancy, preexisting diabetes, gastrointestinal disorders, and asthma. Most of these factors are medical and fetal factors that are not modifiable.

○ **What are the fetal complications of hyperemesis gravidarum?**

Infants born of women who had been admitted for hyperemesis gravidarum are more likely to be low birth weight, small for gestational age, born prematurely, and have a 5-minute APGAR less than 7. These effects are largely attributable to poor maternal weight gain, defined as less than 7 kg.

○ **What are some common treatments for hyperemesis gravidarum?**

Management for hyperemesis gravidarum is supportive, with intravenous fluid resuscitation. No antiemetic has been approved for treatment, although they have been widely used. Antihistamines, phenothiazines, and combination doxylamine + pyridoxine have all been shown to effectively reduce nausea and vomiting. Pyridoxine alone has no effect on vomiting but reduces the severity of nausea. Ginger capsules reduce both nausea and vomiting. Multivitamin supplements taken during the time of conception may decrease the severity of nausea and vomiting. Oral methylprednisolone reduces hospital readmission rates. Acupuncture and acupressure have no significant treatment effect.

Thyroid function should also be assessed because high serum beta hCG may stimulate the thyroid and therefore cause clinical hyperthyroidism. However, treatment for hyperthyroidism should not be started unless there is evidence of intrinsic thyroid disease, even if TSH levels are suppressed.

○ **T/F *Helicobacter pylori* infection is responsible for symptomatic dyspepsia in pregnancy.**

False. In a study of 416 pregnant patients, although 42% were found to be seropositive for *H. pylori*, they were no more likely to experience dyspepsia than seronegative controls.

○ **Describe the factors that lead to the decreased risk of peptic ulcer disease in pregnant women.**

(1) Avoidance of NSAIDs and smoking during pregnancy.

(2) Protective effect of estrogen on gastric and duodenal mucosa.

(3) Immunological tolerance to *H. pylori*, thus decreasing the inflammatory response.

○ **What antisecretory medications are safe for use during pregnancy?**

H_2 receptor antagonists are pregnancy category B. Proton pump inhibitors have documented safety and are category B, except for omeprazole (category C). Regarding other drugs, metoclopramide and sucralfate are both category B.

○ **What effect does inflammatory bowel disease have on fertility?**

Women with ulcerative colitis have a similar fertility rate compared to the general population. An exception is women who have undergone proctocolectomy with ileoanal anastomosis and J-pouch. This group has a longer time to pregnancy, probably stemming from surgery-related pelvic adhesions. Women with Crohn disease may have a lower fertility compared to the general population. Fertility is highest in those in remission or following surgical resection of active disease.

○ **What is the risk of relapse of ulcerative colitis in a patient with inactive disease during pregnancy and the puerperium?**

The same as it is in the nonpregnant state. The most likely time for relapse of inflammatory bowel disease during pregnancy is the first trimester. The postpartum period is not necessarily a high-risk time for relapse; the degree of postpartum disease activity correlates with activity at term.

○ **What are the risks to the pregnancy when Crohn disease is active at the time of conception?**

Increased rates of spontaneous abortion, premature delivery, low birth weight, and neonatal vitamin K deficiency. A case report published in 2001 linked a fetal subdural hematoma diagnosed at 22 weeks to maternal vitamin K deficiency secondary to Crohn disease.

○ **T/F: An ileostomy precludes a vaginal delivery.**

False. The rate of cesarean section is not affected by the diagnosis of inflammatory bowel disease, and the decision should generally be based on obstetric indications. One exception is women with active or inactive perirectal, perianal, or rectovaginal fistulas who may have poor wound healing at the episiotomy site.

○ **What medications for inflammatory bowel disease are safe in pregnancy?**

(1) 5-ASA drugs: sulfasalazine, mesalamine, and balsalazide are category B. Olsalazine is category C.

(2) Azathioprine and 6-mercaptopurine (both category D) have been reported safe in pregnancy; the attendant increased risk of IUGR and prematurity should be weighed with the benefits of inducing remission.

(3) Corticosteroids: prednisone and prednisolone (category C) are widely used in pregnancy; budesonide (category C) is formulated to exert a local effect and is theoretically safe.

(4) Cyclosporine (category C) is controversial because of its side-effect profile.

(5) Infliximab (category C) is not currently being used and lacks pregnancy data.

(6) Methotrexate (category X) is teratogenic and should not be used.

(7) Metronidazole is category B.

○ **What are the normal changes in liver function tests that occur in pregnancy?**

Albumin may decrease by 1 g/dL, while bilirubin and the transaminases may be normal or decreased. These changes are because of hemodilution caused by the increased plasma volume between the 6th and 32nd weeks of gestation. Alkaline phosphatase (ALP) is increased because of both increased bone turnover and the leakage of placental ALP into the maternal circulation. Fibrinogen, transferrin, ceruloplasmin, and cholesterol are all increased.

○ **T/F Spider angiomata and palmar erythema are signs of liver disease in pregnancy.**

False. These are normal findings in up to 60% of pregnant women, and disappear rapidly after delivery. Their etiology is thought to be related to the hyperestrogenemia of pregnancy.

○ **T/F: Hepatomegaly is normal during pregnancy.**

False. Pregnancy has little effect on liver size and architecture; therefore, a finding of hepatomegaly should prompt a search for an underlying pathology.

○ **What is the differential diagnosis of hepatomegaly in pregnancy?**

(1) Infiltrative disease: acute fatty liver of pregnancy

(2) Inflammatory condition: hepatitis

(3) Passive congestion: right-sided heart failure or Budd-Chiari syndrome

(4) Malignancy (rare)

○ **What is the differential diagnosis of jaundice in pregnancy?**

(1) Viral hepatitis: serum transaminases increased mild-to-moderate range, positive serology, prominent inflammatory infiltrate on liver biopsy with cellular disarray.

(2) Acute fatty liver of pregnancy: serum transaminases minimally increased, prominent microvesicular fat deposition on liver biopsy.

(3) Toxic injury: history of exposure to tetracycline, isoniazid, erythromycin, or methyldopa.

(4) Cholestasis of pregnancy: pruritus, bile salt elevation.

(5) Severe preeclampsia: hypertension, proteinuria, thrombocytopenia, elevated creatinine, uric acid, and transaminases.

(6) Mononucleosis: flu-like symptoms, elevated transaminases, positive heterophile antibody.

(7) CMV hepatitis: elevated transaminases, positive viral culture or PCR, CMV antibodies.

(8) Autoimmune hepatitis: elevated transaminases, ANA, liver-kidney microsomal antibodies.

○ **What is the rate of maternal-fetal transmission of hepatitis B?**

Several factors modify the perinatal transmission rate of hepatitis B. In the absence of immunoprophylaxis, 10% to 20% of women who are seropositive for HBsAg alone will transmit the virus to their fetus. This rate increases to 90% in women who are seropositive for both HBsAg and HbeAg. The age of gestation when the illness occurs also affects transmission rates for acute hepatitis B. It is 10% during the first trimester, and increased to 80% to 90% during the third trimester. Intrapartum transmission of the infant via exposure to contaminated blood and genital secretions accounts for 85% to 95% of cases of perinatal transmission; the rest comes about from hematogenous dissemination, breastfeeding, and close physical contact between the mother and her neonate.

○ **T/F: Immunoprophylaxis of hepatitis B is necessary for the infants of HbeAg-negative, HBsAg-positive mothers.**

True. While on average the risk of transmission is lower in this group, it is still significant. Therefore, infants of HBsAg-positive mothers, regardless of HbeAg status, should receive both hepatitis B immune globulin and hepatitis B vaccine within 12 hours after birth, followed by two injections of hepatitis B vaccine during the first 6 months of life.

○ **T/F: Cesarean section should be performed in all pregnant women with chronic hepatitis B.**

False. Appropriate immunoprophylaxis of the infant after delivery is sufficient.

○ **T/F Breastfeeding is contraindicated in chronic hepatitis B carriers.**

False. After neonatal hepatitis B vaccination and immunoprophylaxis, chronic hepatitis B carriers have a less than 4% risk of HBV transmission. This risk is approximately equivalent to the vertical transmission rate in chronic hepatitis B carriers who do not breast feed. Women with high viral loads or who are HBeAg positive could be at higher risk for transmission, although the exact risk is unknown.

○ **What is the rate of maternal-fetal transmission of hepatitis C?**

The rate of perinatal transmission of hepatitis C is proportional to the maternal viral titers. The overall risk of vertical transmission is 7% to 8%, and is higher in women who are also infected with HIV. Furthermore, the presence of antibodies is not protective against transmission. The transmission rate by breastfeeding is 2% to 3%.

○ **Does cesarean section decrease the risk of perinatal transmission of hepatitis C?**

There are no randomized control trials regarding the preferred mode of delivery of pregnant women with hepatitis C. One observational study reported a decreased perinatal transmission rate with cesarean delivery, but this has not been confirmed by other studies.

○ **What is the role of interferon alpha therapy for hepatitis during pregnancy?**

Interferon alfa has been shown to produce clinical improvement in 28% to 46% of patients with hepatitis C, and has also been shown to alter the natural history of hepatitis B and D infection. However, it has abortifacient properties and should be avoided in pregnancy.

○ **What are typical features of fulminant hepatic failure because of herpes simplex occurring during the third trimester of pregnancy?**

Herpes simplex hepatitis can result in fulminant hepatic failure with a 40% mortality rate, with half the reported adult cases occurring during pregnancy. The clinical and biochemical features are usually indistinguishable from other causes of acute liver failure; however, jaundice is characteristically absent. Typical skin lesions are evident in less than half of patients, and diagnosis may ultimately rest on liver biopsy, cultures and serology.

○ **T/F: Treatment for Wilson disease should be discontinued during pregnancy.**

False. Discontinuing penicillamine treatment for Wilson disease increases the risk of maternal hepatic and neurologic failure and hemolysis, and has been associated with fatal relapses. The drug itself is usually well tolerated by both the mother and her fetus. Trientene seems to be safe as well, although a few data are available. Zinc therapy is also effective in preventing relapse in pregnancy.

○ **T/F: A history of Budd-Chiari syndrome precludes a subsequent normal pregnancy.**

False.

○ **List the cholestatic disorders of pregnancy.**

Hyperemesis gravidarum, intrahepatic cholestasis of pregnancy, acute fatty liver of pregnancy, preeclampsia and HELLP (hemolysis, elevated liver tests, low platelets) syndrome.

○ **T/F: Pregnancy is contraindicated in patients with chronic cholestatic liver diseases.**

False. Cholestasis may worsen but can be managed and usually returns to baseline after delivery in primary biliary cirrhosis, Dubin-Johnson syndrome, and the familial intrahepatic cholestatic syndromes such as Alagille syndrome.

○ **T/F Liver transplant is a contraindication to pregnancy.**

False. Pregnancy planned at least two years after liver transplant with stable allograft function can have excellent maternal and neonatal outcomes although the risks are significant. Transplant recipients considering pregnancy should be counseled that pregnancy complications include preterm delivery (19%–20%), fetal growth restriction (10%), congenital malformations (4%–16%), spontaneous abortions (11%), graft rejection (10%), HELLP syndrome (8%), hypertension (up to 20%), preeclampsia (4%–20%), cesarean delivery (45%), maternal deaths (up to 3%). These numbers are higher than in the general population but lower than the corresponding outcomes quoted before 1998.

○ **Which malformations are associated with immunosuppressive therapy after liver transplantation?**

The occurrence of meningocele, urogenital defects, cleft palate, hypospadias, multicystic dysplastic kidneys, and membranous ventricular septal defect have been associated with immunosuppression after a liver transplant. No consistent pattern has, however, been identified in these patients.

○ **What is the most common cause of upper gastrointestinal hemorrhage during pregnancy?**

Mallory-Weiss tear, followed by erosive esophagitis.

○ **What is the most common cause of lower gastrointestinal bleeding during pregnancy?**

Hemorrhoids.

○ **What are the abdominal causes of acute volume loss (with or without abdominal pain) during pregnancy?**

(1) Ruptured ectopic pregnancy.
(2) Placental abruption.
(3) Ruptured liver.
(4) Ruptured splenic artery aneurysm.

○ **What causes of pancreatitis may be exacerbated during pregnancy?**

The incidence of gallstones is increased during pregnancy although pancreatitis is rare. Pregnancy may worsen underlying hypertriglyceridemia and precipitate pancreatitis.

Hyperparathyroidism may first become manifest during pregnancy and cause pancreatitis.

○ **At what stage of pregnancy is pancreatitis most likely to occur?**

During the third trimester and the postpartum period.

○ **What presentations of gallstone disease are common during pregnancy? Which are rare?**

Biliary colic and acute cholecystitis are common; jaundice and acute pancreatitis are rare.

○ **When is cholecystectomy safe during pregnancy?**

Laparoscopic cholecystectomy is the most common laparoscopic procedure in pregnancy. Several studies have shown no increased risk of preterm delivery or adverse outcome after first trimester laparoscopic cholecystectomy. The laparoscopic approach is also feasible in the third trimester. Nonoperative management of symptomatic cholelithiasis is associated with higher recurrence of symptoms necessitating hospitalization, increased risk of gallstone pancreatitis (associated with a 10%–20% rate of fetal loss,) increased risk of miscarriage, preterm labor and preterm delivery compared to those undergoing laparoscopic cholecystectomy. Furthermore, such non-surgical approaches like bile acid therapy, lithotripsy, and dissolution with methyl terbutyl ether are not recommended during pregnancy because of the lack of safety data.

○ **What is the most frequent cause of an acute abdomen in pregnancy?**

Acute appendicitis, which approximates 1 in 1500 deliveries, can occur at any time, with a slight predominance during the second trimester. Maternal mortality is rare, but the rate of fetal loss is 10% to 20%, because of preterm labor or IUFD. Preterm labor usually occurs within 5 days of surgery, and could either be because of the disease or the inflammatory response to surgery. The differential diagnosis includes pyelonephritis, cholecystitis, renal or ureteral calculi, adnexal torsion, degenerating myoma, extrauterine pregnancy, and placental abruption.

○ **What is the most common symptom of appendicitis in pregnancy?**

Right lower quadrant pain is the most common presentation in all three trimesters. The dictum that appendicitis presents as right upper quadrant pain during the third trimester has not been validated by studies.

○ **Why is acute appendicitis more hazardous to the mother during pregnancy than in the nonpregnant state?**

Local perforation may be contained by the uterine wall on one side and may result in premature delivery with free perforation and generalized peritonitis after the uterus empties and pulls away from the appendiceal abscess.

○ **Why should a normal appendix found at laparotomy during pregnancy not be removed?**

Removal of a normal appendix has been associated with a tripling of the risk of fetal loss.

○ **What is the cause of acute granulomatous peritonitis in pregnancy or the puerperium?**

Rupture of fetal contents into the peritoneum or meconium spillage during cesarean delivery.

○ **Name the pregnancy complications experienced by obese women.**

Class I (BMI 30–34.9) and class II (BMI 35–39.9) obesity is associated with increased risk for gestational hypertension, preeclampsia, gestational diabetes, and fetal macrosomia, as well as a progressively increased rate of cesarean delivery. Women in this group who undergo cesarean delivery are more likely to have wound dehiscence and infections. The risk of stillbirth and neonatal death is doubled in this group as well.

○ **What is the benefit of exercise for obese pregnant women?**

Exercise is beneficial for the primary prevention of gestational diabetes, especially in women with a BMI ≥ 33. It is also useful in maintaining euglycemia in gestational diabetes patients who fail diet control alone. The following relative contraindications to aerobic exercise should be kept in mind: extreme morbid obesity, poorly controlled type 1 diabetes, history of extremely sedentary lifestyle, and orthopedic limitations.

○ **What are the benefits of bariatric surgery for obese women contemplating pregnancy?**

Obese women who have undergone bariatric surgery are less likely to have gestational diabetes, hypertension, macrosomia, or cesarean delivery. Bariatric surgery itself is not associated with adverse perinatal outcomes, despite earlier reports of increased rates of GI bleeding, anemia, IUGR, and neural tube defects. It is advisable to wait 12 to 18 months after surgery before attempting to conceive as well as to supplement with vitamin B_{12}, folate, iron, and calcium.

CHAPTER 16 First Trimester Ultrasound

David Peleg, MD

○ **What techniques may be applied to perform a first trimester ultrasound?**

Transabdominal
Transvaginal
Transperineal

○ **What are the advantages of using transvaginal ultrasound (TVUS) vs transabdominal ultrasound?**

The probe is closer to the pelvic organs, allowing a higher frequency (5–7 MHz), which improves resolution and a full bladder is not required.

○ **What are the disadvantages of using transvaginal ultrasound vs transabdominal ultrasound?**

At higher resolution, a shorter distance from the probe is seen.
Transvaginal ultrasound is more invasive.

○ **What is the difference between a threshold level and a discriminatory level?**

The threshold level is the lowest value for which certain observation can be detected by ultrasound.
The discriminatory level is the lowest value for which a certain observation should always be detected.

○ **What is the first ultrasound landmark of pregnancy?**

Gestational sac.

○ **Using TVUS, what size is the threshold for detecting a gestational sac?**

2 to 3 mm.

○ **Does the presence of an intrauterine fluid-filled area confirm an intrauterine pregnancy?**

No, it could be a decidual reaction or "pseudogestational sac."

○ **How is the mean sac diameter (MSD) calculated?**

Adding the three orthogonal dimensions and dividing by 3.

○ **How can one calculate the gestational age from the mean sac diameter (MSD) from 5 to 11 weeks gestation?**

MSD (in mm) + 30 = gestational age in days.

○ **What is the discriminatory size of the gestational sac (MSD) at which one would expect to see the yolk sac?**

MSD = 8 mm via transvaginal ultrasound (5.5 weeks).
MSD = 20 mm via transabdominal ultrasound (7 weeks).

○ **What are the three known functions of the yolk sac?**

(1) Provides nutrients for the embryo.

(2) Initial site of hematopoiesis.

(3) Contributes to developing gut and reproductive systems.

○ **Which is superior in confirming an intrauterine pregnancy (IUP): a yolk sac within the gestational sac or the double decidual sac sign (DDSS)?**

The yolk sac within the gestational sac.

○ **After identification of a gestational sac, what is the next visible landmark for pregnancy dating?**

The yolk sac.

○ **At what hCG level will you typically see an intrauterine gestational sac?**

1000 to 2000 mIU/mL.

○ **The embryonic phase of development is from _____ to _____ weeks gestation?**

6 to 10.

○ **The chorionic cavity normally obliterates from _____ to _____ weeks gestation?**

12 to 16.

○ **What is the discriminatory size of the gestational sac (MSD) at which one would expect to see the embryo?**

MSD = 20 mm via transvaginal ultrasound.
MSD = 25 mm via transabdominal ultrasound.

○ **How can one calculate the gestational age from the CRL from 6 to 9.5 weeks gestation?**

CRL (in mm) + 42 = gestational age in days.

○ **What is the approximate growth rate of the embryo (CRL) and the gestational sac diameter between 6 and 10 gestational weeks?**

1 mm/d

○ **Which is a more accurate indicator of gestational age: crown-rump length or mean gestational sac diameter?**

Crown-rump length.

○ **How accurate is the first trimester CRL measurement in predicting gestational age?**

Within 5 days.

○ **What is the discriminatory size of the embryo (CRL) at which one would expect to see cardiac activity via transvaginal ultrasound?**

CRL = 5 mm via transvaginal ultrasound (6+ weeks).

○ **Is it true or false that cardiac pulsations may be seen when performing TVUS before the embryo itself is identified?**

True.

○ **Cardiac activity should normally be seen when the embryonic pole has achieved what size? This corresponds to what gestational age and what MSD?**

4 to 5 mm; 6.0 to 6.5 weeks; 13 to 18 mm.

○ **How does the fetal heart rate change in the first trimester?**

It increases from 100 to 115 beats per minute (bpm) before 6 weeks to 145 to 160 bpm at 8 weeks gestation after which it plateaus at 135 to 145 bpm. The variability also increases during this time.

○ **The term "missed abortion" has been replaced by what term(s)?**

Embryonic or fetal demise.

○ **What is the percent chance for miscarriage after cardiac activity is seen in an 8-week gestation?**

2% to 3%.

○ **What are some common synonyms for an intrauterine blood collection in the first trimester?**

Subchorionic hemorrhage or hematoma, implantation hemorrhage, and perigestational hemorrhage.

○ **In the presence of an intrauterine hematoma, the risk of a spontaneous abortion is associated with:**

(1) Increasing size of the hematoma

(2) Advanced maternal age

(3) Earlier gestational age

(4) Structural uterine anomalies

(5) History of miscarriage

○ **True or False: An abnormal appearing yolk sac is associated with early pregnancy failure?**

True.

○ **Recurrent miscarriage is defined as:**

Three or more consecutive first trimester spontaneous losses.

○ **What is the arrow in this first trimester ultrasound pointing to?**

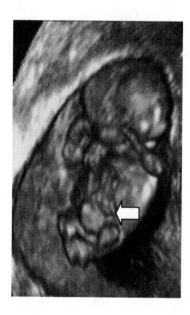

Physiologic herniation of the midgut.

○ **Is this a normal or abnormal finding?**

Normal.

○ **What abnormality could it be mistaken for?**

Abdominal wall defects, such as omphalocele and gastroschisis (which should not be diagnosed until the second trimester).

○ **The midgut typically returns to the abdomen at what week gestation?**

11 to 12 weeks.

○ **When can the midgut be seen?**

Seen from 8 to 11 weeks with herniation of the fetal bowel into the base of the umbilical cord and 90 degree counter-clockwise rotation of the bowel around the base of the superior mesenteric artery.

○   **What is the arrow in this first trimester ultrasound pointing to?**

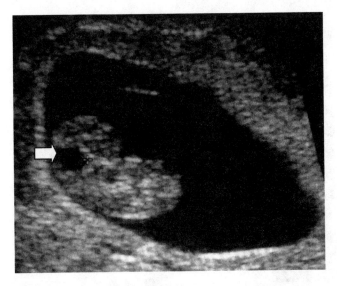

The developing rhombencephalon.

○   **Is this a normal or abnormal finding?**

Normal.

○   **What abnormality could it be mistaken for?**

Dandy-Walker malformation or hydrocephalus (which should not be diagnosed until the second trimester).

○   **When can it be seen?**

Seen from 7 to 9 weeks, it will eventually contribute to the fourth ventricle, brain stem, and cerebellum.

○   **What sign are the large arrows pointing to in this first trimester ultrasound?**

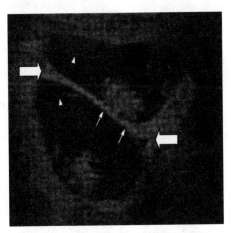

Lambda sign or twin peaks sign.

○ **What does this sign tell us about the chorionicity and amnionicity of this twin gestation?**
It is dichorionic (and diamnionic)

○ **How would you describe the amnionicity and chorionicity of this first trimester pregnancy?**

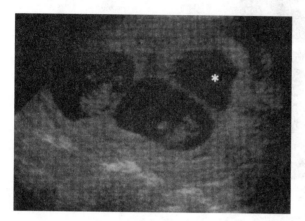

Trichorionic, triamniotic.

○ **How would you describe the amnionicity and chorionicity of this first trimester pregnancy?**

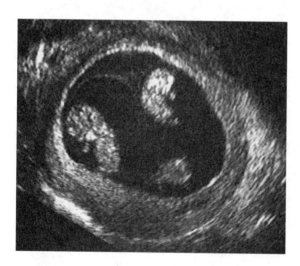

Monochorionic, triamniotic.

○ **How are the number of yolk sacs and amnionicity related?**
The number of yolk sacs equals the number of amniotic sacs.

○ **When is the best time to determine amnionicity and chorionicity in a multiple gestation?**
8 to 10 weeks (the earlier the better).

○ **What is the most common adnexal mass visualized during a first trimester ultrasound?**

The corpus luteum.

○ **The resistance index (RI) and pulsatility index(PI) of the uterine artery decline from 6 to 12 weeks gestation due to:**

Establishment of the intervillous circulation.

○ **Name some fetal anomalies that can be detected with reliability in the first trimester.**

Large encephalocele, holoprosencephaly, ectopia cordis, and conjoined twins

○ **Name a few major malformations, which should not be diagnosed in the first trimester.**

Renal agenesis, anencephaly, Dandy-Walker malformation, hydrocephalus, omphalocele.

○ **Nuchal translucency (NT) is performed between which gestational weeks?**

Between 10 and 14 weeks.

○ **What variables are used to calculate the Down syndrome risk when performing NT?**

The NT measurement, the CRL, the gestational age, and the age of the mother.

○ **What value for NT is generally considered abnormal?**

3 mm or greater.

○ **What percentage of fetuses with an abnormal NT will have aneuploidy?**

About 75%.

○ **Which congenital abnormality is associated with an abnormal NT, but normal karyotype?**

Congential heart disease (in 27%).

○ **Fetuses with abnormal NT and normal karyotype and anatomy may be at increased risk of what?**

Preterm delivery and growth restriction.

○ **What are the advantages for first trimester aneuploidy screening?**

The potential for earlier diagnosis, which can be confirmed by CVS, allowing for earlier, less traumatic termination with more privacy.

○ **What is the difference between nuchal translucency (NT) and nuchal skin fold (NSF) measurements?**

NT is a first trimester measurement, while NSF is a second trimester measurement.

○ **How does the NT change with gestational age?**

It increases from 10 to 14 weeks gestation.

○   **What are the requirements for a good NT image?**

CRL between 45 and 84 mm.

Fetus in midsagittal plane in neutral position.

Distinguish between fetal skin and amnion.

Magnified so fetus occupies 75% of the screen.

Place calipers on inner margins of skin to soft tissue.

○   **Is transvaginal ultrasound required for NT measurement?**

No, often abdominal ultrasound is successful in 80% of cases.

○   **How does neck flexion and extension affect the NT?**

Neck flexion decreases the NT by about 0.4 mm, while hyperextension increases the NT by about 0.6 mm.

○   **What first trimester biochemical analytes, along with NT, constitute an effective screening strategy for aneuploidy?**

PAPP-A (Pregnancy associated plasma protein A) and hCG (free or total Human chorionic gonadotropin).

○   **What NT is greater than the 99th percentile throughout the measured gestational ages?**

3.5 mm.

○   **While performing NT, what structure pictured below may be a useful marker for detection of aneuploidy?**

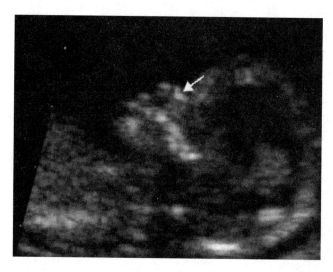

Nasal bone.

○   **What technique should be used for nasal bone (NB) measurements?**

Fetus magnified so that only the head and upper thorax are in the screen.

Precise midsagittal view of the fetal profile.

Fetal spine down with slight neck flexion.

Transducer parallel to the direction of the fetal nose (45–135 degrees).

Three distinct lines should be seen.

○ **What is ductus venosus?**

A trumpet-shaped vein connecting the umbilical sinus to the hepatic veins and the IVC, directing high-velocity oxygenated blood returning from the placenta to the left atrium via the foramen ovale.

○ **What is the normal Doppler waveform pattern in the ductus venosus?**

Biphasic pulsatile continuously forward flow.

○ **What heart abnormalities might not develop until the third trimester?**

Cardiac rhabdomyomas
Cardiomyopathies

○ **What heart abnormalities may be apparent in the first trimester, but may resolve by the third trimester?**

Muscular ventricular septal defect.

CHAPTER 17

Obstetrical Ultrasound and Fetal Abnormalities

Hima Bindu Tam Tam, MD

○ **What percentage of pregnant women in the US undergoes at least one ultrasound?**

According to ACOG this number was 65% in 2002.

○ **How is ultrasound produced?**

It is the vibrations of crystals in response to electrical current generate sound waves. This is known as the piezoelectric effect.

○ **The frequencies of the transvaginal transducers are typically higher than the transabdominal.**

True. The transabdominal probes are typically 3 to 7 MHz and the transvaginal probes 5 to 9 MHz. With higher frequencies there is greater resolution but decreased penetration.

○ **Is ultrasound safe?**

With the widespread use, no biological effects have been confirmed on the fetus with the frequencies used in obstetrical ultrasound. The level of ultrasound intensity that is defined as safe is ≤ 100 mW/cm^2. It has been shown to cause thermal effects and mechanical changes via cavitation in animal studies.

○ **What serum analytes are used in conjunction with ultrasound to screen for aneuploidy?**

In the first trimester, serum PAPP-A and free beta-hCG levels and in the second trimester unconjugated estriol, beta-hCG and inhibin A are also measured. In Down syndrome, the serum beta-hCG (free and total) and inhibin-A levels are increased and the levels of PAPP-A, uE3, and AFP are decreased.

○ **What is the most accurate predictor of gestational age in first trimester?**

Crown-rump length is better than the gestational sac and yolk sac measurements.

○ **If only one ultrasound can be done, what is the optimal gestational age at which it should be done?**

16 to 20 weeks.

○ **What parameters are commonly used to assess gestational age in the second and third trimester?**

Biparietal diameter, head circumference, abdominal circumference, and femur length.

○ **How is the biparietal diameter measured?**

The image should show the oval shape, falx cerebri and the cavum septum pellucidum at the level of the thalami measure, then measure two-thirds from the frontal area the outer to inner edge. The head circumference is also measured at this level.

○ **Dolichocephaly is associated with:**

Breech presentation. There is decreased parietal to occipital frontal diameter (cephalic index).

○ **At what level is the abdominal circumference measured?**

The image should be at the level of the junction of the umbilical vein and portal sinus.

○ **Why does femur appear to be bowed in normal fetus?**

It is the inability to see the full thickness of the femoral diaphysis that gives the impression that the femur farther away from the transducer is bowed. The femoral length should only include the diaphysis and metaphysis.

○ **Asymmetric IUGR is associated with?**

Decreased abdominal circumference to head circumference.

○ **Which Doppler study is used to follow fetuses with IUGR?**

Umbilical artery velocimetry. It has also been shown that the increase in flow resistance in the umbilical artery is correlated with decreased flow resistance in the MCA, and this has been attributed to the brain sparing response of the IUGR fetus.

○ **Which Doppler measures fetal anemia?**

MCA Doppler. With anemia there is increased fetal cardiac output, which is attributed to decreased blood viscosity and decreased peripheral vascular resistance. These allow for delivery of larger volume of less oxygenated blood. Hence, the blood flow velocity in the MCA is increased. The Doppler is used to follow fetuses at risk for anemia from isoimmunization.

○ **What Doppler measurement must be followed when indomethacin is given for preterm labor?**

Ductus arteriosus. Indomethacin has been shown to cause premature constriction of the ductus arteriosus. This is seen by increase in PSV and decrease in PI. The effect is considered reversible and abnormal Doppler should lead to discontinuation of the indomethacin.

○ **Which Doppler measurement in the second trimester has been suggested as a screening test for development of preeclampsia?**

Uterine artery.

○ **The evaluation of placenta accreta is improved by:**

Color Doppler and MRI.

○ **Macrosomia caused by maternal diabetes is associated with?**

Increased abdominal circumference to head circumference.

○ **Evaluation of amniotic fluid volume:**

Single vertical pocket with normal being between 2 and 8 cm and the amniotic fluid index with is the sum of the largest vertical pockets in four quadrants.

○ **What abnormalities cannot be ruled out on four-chamber view of the heart?**

Small ASDs and VSDs and abnormalities of the great vessels. Hence, the RVOT and LVOT should also be visualized. The chamber closest to the spine is the left atrium. The mitral valve appears to be at a higher level than the tricuspid valve. Important information regarding the size, position and the axis of the heart can be obtained from this single view.

○ **What follow-up study should be performed on a fetus with increased NT?**

Fetal echocardiogram, as there is an increased risk of cardiac defects even in fetuses with normal karyotype.

○ **Multicystic mass posterolateral to the fetal neck:**

Cystic hygroma and risk of aneuploidy is 60% to 75%, the most common being Turner syndrome.

○ **What is potter's sequence?**

A single factor oligohydramnios resulting from bilateral renal agenesis (BRA) or PPROM leads to multiple secondary effects such as hypoplastic lungs, limb deformities, and abnormal facies. Kidneys should be visualized by 16 to 18 weeks. In BRA bladder is not seen.

○ **Single umbilical artery is associated with?**

15% to 20% incidence of cardiovascular abnormalities. It is seen in more than 50% of fetuses with trisomy 18. Found in 1/200 newborns. Color flow Doppler of the umbilical arteries at the level of the fetal bladder is used to confirm a three-vessel cord.

○ **Cervical length of greater than ___ mm has good negative predictive value of preterm labor**

25.

○ **When is funneling of membranes considered to be significant?**

Greater than 50% of the cervical length.

○ **Ultrasound at seventh week demonstrates a midgut herniation. This finding is most likely?**

Normal.

○ **At which gestational age should the fetal abdomen be intact?**

12 weeks.

○ **Which anterior abdominal wall defect is associated with aneuploidy?**

With an omphalocele there is a 30% to 40% risk of aneuploidy. It is a midline defect resulting in the herniation into the base of the cord, which is unlike gastrochesis (where the herniation is lateral to the cord insertion) not associated with aneuploidy.

○   **What is an Arnold Chiari malformation and what is it associated with:**

Displacement of the cerebellum, fourth ventricle, and the medulla. It is associated with open neural tube defects.

○   **Characteristic ultrasound findings associated with Arnold Chiari malformation:**

Lemon sign and Banana sign.

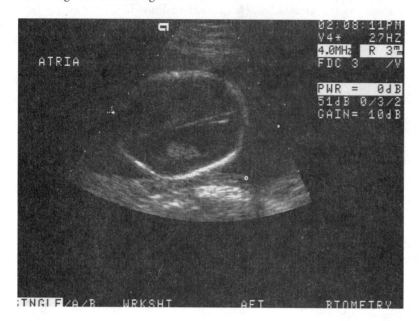

○   **What substances are elevated in the amniotic fluid of a fetus with open neural tube defect?**

AFP and acetyl cholinesterase.

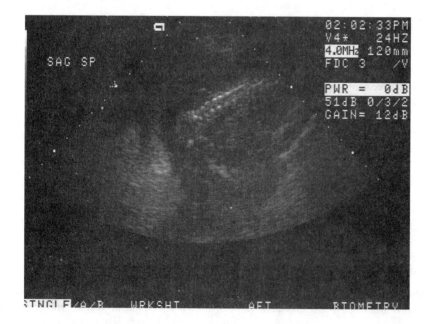

○   **3D/4D ultrasound is useful in the assessment of:**

Fetal facial abnormalities. Cleft lip and palate when found as an isolated anomaly follow a multifactorial inheritance. They have been associated with folate deficiency.

○   **At what maternal age is an amniocentesis recommended for this isolated finding?**

With an isolated choroid plexus cyst, testing is indicated only if maternal age will be greater than 32 at delivery.

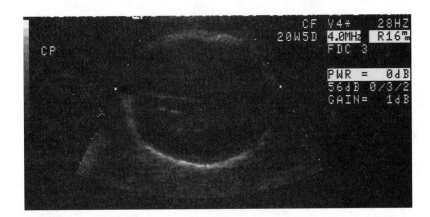

○   **This ultrasound demonstrates:**

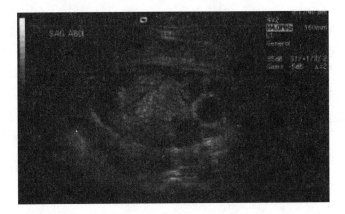

Fetal hydrops.

○   **This ultrasound in association with fetal isoimmunization indicates:**

Severe fetal anemia leading to cardiac failure.

○   **What are some of the causes of nonimmune hydrops?**

Chromosomal anomalies, TTTS, cystic hygroma, cardiac anomalies, CCAM, TORCH infections, and hemoglobinopathies.

○ **Echogenic bowel is associated with:**

Cystic fibrosis, abnormal karyotype, TORCH infections, and fetal ingestion of bloody amniotic fluid.

○ **What type of defect is anencephaly?**

It is an open neural tube defect resulting from the failure of the rostral neuropore. The recurrence risk is 2% to 3% and patient should receive 4 mg of folic acid supplementation prior to next pregnancy.

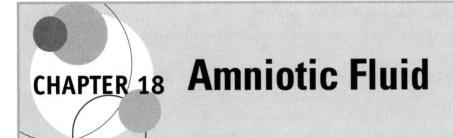

CHAPTER 18 Amniotic Fluid

Kristen Quinn, MD

○ **What are the five major functions of amniotic fluid?**

(1) Helps to protect the fetus from trauma.

(2) Cushions the umbilical cord from compression between the fetus and the uterus.

(3) Antibacterial properties that provide some protection from infection.

(4) Serves as a reservoir of fluid and nutrients for the fetus.

(5) Provides the necessary fluid, space, and growth factors to permit normal development of the fetal lungs and musculoskeletal and gastrointestinal systems.

○ **What is the major source of amniotic fluid production in the second half of pregnancy?**

Fetal urination.

○ **What other sources contribute to amniotic fluid production in the second half of pregnancy?**

Secretions from the fetal respiratory tract, including the lungs and oral–nasal cavity and intramembranous flow.

○ **What is the major pathway of clearance of amniotic fluid in the last half of pregnancy?**

Fetal swallowing.

○ **Significant amounts of water and solutes are not transferred across the fetal skin after keratinization occurs. At what gestational age does this occur?**

Between 22 and 25 weeks gestation.

○ **When is amniotic fluid volume at its peak?**

34 to 36 weeks gestation.

○ **What is the average peak of amniotic fluid volume?**

1 L (1000 cc).

○   **What is the composition of amniotic fluid in the first trimester?**

The electrolyte composition and osmolality is essentially the same as fetal and maternal blood.

○   **When does fetal urine first enter the amniotic sac?**

8 to 11 weeks.

○   **Is amniotic fluid hypertonic, isotonic, or hypotonic in the third trimester as compared to maternal plasma?**

Hypotonic.

○   **What causes amniotic fluid osmolality to decrease as pregnancy progresses?**

Inflow of markedly hypotonic fetal urine.

○   **Under normal conditions, what is the average increase in amniotic fluid volume late in gestation?**

30– to 40 mL/d.

○   **What are the six major pathways that help to regulate amniotic fluid volume late in pregnancy?**

(1) Fetal urination

(2) Fetal swallowing and reabsorption by the intestine

(3) Secretion from the respiratory tract

(4) Secretions from the fetal oral-nasal cavities

(5) Intramembranous pathway

(6) Transmembranous pathway.

○   **What are the three major determinants of amniotic fluid volume (when fetal anomalies are excluded)?**

(1) Movements of water and solutes within and across the membranes.

(2) Physiologic regulation by the fetus of flow rates such as urine production and swallowing.

(3) Maternal effects on transplacental fluid movement.

○   **Approximately what volume of amniotic fluid is swallowed daily by the fetus near term?**

200– to 500 mL/d.

○   **How many milliliters of fluid does the fetal lung secrete per day in the third trimester?**

300– to 400 mL/d.

○   **Over the course of 1 day, what is the net turnover volume of the amniotic fluid?**

95% of the total amniotic fluid volume is turned over daily.

○   **What is the source of meconium in the amniotic fluid?**

Fetal bowel movements associated with fetal stress and /or postmaturity.

○ **How is amniotic fluid volume most commonly measured?**

Ultrasound.

○ **What are the two most commonly used objective methods to measure amniotic fluid volume via ultrasound?**

Measurement of the maximum vertical pocket (MVP) and calculation of the amniotic fluid index (AFI).

○ **How is the MVP obtained?**

Measurement of the vertical depth of the largest cord- and limb-free pocket of amniotic fluid.

○ **How is the AFI calculated?**

Summation of the depths of the largest vertical pocket in each of the four quadrants.

○ **When calculating the AFI, what anatomical landmarks are used to divide the uterus into quadrants?**

Linea nigra and umbilicus.

○ **How is the AFI calculated before 20 weeks gestation?**

Summation of the two maximum vertical pockets on each side of the linea nigra.

○ **How might the measurement of amniotic fluid volume be artificially increased?**

By not maintaining the transducer perpendicular to the floor.

○ **How might the measurement of amniotic fluid volume be artificially decreased?**

By applying excessive pressure on the maternal abdomen with the transducer.

○ **What is oligohydramnios?**

Less than normal or diminished amniotic fluid volume.

○ **What is the incidence of oligohydramnios?**

0.5% –to 8% of all pregnancies.

○ **What MVP is consistent with oligohydramnios?**

Less than 2 cm.

○ **What AFI is consistent with oligohydramnios?**

0 to 5 cm or less than fifth percentile for a particular gestational age.

○ **What AFI is consistent with severe oligohydramnios?**

Less than 2 cm.

○   **What are some clinical findings pointing toward the possibility of oligohydramnios?**

Fundal height less than estimated gestational age.

Fetal parts easily palpated through maternal abdomen.

Ultrasound exam demonstrates fetal crowding and poor visualization of fetal anatomy.

○   **What subjective ultrasound criteria have been used to determine oligohydramnios?**

Absence of fluid pockets throughout the uterine cavity.

Crowding of fetal limbs.

Absence of pockets surrounding the fetal legs.

Overlapping of the fetal ribs (in severe cases).

○   **Name some causes of oligohydramnios:**

Congenital anomalies, especially related to renal system dysfunction (e.g., renal agenesis, polycystic kidneys, genitourinary obstruction, dysplastic multicystic kidneys, or posterior urethral valves in males).

Chromosomal anomalies.

Fetal anuria or oliguria as a result of decreased renal perfusion.

Intrauterine growth restriction.

Side effect of certain drugs (e.g., indomethacin, ACE inhibitors).

Maternal dehydration.

Severe preeclampsia.

Postdate pregnancy.

Ruptured membranes.

○   **What is the most common cause of oligohydramnios?**

Premature rupture of the membranes.

○   **What serious complications are associated with oligohydramnios occurring before 22 weeks?**

Pulmonary hypoplasia

Amniotic band syndrome

Fetal compression syndrome

○   **Why is second trimester oligohydramnios associated with pulmonary hypoplasia?**

Amniotic fluid inspired at regular intervals and the distending force it creates is needed for proper terminal alveolar development.

○   **What is the most likely cause of second trimester oligohydramnios in the absence of ruptured membranes?**

Congenital anomalies.

○   **What is the most likely cause of third trimester oligohydramnios in the absence of ruptured membranes?**

Intrauterine growth restriction.

○ **What is the mechanism of oligohydramnios in fetuses with intrauterine growth restriction?**

Chronic hypoxia resulting in shunting of fetal blood flow from the kidneys, thereby decreasing GFR and decreasing fetal urine output.

○ **A large bladder in the presence of oligohydramnios is associated with what cause for the oligohydramnios?**

Urethral obstruction.

○ **A fluid-filled bladder seen on ultrasound is used to rule out what potential congenital abnormality cause of oligohydramnios?**

Bilateral renal agenesis.

○ **What drugs can cause oligohydramnios?**

Prostaglandin synthetase inhibitors and angiotensin-converting enzyme inhibitors.

○ **What is the mortality rate of oligohydramnios in the second trimester?**

Fetal mortality rate has been reported as high as 80% to 90%. The earlier the diagnosis, the worse the prognosis.

○ **Why is the gestational age at which oligohydramnios occurs, important?**

The earlier that oligohydramnios occurs, the poorer the prognosis.

○ **What is a common fetal heart rate tracing finding in patients with oligohydramnios?**

Variable decelerations.

○ **Why are variable decelerations more commonly seen with oligohydramnios?**

Cord compression as a result of less cushioning effect of normal amniotic fluid volume.

○ **What is oligohydramnios associated with asymmetric growth restriction most likely due to?**

Uteroplacental insufficiency.

○ **What is the mechanism by which uteroplacental insufficiency might cause oligohydramnios?**

Chronic hypoxia causes shunting of fetal blood away from the kidneys to more vital organs, leading to decreased fetal urine output, thus decreasing amniotic fluid production.

○ **What is oligohydramnios associated with symmetric growth restriction most likely due to?**

Chromosomal abnormalities.

○ **How does oligohydramnios make ultrasound assessment of the fetus more difficult?**

Amniotic fluid easily transmits sound waves; therefore, ultrasound visualization of fetal anatomy is impaired by less amniotic fluid.

○   **What can be done to improve the quality of diagnostic ultrasound in a pregnancy complicated by oligohydramnios?**

Intra-amniotic placement of sterile saline (i.e., amnioinfusion) may enhance visualization of the fetal anatomy.

○   **How does amnioinfusion help pregnancies complicated by oligohydramnios?**

Amnioinfusion decreases the incidence of variable decelerations, and consequently decreases the cesarean section rate for nonreassuring fetal heart rate tracing.

○   **Has delivery of postdate pregnancies complicated by oligohydramnios been shown to result in improved perinatal outcomes by randomized investigation?**

No.

○   **When might delivery be safely postponed in a term pregnancy complicated by oligohydramnios?**

In an otherwise uncomplicated pregnancy with an AFI close to five, reassuring fetal testing and an unfavorable cervix at 37 weeks gestation.

○   **What is polyhydramnios?**

Synonymous with hydramnios, means abnormally excessive amounts of amniotic fluid.

○   **What is the clinical definition of polyhydramnios?**

>2 L of amniotic fluid measured at time of delivery.

○   **What is the incidence of polyhydramnios?**

1% to 4% of all pregnancies.

○   **What MVP is consistent with polyhydramnios?**

>8 cm.

○   **What AFI is consistent with polyhydramnios?**

>25 cm or greater than 95th percentile for a particular gestational age.

○   **What is the incidence of polyhydramnios?**

1% of pregnancies.

○   **What is one of the first clinical findings that might indicate a diagnosis of polyhydramnios?**

Fundal height greater than dates.

○   **What is the differential diagnosis for polyhydramnios?**

Diabetes—gestational and insulin dependent
Congenital anomalies

Multiple gestations

Immune and nonimmune fetal hydrops

Idiopathic

○ **What is the most likely etiology of polyhydramnios?**

Idiopathic; accounts for 66% of all cases of polyhydramnios

○ **What specific congenital anomalies are associated with polyhydramnios?**

Central nervous system anomalies (e.g., anencephaly)

Skeletal dysplasias (e.g., achondroplasia)

Gastrointestinal atresias (e.g., esophageal, duodenal)

Tracheoesophageal fistulas

Facial clefts

Neck masses (such as cystic hygroma), which may interfere with fetal swallowing

Cystic malformations of the lung

Diaphragmatic hernia

○ **What five tests are included in the initial work-up of a patient with polyhydramnios?**

Glucola screen

Antibody screen

Screen for maternal hemoglobinopathies

Maternal viral titers (e.g., parvovirus)

Targeted ultrasound

○ **Does excess fetal urine production play a major role in polyhydramnios?**

No.

○ **What percentage of patients with polyhydramnios in the second trimester have spontaneous resolution?**

40%– to 50% of cases.

○ **What obstetrical complications are associated with polyhydramnios?**

Maternal respiratory compromise

Preterm labor

Premature rupture of membranes

Fetal malposition

Umbilical cord prolapse and/or postpartum uterine atony

○ **What are two therapeutic options that might ameliorate polyhydramnios?**

Therapeutic amniotic fluid drainage via amniocentesis

Maternal indocin administration

○   **What is the mechanism of action of prostaglandin synthetase inhibitors in decreasing amniotic fluid?**

These medications stimulate fetal secretion of arginine, vasopressin, and facilitate vasopressin-induced renal antidiuretic responses, as well as reduced renal blood flow, thereby reducing fetal urine flow. These medications may also impair production or enhance reabsorption of liquid in the lungs.

○   **What is the primary fetal concern with use of indomethacin?**

Constriction of the ductus arteriosus.

○   **Why should rapid decompression of a gravid uterus with polyhydramnios be avoided?**

Rapid decompression may result in cord prolapse or placental abruption.

CHAPTER 19

The Placenta and Umbilical Cord

Ruby Shrestha, MD

○ **Molecules with what characteristics most easily cross the placenta?**

Those with molecular weight less than 5,000 d and with high lipid solubility.

○ **When does the placenta take over as the major source of progesterone?**

After 7 to 9 weeks.

○ **What cells of the placenta produce most of the progesterone?**

The synctiotrophoblast.

○ **What cell is the precursor of placenta?**

Trophoblast.

○ **What serves as the precursor for the placental progesterone?**

Maternal cholesterol precursors.

○ **What enzyme activity is lacking in the placenta, thus limiting direct production of estrogen from cholesterol via the common pathway?**

17-hydroxylase activity.

○ **What hormone, produced by the placental endocrine unit, functions to maintain the corpus luteum in early pregnancy?**

hCG, human chorionic gonadotropin.

○ **What other hormones are produced by placenta?**

Progesterone, estrogen, ACTH, parathyroid hormone-related protein (PTH-rP), growth hormone variant (hGH-V), hypothalamic-like releasing hormones, leptin, neuropeptide Y, inhibin, activin, relaxin.

○ **When does the hCG level peak?**

Between 8 and 10 weeks gestation.

○ **What is hPL and what is its function?**

Human placental lactogen; it promotes lipolysis and directs nutrients to the fetus by an anti-insulin effect.

○ **What is the principal substrate for oxidative metabolism by placental tissue?**

Glucose.

○ **At what gestational age does the amnion and chorion fuse?**

Between 14 and 16 weeks.

○ **What are the five different layers of amnion?**

(1) Innermost uninterrupted single layer of cuboidal epithelial cells.

(2) Basal layer.

(3) A cellular compact layer composed of interstitial collagen.

(4) Outer compact layer of row of fibroblast-like mesenchymal cell.

(5) Outermost layer of acellular zona spongiosa.

○ **What early ultrasound finding is seen at the placenta-membrane junction with twin dichorionic placentas?**

Lambda sign or "twin peak" sign.

○ **What kind of placenta can cause twin-twin transfusion?**

Only monochorionic.

○ **What information about the placenta should be noted on a routine second or third trimester ultrasound?**

Placental location, relationship to the internal cervical os, grade, and any evidence of placental abruption.

○ **Increasing placental maturity is associated with what ultrasound finding?**

Increased echogenicity secondary to increased calcium deposits.

○ **What conditions are associated with abundant placental calcifications prior to 36 weeks?**

IUGR, oligohydramnios, maternal hypertension, diabetes, and smoking.

○ **What is the average weight of the term placenta?**

450 g.

○ **What defines placentomegaly?**

Weight greater than 600 g or thickness greater than 4 to 4.5 cm by ultrasound antenatally.

○ **What conditions are associated with placentomegaly?**

Maternal diabetes, maternal or fetal anemia, chronic infection, hydrops fetalis, and Beckwith-Wiedemann syndrome.

○ **What conditions are associated with small placentas?**

Maternal hypertension, preeclampsia, polyhydramnios, and fetal IUGR.

○ **What percentage of the fetal biventricular cardiac output goes to the placenta?**

40%.

○ **What are the small white lesions that can be scraped away from the fetal surface of the placenta called? What are they formed by?**

Amnion nodosum, formed by desquamated skin cells.

○ **What condition is amnion nodosum associated with?**

Long-standing oligohydramnios.

○ **What is the pathological finding of placental microabscesses pathognomonic for?**

Listeriosis.

○ **What are the fetal macrophages, with scavenger and immunologic functions, found within the chorionic villi called?**

Hofbauer cells.

○ **What is the mesenchyme of the umbilical cord called?**

Wharton's jelly.

○ **Where is the preferred site for ultrasound-guided cordocentesis?**

The umbilical vein at its placental origin.

○ **What length is defined as a short umbilical cord?**

Less than 30 cm.

○ **What complications are associated with a short umbilical cord?**

Avulsion of the cord, abruption, and uterine inversion.

○ **What length is defined as a long umbilical cord?**

More than 70 cm.

○ **What complications are associated with a long umbilical cord?**

Cord prolapse, cord entanglement of the fetus, and true knots in the umbilical cord.

○ **What percentage of true knots are associated with intauterine fetal demise?**

About 10%.

○ **What are the risk factors for cord prolapse?**

Excessive cord length, malpresentation, low birth weight, grand multiparity, multiple gestation, obstetric manipulation like AROM, and polyhydramnios.

○ **What is the fetal heart tracing abnormality seen with cord prolapse?**

Sustained bradycardia or less frequently profound variable deceleration.

○ **What is the management of cord prolapse?**

Patient is placed in trendelenberg or knee-chest position, presenting part is manually elevated, avoid manual palpation of the cord, confirm viability of the fetus, cesarean delivery as soon as possible.

○ **What is the perinatal mortality rate with cord prolapse?**

Approximately 5%.

○ **What is the incidence of nuchal cord?**

25% overall, 21% with one nuchal cord, 4% with two or more nuchal cords.

○ **What is the incidence of true knot in a cord?**

1.0%.

○ **What are some of the possible consequences of a nuchal cord?**

Decreased 1-minute Apgar, no change in 5-minute Apgar, perinatal mortality or abnormal neonatal development.

○ **What is the recommended method of delivery for monoamniotic monochorionic twins?**

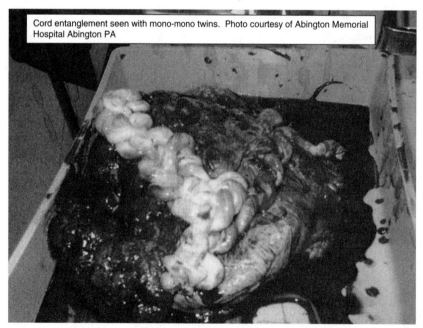

Cord entanglement seen with mono-mono twins. Photo courtesy of Abington Memorial Hospital Abington PA

Cesarean section secondary to high risk of cord entanglement.

○ **What is the normal number of vessels found in the umbilical cord?**

Three; two arteries and one vein.

○ **What proportion of pregnancies have only one umbilical artery?**

1% of singletons and 7% of twins.

○ **How often are additional congenital malformations seen when only one umbilical artery is present?**

25% to 50%.

○ **What time period denotes the third stage of labor?**

From delivery of the infant to delivery of the placenta.

○ **Name three signs of placental separation during the third stage of labor.**

Increased vaginal bleeding.
Lengthening of the umbilical cord.
Changing of the shape of the abdominally palpated uterus to a more globular shape.

○ **What duration of time of the third stage of labor defines a retained placenta?**

≥30 minutes.

○ **What are the complications of retained placenta?**

Infection and postpartum hemorrhage.

○ **What location of the placenta is associated with uterine inversion?**

Fundal implantation of the placenta.

○ **What is the name of the 10 to 30 lobes comprising the basal surface of a normal placenta?**

Maternal cotyledons.

○ **What characteristics of the placenta should be noted once the placenta is delivered?**

Time of delivery, cord insertion, confirmation of three-vessel cord, clinical evidence of infection or meconium-staining, and completeness of the placenta and membranes.

○ **What is an accessory lobe of the placenta called?**

A succenturiate lobe.

○ **What is its clinical significance?**

If left within the uterus after delivery, infection or postpartum hemorrhage may result.

○ **What is the name of a placenta with the umbilical cord insertion at the margin of the placenta?**

Battledore placenta.

○ **What insertion of membranes into the placental disc is characterized by a curved border of folded membranes at the margin, elevating the membranes in a white rim above the placental surface?**

Circumvallate insertion.

○ **Why is it important?**

It results in placental villi around the border of the placenta that are not covered by the chorionic plate, and is associated with hemorrhage and premature rupture of the membranes.

○ **What is the term used to describe a cord that begins its branching to major stem vessels before it inserts into the placenta?**

A furcate insertion.

○ **What are pregnancies with furcate insertions predisposed to?**

Distress during delivery and fetal hemorrhage, if these vessels were to tear during delivery.

○ **What is a velamentous placenta?**

An abnormality complicating approximately 1% of singleton deliveries, in which, the umbilical cord inserts into the membranes.

○ **What is a vasa previa?**

Velamentous insertion of the cord in the lower uterine segment such that the cord vessels course unsupported through the membranes in advance of the fetal presenting part, and often across the cervical os.

○ **What is the incidence of vasa previa?**

Approximately 1 per 3000 deliveries.

○ **What is the perinatal mortality rate associated with vasa previa?**

$\geq 75\%$.

○ **Why is the perinatal mortality rate of vasa previa so high?**

Rupture of the membranes leads to rapid fetal exsanguination.

○ **How is the diagnosis of vasa previa made prior to delivery?**

By color flow Doppler techniques.

○ **Define placenta previa.**

When the placenta covers the internal os of the cervix in the third trimester.

○ **What is the incidence of placenta previa at the time of delivery?**

0.5% (1 in 200).

○ **Name the factors that increase the risk of placenta previa:**

Advancing maternal age
Multiparity
Multiple gestation
African or Asian ethnic background
Smoking
Cocaine use
Prior previa
Prior cesarean section
Prior suction curettage for spontaneous or induced abortion

○ **What is the incidence of placenta previa in nulliparas at the time of delivery?**

1 in 1500.

○ **What is the incidence of placenta previa in grand multiparas at the time of delivery?**

Up to 1 in 20.

○ **How are placenta previa classified?**

Complete: The internal os is entirely covered by placenta.
Partial: The os is partially covered.
Marginal: The placenta edge just reaches the internal os.

○ **What percentage of women with second trimester bleeding have a low-lying placenta diagnosed by ultrasound at that time?**

Up to 45%.

○ **What percentage of placenta previa diagnosed in the second trimester are no longer previa at the time of delivery?**

≥90%.

○ **What is the classic presentation for placenta previa?**

Sudden onset of painless vaginal bleeding in the second or third trimester.

○ **What is the most accurate method for diagnosing placenta previa?**

Transvaginal or translabial ultrasound.

○ **Is placenta previa associated with fetal growth restriction?**

No, recent studies do not show an association.

○ **How has maternal mortality from placenta previa changed since the 1950s?**

From 25% to ≤1%.

○ **How has perinatal mortality from placenta previa changed since the 1950s?**

From 60% to ≤5%.

○ **What is the method of delivery for placenta previa?**

Cesarean section.

○ **What two factors have been responsible for the reduction in maternal and perinatal mortality rates with placenta previa?**

The expectant management approach and the liberal use of cesarean section.

○ **What is the management of bleeding from placenta previa in the third trimester?**

If the mother and the fetus are stable then immediate delivery is not necessary; steroids should be given if between 24 and 34 weeks of gestation. Continuous monitoring of the fetus until bleeding is stable, then daily fetal assessment. Prolonged bedrest and observation. It is not unreasonable to consider hospitalization until delivery.

○ **What are the complications of placenta previa?**

Longer hospital stay, cesarean delivery, abruptio placenta, postpartum hemorrhage, fetal malpresentation, DIC, and maternal death.

○ **Why is magnesium sulfate a better choice of tocolytic than beta-mimetics and calcium channel blockers in patients with placenta previa and preterm labor?**

Beta-mimetics produce tachycardia and hypotension and calcium channel blockers can cause hypotension, making evaluation of maternal blood volume status difficult. Tocolytics should not be administered to actively bleeding patients.

○ **What is the zone of fibrinoid degeneration between the invading trophoblast and the decidua basalis?**

Nitabuch's layer.

○ **Define placenta accreta.**

Trophoblastic invasion beyond the normal boundary established by Nitabuch's layer.

○ **Define placenta increta.**

Placental invasion extends into the myometrium.

○ **Define placenta percreta.**

Placental invasion beyond the uterine serosa, sometimes involving the bladder.

○ **What are the risk factors associated with placenta accreta?**

Placenta previa, prior uterine surgery, advanced maternal age, multiparity, Asherman syndrome, and submucous leiomyomata.

○ **What is the frequency of placenta accreta?**

1 in 2500 deliveries.

○ **What is the risk of placenta accreta in a patient with placenta previa, with no history of prior cesarean section?**

4% to 6%.

○ **What is the risk of placenta accreta in a patient with placenta previa and one prior cesarean section?**

10% to 25%.

○ **What is the risk of placenta accreta in a patient with placenta previa and two or more prior cesarean sections?**

≥50%.

○ **What are the most promising methods of diagnosing placenta accreta prior to delivery?**

Ultrasound (gray-scale, color Doppler, and power Doppler) and MRI.

○ **What gray-scale ultrasound findings have been associated with placenta accreta?**

Placental lacunae (lakes)
Loss of the retroplacental clear zone
Uterine serosa-bladder line interruption.

○ **What is the standard of care treatment for placental accreta?**

Hysterectomy after delivery.

○ **What is the definition of abruptio placentae?**

Premature separation of the normally implanted placenta prior to the birth of the fetus, secondary to bleeding into the decidua basalis.

○ **What is the incidence of placental abruption?**

Approximately 1 in 120 deliveries (but varies with population under study).

○ **What risk factors are associated with placental abruption?**

Maternal hypertension (both chronic and pregnancy-induced)
Advanced maternal parity and age
Smoking
Cocaine use
Trauma
Short umbilical cord
Sudden decompression of the uterus (either by rupture of the membrane in a patient with polyhydramnios or by delivery of the first twin)
Uterine anomalies or myomas
Pregnancies with PPROM managed expectantly

○ **What are the classic signs and symptoms of placental abruption?**

Vaginal bleeding, abdominal pain, uterine contractions, and uterine tenderness.

○ **What is the characteristic uterine contraction pattern associated with placental abruption?**

High frequency and low amplitude with increased baseline tone.

○ **What is a placental abruption without vaginal bleeding called?**

Concealed abruption.

○ **What percentage of placental abruptions are concealed?**

10% to 20%.

○ **How long should a patient be monitored after significant abdominal trauma late in pregnancy?**

4 to 6 hours if fetal heart-rate tracing is reassuring and uterine contractions are absent.

○ **How long should a patient be monitored after significant abdominal trauma late in pregnancy with uterine activity present?**

At least 24 hours of continuous electronic fetal monitoring.

○ **In late pregnancies complicated by maternal cocaine use, what proportion terminate in abruption?**

10%.

○ **What is the recurrence risk of placental abruption?**

5.5% to 16.6% of subsequent pregnancies, 25% of pregnancies if preceded by two consecutive abruptions.

○ **How often is ultrasound demonstration of a retroplacental mass used to confirm abruption?**

Only 20% to 25%.

○ **What laboratory studies are useful in the management of abruption?**

Hemoglobin, hematocrit, platelets, and coagulation studies (PT, PTT, fibrinogen, and FSP).

○ **What is the term used to describe extravasation into and through the myometrium to the serosal surface of the uterus?**

Couvelaire uterus.

○ **Abruptions account for what percentage of perinatal deaths?**

15%.

○ **What proportion of abruptions result in fetal death?**

4 in 1000 abruptions.

○ **What is the most common metastatic tumor to the placenta?**

Malignant melanoma.

○ **What are the most common benign tumors of the placenta?**

Chorioangiomas.

○ **What are placental site trophoblastic tumors?**

Very rare trophoblastic neoplasms characterized by absence of chorionic villi and proliferation of intermediate cytotrophoblast cells; they secrete beta-hCG in amounts small in relation to tumor volume.

○ **Are placental site trophoblastic tumors sensitive to chemotherapy?**

No.

○ **What is the treatment of choice for placental site trophoblastic tumors?**

Hysterectomy, although D & C alone has cured some patients.

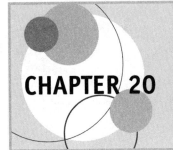

CHAPTER 20 Rh Isoimmunization

Gretchen Glaser, MD and
Frank J. Craparo, MD

○ **What is Rh factor?**

An antibody directed against an erythrocyte surface antigen of the rhesus blood group system.

○ **What is isoimmunization?**

The development of maternal antibodies to the fetal red blood cell antigens.

○ **Rh isoimmunization is a result of...**

Fetal inheritance of the paternal D erythrocyte surface antigen in an Rh-negative mother.

○ **What type of maternal antibody can cross the placenta?**

IgG.

○ **Name three systems of nomenclature for the Rh blood group system.**

Fischer-Race, Weiner, HLA.

○ **What is the Fisher-Race nomenclature with respect to Rh isoimmunization?**

The nomenclature assumes that there are three genetic loci with two major alleles each. The antigens produced by these alleles have a letter—C, c, D, E, and e (no "d" has been identified, but it is used to indicate an absence of an allele product). The most common genotypes are Cde/cde and CDe/Cde. The majority of Rh isoimmunization is caused by D antigen. Thus, Rh positive has come to represent the presence of the D antigen and Rh negative indicates the absence of D antigen on erythrocytes.

○ **This system can assist in predicting...**

Paternal zygosity.

○ **On what chromosome is the genetic locus of the Rh antigen?**

Chromosome 1.

○   **What percent of Rh-positive individuals are heterozygous?**

Approximately 60% of Rh-positive individuals are heterozygous.

○   **What is hemolytic/Rh disease of the newborn?**

Maternal IgG binds to the Rh D antigen on the fetal red blood cells causing hemolysis, which results in the fetus becoming anemic and hydropic.

○   **What must occur for Rh isoimmunization to develop in pregnancy?**

(1) Fetus must have Rh-positive erythrocytes and mother must have Rh-negative erythrocytes.

(2) Fetal erythrocytes must enter maternal circulation.

(3) Mother must be able to produce antibodies against the D antigen.

○   **Why are most first pregnancies unaffected by hemolytic/Rh disease of the newborn?**

The mother's antibody response mounts slowly (over 2–6 months). Exposure during pregnancy is mostly likely to occur after 28 weeks gestation, meaning that a first child will likely be delivered before he or she is affected. In addition, transplacental fetomaternal hemorrhage is most common at delivery.

○   **Does a maternal antibody response occur in all cases of Rh incompatible pregnancies?**

No.

○   **What is the primary factor influencing severity of fetal anemia in Rh disease?**

Antibody concentration.

○   **How do fetal cells enter maternal circulation?**

Fetal-maternal hemorrhage, transplacental passage of fetal red blood cells into the maternal circulation.

○   **What is the most common time for a fetal-maternal hemorrhage to occur?**

At the time of delivery. Approximately 15% to 50%.

○   **What percentage of fetal-maternal hemorrhages at the time of delivery is thought to be sufficient to cause isoimmunization?**

15% to 20%.

○   **An estimated fetal-maternal hemorrhage of greater than 30 mL occurs in what percentage of cases?**

Approximately 1%.

○   **What are some common clinical factors associated with an increased risk of a substantial fetal-maternal hemorrhage?**

Cesarean delivery, multiple gestation, manual removal of the placenta, placenta previa, placental abruption, intrauterine manipulation.

○ **How frequently is a fetal-maternal hemorrhage noted in the first trimester?**

Approximately 7%.

○ **How frequently is a fetal-maternal hemorrhage noted in the second trimester?**

16%.

○ **What percentage of Rh-negative mothers becomes sensitized prior to delivery?**

1% to 2%.

○ **How early does the Rh antigen develop?**

Rh antigens can be detected 38 days postconception.

○ **Can CVS performed in an Rh-negative patient result in sensitization?**

Yes.

○ **What are two mechanisms thought to impact the risk of sensitization?**

Approximately 30% of Rh-negative individuals are thought to be immunologic "nonresponders." ABO incompatibility exerts a protective effect against developing Rh sensitization.

○ **ABO incompatibility is thought to be associated with a decreased risk of sensitization from 10% to ...**

1% to 2%.

○ **What combination of ABO incompatibility is associated with the most protective effect?**

Mother blood type O, fetal blood type A, B, AB.

○ **What is the definition of fetal hydrops?**

Fetal hydrops is defined as having fluid within at least two areas in the fetal-placental unit.

○ **These fluid collections used in the definition of hydrops include ...**

Pericardial effusion, pleural effusion, abdominal ascites, skin edema, increased amniotic fluid, or placentomegaly.

○ **What is thought to be the cause of anemia leading to hydrops in the sensitized pregnancy?**

Severe anemia causes increased production of red blood cells in the fetal liver and spleen, which disrupts the portal venous circulation leading to hepatomegaly, ascites, edema of the placenta, and hyperbilirubinemia.

○ **What process can lead to nervous system damage?**

Hyperbilirubinemia can lead to kernicterus. When levels of total serum bilirubin exceed 25 mg/dL, unconjugated bilirubin can enter brain tissue and cause apoptosis and necrosis. This leads to acute bilirubin encephalopathy, which may result in permanent neurologic damage (kernicterus).

○ **What is the percentage of Rh-negative European white women, American black women, and Asians and Native Americans?**

European white = 15%

American black = 5% to 8%

Asian and Native American = 1% to 2%

○ **What percentage of pregnancies is Rh incompatible?**

10%.

○ **What percentage of pregnancies develop maternal sensitization (not taking into account Rh-immune globulin prophylaxis)?**

≤20%.

○ **There are 0.1% to 0.2% of susceptible Rh D-negative women who still become alloimmunized despite recommendations for immunoprophylaxis. Why is this?**

(1) Failure to administer anti-D immune globulin at 28 to 29 weeks gestation.

(2) Failure to recognize clinical events that place patients at risk for alloimmunization and failure to administer anti-D immune globulin appropriately.

(3) Failure to administer or failure to administer timely anti-D immune globulin postnatally when indicated.

○ **What amount of fetomaternal hemorrhage is necessary to cause isoimmunization?**

The exact amount varies. Isoimmunization has been shown to occur with as little as 0.1 mL of Rh-positive red cells.

○ **How many Rh-negative women will become isoimmunized by their first Rh-incompatible pregnancy if not treated?**

16%.

○ **What is the associated risk of Rh isoimmunization with the following: spontaneous abortion, induced abortion, and amniocentesis?**

Spontaneous 1st trimester abortion = 3% to 4%

Induced abortions = 5%

Amniocentesis in 2nd or 3rd trimester = fetomaternal hemorrhage in 15% to 25%

○ **What laboratory studies should every woman have at the first prenatal visit (with regards to isoimmunization)?**

ABO blood group

Rh type

Antibody screen

○ **Who should be given Rh-immune globulin during pregnancy?**

Mothers who are Rh negative with a father who is Rh positive or has unknown status.

○ **When is Rh-immune globulin given during an otherwise uncomplicated pregnancy?**

At 28 weeks (and postpartum if fetus is Rh positive).

○ **What is the standard dose of Rh-immune globulin used in the United States?**

300 μg.

○ **How does Rh-immune globulin work?**

It absorbs fetal Rh D-positive antigen, which inhibits the formation of antibodies.

○ **How is anti-D immune globulin obtained?**

It is collected by apheresis from Rh D-negative male volunteer donors who are given multiple injections of Rh D-positive red cells and thus have high titers of circulating anti-Rh D antibodies. A search is currently underway for a synthetic anti-D immune globulin and some progress has been made on this front.

○ **Is anti-D immune globulin indicated in a sensitized pregnancy?**

No.

○ **How many mL of fetomaternal hemorrhage does the 300 μg dose cover?**

30 mL of fetal blood or 15 mL of D-positive red cells (only 1% of women have ≥5 mL of fetal blood mixing with maternal blood after delivery).

○ **What test can quantitate the volume of fetal red cells in the maternal circulation?**

Kleihauer-Betke.

○ **Name the qualitative test for fetomaternal hemorrhage.**

Rosette test. If this test is negative, a standard dose of anti-D immune globulin should be given. If this test is positive, further evaluation is recommended using the Kleihauer-Betke test to evaluate the percentage of fetal cells in maternal circulation.

○ **How is the dose of Rh-immune globulin calculated if the volume of hemorrhage is estimated to be greater that 30 mL of whole blood?**

A dose of Rh-immune globulin is given at 10 μg/mL.

○ **When should a larger amount of fetomaternal hemorrhage be suspected (≥15 mL fetal red blood cells)?**

Multiple gestation
Placenta previa with bleeding
Placental abruption
Manual extraction of placenta
Fetal death in the second or third trimester
Blunt abdominal trauma
Clinically significant vaginal bleeding after 20 weeks gestation

○ **Within what time limit should Rh-immune globulin be given after delivery?**

Standard is within 72 hours, however, this is just a by-product of how the original studies were performed because women had to return within 3 days. Rh-immune globulin should be given before a primary immune response occurs, and it can be given up to 14 to 28 days after delivery.

○ **How long does the effect of anti-D immune globulin last?**

The half-life of anti-D immune globulin is 24 days, and a woman can be considered fully protected for 12 and 3/7 weeks after injection. There are scattered case reports of maternal sensitization from decreasing antibody concentrations.

○ **If standard antenatal anti-D immune globulin administration is given within 3 weeks of delivery, can the postnatal dose be withheld in the absence of excessive fetomaternal hemorrhage?**

Yes.

○ **What percentage of women has evidence of fetomaternal hemorrhage after delivery?**

75%.

○ **For which gestational events is Rh-immune globulin indicated?**

Fetomaternal hemorrhage with ectopic pregnancy or abortion, chorionic villus sampling, amniocentesis, external cephalic version, significant antepartum bleeding, molar pregnancy (complete mole controversial), blunt abdominal trauma, fetal death in the second or third trimester, or multifetal reduction.

○ **Is threatened abortion before 12 weeks gestation an indication for anti-D immune globulin prophylaxis?**

Controversial. The Rh D antigen has been reported on fetal erythrocytes as early as 38 days of gestation, but alloimmunization rate is low in threatened abortions before 12 weeks.

○ **What dose of anti-D immune globulin, if indicated, should be given in the first trimester?**

50 μg.

○ **At what anti-D antibody titer is a patient considered to be sensitized?**

1:4.

○ **It has been suggested that severe erythroblastosis or perinatal death does not occur when antibody levels remain below a "critical titer." What is this critical titer level?**

1:16. This number may vary depending on the laboratory studies.

○ **In which situation is measuring maternal anti-D antibody titers not indicated?**

If a previous affected pregnancy included severe fetal anemia (perinatal loss or intrauterine/neonatal transfusion).

○ **If a mother had a hydropic fetus, what is the recurrence risk?**

80%.

○   **What is the initial management for a subsequent pregnancy following an affected fetus/infant?**

First check the paternal genotype. If the father is a heterozygote, perform amniocentesis at 15 weeks gestation to determine fetus's Rh D status. If fetus is Rh D negative, no further follow-up is needed. If fetus is Rh D positive or father is a homozygote, begin serial middle cerebral artery (MCA) Doppler or amniocentesis (if Doppler not available) at 18 weeks.

○   **What noninvasive test is known to be the most accurate way to document fetal anemia in at-risk pregnancies?**

Middle cerebral artery Doppler blood flow studies.

○   **What is the sensitivity and specificity of MCA Doppler?**

Up to 90% sensitive and 98% specific.

○   **What MCA Doppler measurement corresponds with severe fetal anemia?**

An MCA peak systolic velocity (PSV) above 1.5 multiples of the median (MoMs).

○   **How often are MCA Dopplers performed during at-risk or affected pregnancies?**

Weekly.

○   **After what gestational age do MCA Dopplers have a higher false-positive rate?**

34 to 35 weeks.

○   **How is amniotic fluid analysis used to estimate the degree of fetal red cell hemolysis?**

Bilirubin causes a shift in spectrophotometric density of the amniotic fluid and the amount of shift from 450 nm (the ΔOD_{450}) is used to estimate the degree of fetal red cell hemolysis. It is useful to follow the trend of these results.

○   **If fetal hydrops is detected on an ultrasound, how low is the fetal hematocrit?**

Probably less than 15%.

○   **The Liley curve is divided into how many zones?**

Three zones.

○   **What does each zone of the Liley curve indicate?**

Zone I usually indicates mildly affected or unaffected fetus with a low risk for severe anemia.
Zone 2 indicates mild to moderate fetal hemolysis but low risk of severe anemia.
Zone 3 indicates severe anemia with fetal death within 7 to 10 days.
Lower zone expected hemoglobin is 11.0 to 13.9 g/dL; upper zone expected hemoglobin is 8.0 to 10.9 g/dL.

○   **Amniocentesis is performed and demonstrates results in zone 1, when would the next amniocentesis be repeated?**

Approximately 2 weeks.

○   **When describing the Liley curve, in addition to zones, what other information is needed to properly plot an amniocentesis result?**

Gestational age, Liley curve is gestational age specific.

○   **In a preterm fetus with a value in Liley zone 3, management would include what?**

Fetal blood sampling and intrauterine transfusion.

○   **If ΔOD_{450} values are in zone I to the lower half of zone II, when is amniocentesis repeated?**

2 to 4 weeks.

○   **What is the proper management of a fetus with severe Rh sensitization and absent lung maturity at 30 to 32 weeks gestation?**

Controversial, but because of excellent outcomes with current neonatal intensive care, transfusion and maternal steroid administration with delivery at 32 to 34 weeks may be considered.

○   **What is the proper management of mild fetal hemolysis and reassuring fetal testing?**

Delivery at 37 to 38 weeks gestation or ealier, if fetal lung maturity documented.

○   **Do the lungs of an infant with Rh sensitization mature more quickly or more slowly than an infant of the same gestational age?**

More slowly. Hydropic changes in the placenta may increase insulin production leading to delayed lung maturation as seen in diabetics.

○   **What ultrasound findings are suggestive of prehydropic fetal anemia?**

Polyhydramnios
Placental thickness ≥ 4 cm
Pericardial effusion
Dilation of cardiac chambers
Enlargement of spleen and liver
Visualization of both sides of fetal bowel wall
Dilation of the umbilical vein

○   **For a fetus with evidence of hemolysis based on MCA Doppler or amniotic fluid bilirubin analysis, what is the next best test to perform?**

Percutaneous umbilical blood sampling to determine fetal hematocrit.

○   **What routine tests, besides assessment of amniotic fluid bilirubin or umbilical cord hematocrit, are undertaken in cases of Rh isoimmunization?**

After 26 to 28 weeks, NST biweekly and ultrasound every 1 to 2 weeks.

○   **What are the two types of transfusions?**

Intrauterine intraperitoneal (needle into peritoneal cavity of fetus)
Intrauterine intravascular (needle into umbilical vein)

○ **What are the advantages of intraperitoneal and intravascular transfusions?**

Intraperitoneal—ease of placement, decreased dislodgement

Intravascular—ability to obtain fetal hematocrit prior to transfusion and after, direct placement of red cells intravascularly

○ **What are the complications of transfusions? Which is the most common?**

Fetal bradycardia, infection, premature rupture of membranes, fetal death (4% to 9%), emergent delivery because of nonreasurring fetal status.

Fetal bradycardia is the most common.

○ **What is the purpose of intrauterine transfusion?**

To correct fetal anemia, which improves oxygenation and hepatic function as a result of fall in portal venous pressure from reduction of extramedullary hematopoiesis.

○ **What type of blood is used for the transfusion?**

O-negative, leukocyte poor, packed erythrocytes cross-matched with the mother.

○ **At what hematocrit level is transfusion considered in the fetus remote from term?**

$\leq 25\%$.

○ **What mode of delivery is recommended for fetus remote from term with evidence of hemolytic disease?**

Cesarean section.

○ **Which antibodies to minor antigens have also been shown to result in fetal anemia and hydrops (the most common ones)?**

Anti-E, anti-Kell, anti-c, anti c + E, anti-Fy (Duffy).

○ **Which minor antigen is the most common?**

Anti-Kell (10% of people are Kell positive).

○ **If a patient presents with anti-Kell antibodies, what two pieces of information should be obtained?**

(1) Paternal Kell status

(2) Question the patient, if she has ever had a transfusion (Kell status is not checked for in transfused blood).

○ **What is the management of patients with antibodies to minor antigens?**

Similar to Rh-isoimmunization, measurement of maternal antibody titers, serial amniocenteses after a critical titer is reached, and transfusion or delivery based on ΔOD_{450} levels and gestational age.

○ **What are the red blood cell surface antigens called that a fetus can inherit from the father?**

Private antigens (mother may become sensitized at first pregnancy and future pregnancies may develop isoimmunization).

○ **What percentage of pregnancies are ABO incompatible?**

20% to 25%.

○ **What blood types (maternal and fetal) cause most cases of ABO incompatibility?**

O mother; A or B infant (mother has anti-A and anti-B IgG).

○ **Does ABO incompatibility require previous sensitization to affect the fetus?**

No, ABO hemolytic disease may affect the first-born child (unlike Rh).

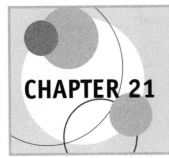

CHAPTER 21

Genetics for the Obstetrician

Rosanne B. Keep, MS, CGC and Darnelle L. Dorsainville, MS, CGC

○ **Meiosis begins with 46 chromosomes, each consisting of two chromatids. At the end of meiosis I how many chromosomes and how many chromatids are present? At the end of meiosis II how many chromosomes and how many chromatids are present?**

Meiosis I—23 chromosomes, 46 chromatids.

Meiosis II—23 chromosomes, 23 chromatids.

○ **What is crossing over and when specifically does it occur?**

The exchange of genetic material between homologous chromosomes, a mechanism for increasing genetic variation. Occurs during meiosis I (during pachytene of prophase I).

○ **When does female meiosis begin?**

At approximately 4 months gestation.

○ **When is meiosis I completed?**

At ovulation.

○ **When is meiosis II completed?**

At fertilization.

○ **What is the most common trisomy in liveborn infants?**

Trisomy 21 (Down syndrome).

○ **Monosomy for an entire chromosome is typically incompatible with life. What condition is an exception to this?**

45, X (Turner syndrome).

○   **What is the only etiologic factor conclusively linked to an increased risk for trisomy?**

Advanced maternal age.

○   **Chromosome analysis on your patient's husband revealed the following: 45,XY, der(14;21)(q10;q10) What would you discuss with this couple?**

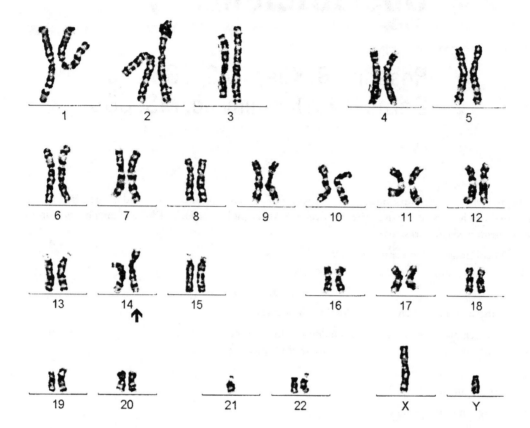

He is a carrier of a balanced 14:21 translocation. There is an increased risk for offspring with Down syndrome, recurrent pregnancy loss, decreased fertility, or UPD (uniparental disomy). Carriers of this translocation do not typically have developmental or phenotypic abnormalities.

○   **Your patient reports that her brother has a son with Trisomy 21 and she is concerned about her risk to have a child with Down syndrome. What would you discuss with her?**

Her risk for Down syndrome would be equal to her age-related risk. Trisomy 21 is typically a sporadic occurrence (and is not inherited in families).

○   **What meiotic process is the major cause of aneuploidy?**

Nondisjunction.

○   **What percentage of fetuses with 45,X (Turner syndrome) spontaneously aborts?**

More than 99%.

○ **Certain genetic disorders occur when both chromosomes of a pair are inherited from the same parent. What is the process called?**

Uniparental disomy.

○ **What percentage of couples who have had two or more SABs will be found to have a chromosome abnormality?**

6% of these couples (or 3% of the individuals).

○ **What are the risks associated with advanced paternal age?**

Men who are 40 to 45 years of age or older are at increased risk for new mutations, associated with autosomal dominant conditions (e.g., neurofibromatosis I, achondroplasia, Marfan syndrome, osteogenesis imperfecta).

○ **At a preconception visit your patient and her husband disclose that they are first cousins. What would their offspring be at risk for?**

Birth defects, autosomal recessive conditions, and conditions that are more common in their ethnic background.

○ **What genetic test should be considered in women with unexplained ovarian failure or elevated FSH prior to 40 years of age?**

Fragile X carrier screening.

○ **A new patient reports that she suffers from depression and had a heart problem as a child. She seems to have difficulty following your conversation. Her mother, who accompanies her to the visit, has a scar over her upper lip. What genetic testing would your order on this patient?**

FISH for 22q11.2 deletion.

○ **A patient of yours reports that her father has Marfan syndrome. What is her risk to have inherited the condition? What features would you look for in your patient and what consults would you recommend?**

50% risk.

Tall, thin body habitus, long, curved fingers (arachnodactyly), pectus, striae.

Patient needs cardiology evaluation with echocardiogram, ophthalmology examination, and genetics evaluation.

○ **A patient reports that her brother died of Canavan disease. What is her risk to be a carrier?**

2/3.

○ **Chromosomes on the products of conception of your 38-year-old patient reveal a karyotype of 47,XX,+18. What is the likely etiology of this result, and what is her recurrence risk?**

The risk of trisomy increases with maternal age and most trisomic conceptions spontaneously miscarry. Her recurrence risk would be equal to her age-related risk at her next pregnancy.

○ **A patient states that she was recently diagnosed with neurofibromatosis I (NF1), following a diagnosis of NF1 in her daughter. She tells you that her daughter has numerous café-au-lait marks, several neurofibromas, and learning difficulties. The patient herself appears clinically normal except for several café-au-lait marks. What genetic concept can explain this?**

Variable expressivity.

○ **What are the potential risks associated with SSRI use during pregnancy?**

Possible increased risk for congenital cardiac anomalies with 1st trimester exposure to Paxil. Exposure to SSRIs in late pregnancy can result in transient neonatal complications including persistent pulmonary hypertension.

○ **A patient reports that she and her partner are of Ashkenazi Jewish ancestry. Which screening tests would you offer and what inheritance pattern would you discuss with them?**

ACOG recommends screening for Tay-Sachs disease, Canavan disease, Familial dysautonomia, and CF. Additionally this couple is at increased risk for Gaucher disease, Niemann-Pick disease, Fanconi anemia, Bloom syndrome, Mucolipidosis IV, Glycogen storage disease 1A, and Maple syrup urine disease. These conditions all have an autosomal recessive inheritance pattern.

○ **Besides the Ashkenazi Jewish population, what other ethnic backgrounds are at increased risk for Tay-Sachs disease?**

French Canadian (1:30), Louisiana Cajun (1:30), and Celtic/Irish (1:50).

○ **Your patient is of Irish and German descent. What is her risk to be a carrier of CF? If she screens negative on the standard CF panel (23 mutations) what is her residual risk to be a CF carrier?**

1:25; 1:240.

○ **For which ethnic group is the detection rate for CF screening the lowest?**

Asian.

○ **An African American couple reports that they have a daughter with CF. Your patient's prenatal CF carrier screen is negative. What explanation can you give this couple?**

The standard CF panel looks for 23 mutations and has a 69% detection rate in the African American population (as compared to a 90% detection rate in the Caucasian population). There are more than 1000 mutations in the CFTR gene; thus, the patient may carry a mutation not screened for in the standard panel.

○ **A patient of yours has sickle cell trait and her partner's hemoglobinopathy evaluation revealed probable β-thalassemia trait. What are the risks to their offspring?**

25% carrier of Hb S; 25% carrier of β-thalassemia; 25% noncarrier/unaffected; 25% affected with sickle β-thalassemia.

○ **A patient's α-thalassemia DNA report shows she is a cis carrier of α-thalassemia; her husband is found on to have one α-thalassemia mutation. What condition is their offspring at risk for?**

Hemoglobin H disease (–/α-).

○ **A pregnant patient with achondroplasia is under your care. Her husband is of typical stature. What is the inheritance pattern of this condition? What is the chance for this couple to have a child with achondroplasia?**

Autosomal dominant; 50%.

○ **Your patient is a Fragile X premutation carrier. What is her risk to have an affected son?**

50%.

○ **Your patient is a Fragile X premutation carrier and is pregnant with a female fetus. What are the clinical possibilities for this patient's daughter?**

She could be a premutation carrier (like her mother), the repeat size could expand to a full mutation (she could have some clinical symptoms of Fragile X), or she could be "normal" if she receives the typical X from her mother.

○ **What analytes are utilized in first trimester screening?**

PAPP-A and Beta HCG.

○ **At what gestational age would you offer first trimester screening?**

Between 10 and 14 weeks (each center may have a slightly different range).

○ **What conditions are screened for by the first trimester screen?**

Down syndrome and Trisomy 18.

○ **If a patient has an increased nuchal lucency in the 1st trimester and a normal fetal karyotype on CVS, what 2nd trimester screening tests would you offer?**

Anatomy scan/level 2 ultrasound, fetal echocardiogram (because of increased likelihood of congenital cardiac anomaly), and MSAFP (as routine screen for ONTD).

○ **What conditions are screened for by the quadruple screen?**

Down syndrome, Trisomy 18, and ONTD.

○ **What analytes are utilized for the quadruple screen?**

AFP, Unconjugated estriol, Dimeric inhibin A, and hCG.

○ **What are the potential causes of an elevated AFP level on a quad screen?**

Multiple gestations, IUFD, ventral wall defect, ONTD, incorrect dating of pregnancy, oligohydramnios, renal agenesis, congenital nephrosis.

○ **What factors affect the interpretation of the quadruple screen?**

Maternal age, race, weight, maternal IDDM, gestational age, multiple gestations, previous pregnancy with ONTD.

○ **What factors affect the interpretation of a first trimester screen?**

Maternal age, race, weight, multiple gestation, maternal IDDM, previous pregnancy with Down syndrome.

○ **Your patient's CVS results show: 47, XY +21[3]/46, XY[17]. What does this mean for the patient's pregnancy?**

Possibilities with this result include true fetal mosaicism for Down syndrome, confined placental mosaicism (CPM)/normal fetus, fetus with full Trisomy 21. Amniocentesis should be offered to distinguish between these possibilities.

○   **An amniocentesis result reveals 46 total chromosomes with an inversion of chromosome 22. What follow-up testing on the parents should be recommended?**

Parental karyotype to determine if the results are de novo or inherited. If one of the parents has the same inversion and is clinically normal, there is a high probability that the fetus will be unaffected (like the parent).

○   **Chromosome analysis on your patient shows the following. [Fig. 21-2] What would be this patient's clinical picture?**

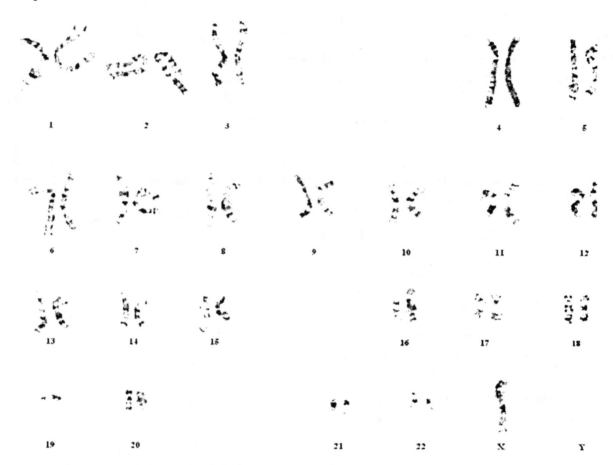

Features of Turner syndrome can include short stature, webbed neck, renal anomalies (e.g., horseshoe kidney), cardiac anomalies (e.g., coarctation of aorta), amenorrhea, difficulty with visual-perceptual skills (overall intelligence is average or above).

○   **On ultrasound, a fetus has bilateral post-axial polydactyly with no additional findings. Neither parent reports a personal history of polydactyly, but the husband says that his father was born with an extra finger on each hand. What inheritance pattern is exhibited by this family history?**

Autosomal dominant inheritance with incomplete penetrance.

○   **What are the usual indications for prenatal diagnosis (e.g., CVS, amniocentesis)?**

Advanced maternal age, abnormal maternal serum screen, ultrasound finding, parental or family history of genetic condition or chromosome abnormality.

○ **What are the common chromosome abnormalities in humans?**

There are aneuploidies, polyploidies, and structural alterations. *Aneuploidy* refers to numeric abnormalities. These can result from (i) nondisjunction: one pair of chromosomes fails to separate at anaphase resulting in one daughter cell having both parts of the pair and the other having none; (ii) anaphase lag: one chromosome of a pair moves slower during anaphase so its material is lost; (iii) polyploidy: the total number of chromosomes is duplicated more than once, e.g., 69 chromosomes. *Structural alterations* include (i) deletion: losing a portion of a chromosome; (ii) duplication: there is an extra portion of a chromosome; (iii) insertion: a portion of a chromosome is attached to another; (iv) inversion: the order of placement of a genetic material is inverted in the chromosome; (v) translocation: portions of genetic material are removed from one chromosome and inserted onto another.

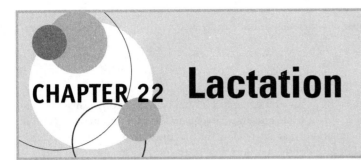

CHAPTER 22 Lactation

Gretchen E. Glaser, MD

○ **When do prolactin levels peak in pregnancy and postpartum?**

Peak levels of 200– to 400 ng/mL are common in the late third trimester. Levels slowly decline after delivery, and by 6 months postpartum, levels are 50 ng/mL.

○ **Why does lactogenesis, or actual lactation, not occur during pregnancy even though the prolactin levels are elevated?**

The receptor sites in the breast are competitively bound by estrogen and progesterone, preventing prolactin from activating lactation. When the placenta is delivered, these levels of estrogen and progesterone rapidly drop and the prolactin floods the receptors.

○ **In the fully lactating mother, at what month postpartum do the baseline prolactin levels return to normal?**

Prolactin levels remain elevated as long as the mother is lactating, even if she breastfeeds for years. The normal prolactin level in a nonpregnant, nonlactating woman is <25 ng/mL.

○ **Suckling produces a pulsatile release of what substance and where does it originate?**

Oxytocin, from the posterior pituitary.

○ **Oxytocin has a direct effect on what cells in the breast?**

Myoepithelial cells, which surround the alveolar cells. When the myoepithelial cells contract, milk is forced into the ductal system.

○ **The let-down reflex is dependent on what hormone?**

Oxytocin.

○ **What is the most common cause of lactation failure?**

Inadequate stimulation is the usual cause of insufficient milk production to adequately nourish and satisfy an infant. This may be secondary to poor technique with inadequate contact with the breast or simply to not nursing frequently enough. The average newborn will nurse 8 to 10 times in 24 hours. True lactation failure not related to poor stimulation is very rare, and may be because of either anatomical defects such as hypoplasia (which may be unilateral) or to absence of prolactin.

○   **What is the definition of tandem nursing?**

The nursing of two children of differing ages during the same time frame. This can be siblings (i.e., a newborn and an older child) or could be adoptive nursing of an infant while nursing a biologic toddler. Of importance is that if both children are biologic, the newborn must be nursed first at any feeding time, as the milk produced will revert to colostrum just after delivery. Colostrum should be given to the newborn first to assure adequate nutrition and hydration. It is presumed that the older child receives most of its nutrition elsewhere and does not rely on the breast.

○   **What are the three major factors used to assess risk of maternal consumption of a drug to the breastfed infant?**

(1) Dose consumed, (2) oral bioavailability of the drug in both mother and infant, and (3) elimination route and timing in both mother and infant.

○   **What is the most common cause of sore nipples in the immediate postpartum period?**

Improper positioning of the infant at the breast, resulting in abnormal friction or traction on the breast and nipple.

○   **What is the most common cause of delayed nipple soreness?**

Yeast. Aggressive, simultaneous treatment of mother and baby is indicated, usually with an antifungal such as nystatin. During treatment, all objects such as pacifiers and toys that enter the baby's mouth must be washed between each use to avoid recontamination.

○   **What is the term used to describe the presence of milky secretions from the breast of a newborn infant?**

Witch's milk. Can be found in both sexes and results from the effect of maternal hormones on the fetal tissue. It generally disappears rapidly postpartum and no treatment is needed.

○   **What is the proper postpartum management of a mother who chooses not to breastfeed?**

A firmly fitting (but not binding) bra, ice packs prn, and decreased stimulation to the nipples such as loose clothes rubbing across the breast or direct contact from a shower. Pharmacologic suppression is frequently ineffective, because it is improperly prescribed and/or used. Bromocriptine is no longer indicated because of severe maternal side effects and should not be prescribed. The introduction of 35 μg or higher oral contraceptives within 2 weeks of delivery may inhibit lactation in some women and may be of use to decrease production of milk.

○   **When does complete involution of the breast occur?**

At menopause. Partial involution occurs at each weaning, but complete involution does not occur until withdrawal of all hormone stimulation. Women who receive postmenopausal hormone replacement will retard this process.

○   **Can an adoptive mother nurse her infant?**

Yes. If the mother has had a prior term pregnancy and lactated with that delivery, her success rate is highest. The breast of a woman who has never been pregnant can be primed with oral estrogen, and then given TRH to stimulate prolactin. If there is then mechanical stimulation and/or suckling, the breast will produce milk. The quantity in the latter circumstance may not be sufficient for total nutrition. The infant should be supplemented with formula.

○ **What is the area of the breast that stores milk in preparation for the infant to extract? Where is this located? What is the clinical significance?**

The lactiferous sinuses are located just behind the areola. The lactiferous ducts, which drain from the alveolar sacs, empty into the sinuses. If the infant is not positioned such that his/her mouth is over the areola, the infant will suck only on the nipple and have to frequently regrasp the breast to suckle. This results in sore nipples and fissures, leading to possible mastitis.

○ **What term describes the maintenance of lactation over time after the initial episode of lactogenesis?**

Galactopoiesis. It is dependent on continued stimulation to the breast and on the presence of at least baseline levels of prolactin.

○ **A 2- week-old infant cries and wants to nurse every 1 to 2 hours around the clock. When at the breast he nurses for approximately 5 minutes and falls asleep so the mother puts him down. She is now exhausted and thinking of bottlefeeding. What can you do to save this breastfeeding experience? What is wrong?**

This mother needs information, guidance, and reassurance. Her infant is not nursing long enough with each episode. The infant is only receiving the "foremilk," which is high in proteins, carbohydrates, and water. He falls asleep before getting the "hindmilk," which is high in fat and satiates the appetite and takes longer to digest. This infant should be stimulated when he dozes off, changed to the opposite breast, and not put down immediately. If this fails, the mother can pump or express the hindmilk at that time and it can be given by another caregiver later so the mother can rest. This process is only a temporary measure as decreased contact time at the breast will ultimately lead to decreased milk production.

○ **What is the caloric content of mature milk?**

Approximately 70 kcal/100 mL in a well nourished mother. Colostrum has a lower caloric content (55 kcal) because of the absence of fats.

○ **What is the primary carbohydrate in human milk?**

Lactose. Cow's milk is primarily sucrose. The lactose in humans is broken down into lactic acid, decreasing stool pH, and giving the breastfed infant the characteristic loose stool. This should not be confused with diarrhea. Using a cloth diaper or smooth towel, the stool can be checked. If there is no ring of water around the stool, this is not diarrhea and should be considered normal.

○ **A mother needs to be anticoagulated postpartum. What is your drug of choice?**

Coumadin is the easiest for the mother and safe for the infant. Even though small quantities reach the infant, therapeutic levels are not reached. Heparin does not get excreted into the milk but is more complicated for mother to receive.

○ **What are the two major medical illnesses in which breastfeeding is truly contraindicated?**

HIV infection and active untreated TB.

○ **What are the recommendations of the American Academy of Pediatrics (AAP) and ACOG regarding the use of oral contraceptives while breastfeeding?**

ACOG suggests a progestin only contraceptive such as the Mini-Pill or Depo-Provera, while the AAP supports use of any low dose (<50 μg estrogen) pill. Falling progesterone levels trigger lactogenesis, so ACOG recommends delaying progestin only pills until 2 to 3 weeks postpartum and Depo-Provera until 6 weeks postpartum. Combined oral contraceptives should be delayed until 6 weeks postpartum, and then only used if lactation is well established and infant growth can be closely monitored.

○   **What is LAM?**

Lactational amenorrhea method. This method of family planning is advocated by the Population Council and other international groups, especially in areas where other methods of contraception are lacking. The method requires the presence of three criteria to reach 98% effectiveness: (1) No menses, (2) fully or nearly fully breastfeeding (i.e., no solids or formula), and (3) infant less than 6 months of age. At 3 months, nearly 87% are anovulatory but this drops to 57% by 6 months. If menses have not returned, it is felt that on the first ovulatory cycle, the luteal phase is usually poor and would not sustain implantation, making it safe to wait for menses to return before using other contraception.

○   **A 26-year-old patient is being treated during pregnancy for a microadenoma of the pituitary. She has had no tumor enlargement and no symptoms. She would like to breastfeed. How do you advise her?**

There is no contraindication, but in some situations, she may have a low milk supply. This is most common after surgery or prior radiation.

○   **Your patient has just delivered. She has received magnesium sulfate for preeclampsia, which will continue for 24 hours, had a general anesthetic for cesarean section, and is on ampicillin and gentamicin for an intrapartum fever. She is now fully alert and wants to breastfeed her infant, but her pediatrician has recommended that she bottlefeed. What can you do to resolve this problem?**

First try to explain to the pediatrician that there is no oral bioavailability to these drugs (except ampicillin). Little colostrum is available to the infant for 24 hours, but stimulation is vital to establishing lactation. If you are unable to convince pediatrician, use an electric breast pump to stimulate the breast until the baby can be nursed.

○   **How long can breast milk be stored in the refrigerator?**

Approximately 48 hours, after which it should be frozen. Breast milk can be stored for up to 3 months in a daily-use freezer and for up to 6 months in a deep freeze or chest freezer. Freezing will decrease the immunologic value, but not the nutritional component. Thaw under warm or hot running water or in a pan. Do not microwave.

○   **A mother calls you to say her pumped breast milk is "spoiling" in the refrigerator. What is wrong?**

The milk has separated! In our modern society, most people have only seen commercial homogenized milk. The separated milk (fat and water) can be reconstituted with gentle shaking.

○   **Of an average 25-lb weight gain in pregnancy, what portion is considered to be lactation stores? What happens to this weight, if the patient does not breastfeed?**

Approximately 8 to 9 lb, or 3 to 4 kg. If she bottlefeeds, she will have to diet it off—a great piece of propaganda to encourage someone to breastfeed!

○   **How much milk should a breastfeeding woman drink?**

There is no minimum amount needed but she should have calcium supplements if she is not getting dairy products. A woman who drinks large quantities (>1 quart/day) of cow's milk runs the risk of sensitizing her infant to cow's milk protein, which can cross into her milk.

○ **What is the proper management of a patient with postpartum mastitis?**

Antibiotics (dicloxacillin is the drug of choice), hydration, rest, and analgesics. It is also essential that the breast continue to be emptied regularly. If unable to nurse because of discomfort, she should pump or manually express milk. Warm compresses will aid the letdown and soothe the breast.

○ **What are Hoffman's exercises?**

Inverted nipples can be everted if found early in the third trimester, in most cases. One technique is Hoffman's exercises where the fingers are placed at 3- and 9-o'clock positions at the base of the nipple and is gently stretched, then this is repeated at 6- and 12-o'clock positions. The use of a perforated breast shell under the bra will also put pressure at the base of the nipple and help evert it.

○ **Can a breastfeeding mother receive postpartum rubella vaccination?**

Yes.

○ **What are the most common misconceptions about breastfeeding that lead a woman to bottlefeed? What arguments can you give to contradict these misconceptions?**

(1) I want to go back to work—upon returning to work, you can pump and save, or gradually wean down to only have milk during the hours you are home. Or you can nurse until you return to work and then wean. Even 2 to 3 weeks is valuable as it delivers colostrum and all its benefits.

(2) I'm too embarrassed—discuss discrete techniques, availability of clothing just for nursing, and refer patient to supportive group.

(3) My husband doesn't want me to—common reasons are that he wants to feed the baby and that he fears sexual activity during lactation. Reassure him that an occasional bottle of pumped milk or even formula is fine after the first 2 to 3 weeks. Also let him know that sexual contact with the breast during lactation is not harmful. Letdown may occur, even during orgasm.

○ **Your patient is an insulin-dependent diabetic. Can she breastfeed?**

Yes. Insulin does not cross. She must watch her diet carefully but can have a very successful experience.

○ **Should a baby with a cleft lip and/or palate be breastfed?**

It can actually be easier. The large surface area of the breast can help occlude the defect. In very large defects, special devices may be needed.

○ **At 4 months postpartum, your patient has an emergency appendectomy and is separated from her infant for 1 week. Her milk supply is gone on return to home. Three weeks later, she calls and says her infant is having an allergy to formulas and can she get her milk supply to return? How do you answer?**

You can have her use an electric pump until her supply returns. She can slowly reintroduce the baby to the breast in the meantime. The support of a lactation consultant during this process would be very helpful.

○ **What is proper treatment for cracked nipples?**

Evaluate the positioning of the baby during nursing and check for pressure points. Vary the positions at each feeding (Madonna—across the chest, football—under the arm, and on the side). Erythromycin ointment may aid healing. Avoid over the counter creams, especially those with lanolin.

○ **When is the most common time for a breastfeeding mother to quit?**

In the first 2 to 3 weeks. This is the time of greatest adjustment. It also coincides with the first growth spurt at approximately 2 weeks, during which the baby may get fussy and nurse often to increase the supply. If she goes beyond 3 weeks, she will generally nurse for 4 to 6 months on the average.

○ **Your patient planned to breastfeed but delivers at 28 weeks. How do you counsel her?**

Encourage her to use an electric pump and take the milk to the NICU. This milk is rich in immunologic value. It is a way for the mother to be actively involved in her infant's care. Most insurance companies will reimburse for the rental (approximately $2/day). She should pump every 3 hours during the day and once at night to maintain a good supply.

○ **For how long does the AAP recommend breastfeeding?**

Exclusive breastfeeding is recommended for the first 6 months after birth. The American Academy of Pediatrics and the World Health Organization recommend continued breastfeeding until at least 1 or 2 years of age and for as long as mutually desired after 2 years of age.

○ **What are some of the most important benefits of breastfeeding?**

Superior nutrition.

Prevention of infection.

Increased intelligence as adults.

Increased uterine contractions and decreased blood loss postpartum.

○ **What are some contraindications for breastfeeding?**

Maternal HIV infection.

Maternal human T-cell lymphotropic virus type 1 infection.

Maternal drug abuse.

Galactosemia in the newborn.

○ **What are some drugs that should not be taken while breastfeeding?**

Antineoplastic or antimetabolic agents (cyclophosphamide, mercaptopurine).

Some anticonvulsants (felbamate, topiramate).

Ergot alkaloids.

Amiodarone.

Radiopharmaceuticals.

○ **What antihypertensives are considered most compatible with breastfeeding?**

Beta blockers such as propranolol, metoprolol, labetalol.

Calcium channel blockers such as diltiazem, nifedipine, verapamil.

○ **Which antihypertensives should be avoided during breastfeeding?**

Acebutolol and atenolol have been reported in cases of infant bradycardia and hypotension. ACE inhibitors should be used cautiously in the first few weeks of life, because neonatal kidneys are very sensitive to these agents.

○ **What is the preferred medication for treatment of postpartum depression while breastfeeding?**

Sertraline (Zoloft).

○ **How long after a woman consumes alcohol is her breast milk free of the substance?**

A single drink (12 oz of beer, 5 oz wine, or 1 oz hard liquor) will clear from maternal circulation in 2 to 3 hours. Alcohol moves freely from maternal milk to plasma, so it is not necessary to express and/or discard milk after this time period in order to avoid infant exposure. Mothers can be advised to refrain from nursing until 2 to 3 hours after alcohol consumption is completed.

○ **Why is galactosemia an absolute contraindication to breastfeeding?**

Galactosemia is an inborn error of metabolism. Infants with this disorder are unable to utilize galactose, a component of the lactose sugar in human milk. Accumulation of galactose may lead to failure to thrive, liver dysfunction, cataracts, and mental retardation.

○ **Are the iron levels in breast milk affected in women who are anemic?**

No, they produce milk with normal iron levels.

○ **What are some factors that may interfere with successful breastfeeding?**

Hypoplastic breast tissue.
Nipple abnormalities.
Previous breast surgery.

○ **How may hypoplastic breast tissue affect lactation?**

Women without sufficient glandular tissue may have no breast enlargement during pregnancy and will produce little or no milk. As a result, their infants are at risk for early failure to thrive.

○ **How does breast augmentation or reduction affect a woman's ability to breastfeed?**

Outcome cannot be predicted in individual cases, but circular incisions around the areola tend to cause the most damage to ducts, blood supply, and nerves and thus the most potential for difficulty with breastfeeding.

○ **What are some factors that promote success and longer breastfeeding duration?**

Nursing immediately following delivery.
Rooming-in.
Skin-to-skin contact.
Frequent demand feedings in the early postpartum period.

○ **What is the average weight gain on infants that are breastfed?**

Once breastfeeding is established, infants gain 15 to 40 g per day.

○ **What is breast engorgement?**

Engorgement refers to swelling of the breast and can occur early or late in the postpartum period. Early engorgement is secondary to edema, tissue swelling, and accumulated milk, while late engorgement is due solely to accumulated milk.

○ **What are some effective treatments for engorgement?**

(1) Frequent breastfeeding with complete breast emptying at each feeding.

(2) Alternating treatment with cold compresses to decrease swelling and warm showers to promote milk release.

(3) Acetaminophen or ibuprofen for pain control.

(4) Avoiding pumping for longer than 10 minutes, as this can increase milk supply.

○ **How are plugged ducts distinguished from mastitis?**

Plugged ducts are localized areas of milk stasis with distention of mammary tissue. Symptoms include a palpable lump with tenderness. They are distinguished from mastitis by the absence of signs of systemic infection such as fever, erythema, or myalgia. Their etiology is unknown.

○ **What is mastitis and what causes it?**

Mastitis is an infection of the breast. It typically presents as a hard, red, tender, swollen area of the breast associated with fever, myalgia, chills, malaise, and flu-like symptoms. Common etiologic agents include *Staphylococcus aureus*, *Streptococcus*, and *Escherichia coli*.

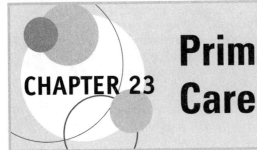

Primary and Preventative Care

CHAPTER 23

Julie Braga, MD and Rachael Cohen, DO

○ **At what age does the American College of Obstetricians and Gynecologists recommend a first visit to an OB/GYN take place?**

Age 13 to 15.

○ **What are the three leading causes of morbidity among teens?**

(1) Acne. (2) Asthma. (3) *Chlamydia* (approximately 5% to 14% of women aged 15 to 20 who are screened for *Chlamydia trachomatis* have positive test results.)

○ **What are the three leading causes of mortality among teens?**

(1) Motor vehicle accidents. (2) Homicide. (3) Suicide.

○ **What are four important periodic vaccinations for teens?**

(1) Tetanus–diphtheria–pertussis (once between 11and16 years of age).

(2) Hepatitis B (if not previously vaccinated).

(3) Human papillomavirus.

(4) Meningococcal.

○ **What four types of HPV does the vaccination protect against?**

HPV 6, 11, 16, 18.

○ **What percentage of American women are overweight or obese?**

Recent estimates indicate that more than 50% of all women aged 20 to 74 are either overweight or obese.

○ **What recommendations should you be making to your patients regarding dietary changes?**

A low-fat, high-fiber diet should be recommended since it has been shown to decrease the risk of coronary artery disease, type 2 diabetes mellitus, and several forms of cancer. It may be helpful to refer a patient to a dietician or nutritionist to help the patient to establish a healthy eating plan, especially if the patient has risk factors for CAD such as a sedentary lifestyle, obesity, or cigarette smoking.

○   **How is anorexia nervosa defined and how prevalent is it?**

Anorexia nervosa is characterized by intentional and continued weight loss in a previously healthy person who perceives herself as overweight but is extremely thin. It is estimated that 0.5% to 1% of women suffer from this disorder; however, this is probably an underestimate because these women usually do not report it to their physicians.

○   **How should you screen for eating disorders?**

First calculate a BMI in every patient.

Then inquire. Some of the following questions may be helpful:

Are you satisfied with your eating patterns?

Do you ever eat in secret?

Does your weight affect the way you feel about yourself?

Have any of your family members had an eating disorder?

Do you have or have ever had an eating disorder?

○   **What is the lifetime risk of developing breast cancer?**

One in eight.

○   **What is the ACOG recommended screening schedule for breast cancer?**

A screening mammogram should be performed every 1 to 2 years from age 40 to 49, and yearly beginning at age 50. Also, all women should have yearly clinical breast examinations. (A study by the National Breast and Cervical Cancer Early Detection Program found that clinical breast examination detected 7.4 cancers per 1,000 women with normal screening mammograms.)

○   **What screening schedule should be offered to patients who are BRCA gene mutation carriers?**

There are no widely accepted guidelines. However, the Cancer Genetics Studies Consortium has offered the recommendations of annual mammography beginning at age 25 to 35 as well as monthly self-breast examinations and yearly clinical breast examinations.

○   **What are appropriate options that you may offer a patient for colorectal cancer screening?**

Any of the following are acceptable:

(1) Yearly patient-collected fecal occult blood test of fecal immunochemical testing.

(2) Flexible sigmoidoscopy every 5 years.

(3) Options 1 and 2 together.

(4) Double-contrast barium enema every 5 years.

(5) Colonoscopy every 10 years.

○   **When should you initiate cholesterol screening in women?**

Beginning at age 45, a lipid profile should be obtained and every 5 years after. Earlier testing is warranted if the patient has a history of heart disease, diabetes, or a family history of coronary artery disease or hypercholesterolemia.

○   **Which test in the lipid profile is continuously correlated with the relative risk of developing coronary artery disease?**

LDL cholesterol.

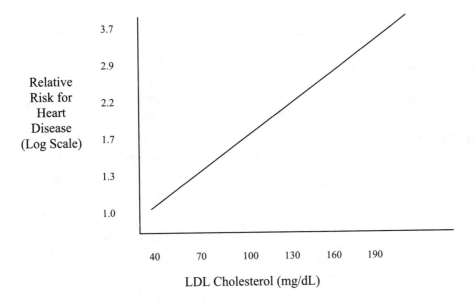

○   **What are the main side effects of the cholesterol lowering agents?**

Statins (HMG-CoA reductase inhibitors) → Myopathy, increased liver enzymes.

Bile acid sequestrants → Gastrointestinal distress, constipation, decreased absorption of other medications.

Nicotinic acid → Flushing, hyperglycemia, gout, upper GI distress, hepatotoxicity.

Fibric acids → Dyspepsia, gallstones, myopathy.

○   **At what age should one be screened for diabetes?**

Beginning at age 45, and repeated every 3 years, unless the patient is considered high risk.

○   **Who is considered high risk for diabetes and therefore warrants earlier screening?**

Overweight (BMI ≥ 25).

Family history of diabetes mellitus.

Habitual physical inactivity.

African American, Hispanic, Native American, Asian, Pacific Islander.

History of having a macrosomic baby or gestational diabetes.

Hypertensive.

HDL ≤ 35.

Triglycerides ≥ 250.

Polycystic ovary syndrome.

Vascular disease.

○ **What are acceptable ways of diagnosing diabetes mellitus in nonpregnant adults?**

(1) If patient has the symptoms of diabetes and a casual plasma glucose of 200 mg/dL or greater. The classic symptoms include polyuria, polydipsia, and unexplained weight loss.

(2) A fasting plasma glucose of 126 mg/dL or greater.

(3) A 2-hour glucose tolerance test value of 200 mg/dL or greater. The two-hour test uses a 75 g glucose load.

○ **How is hypertension in nonpregnant adults classified?**

Blood Pressure Classification	Blood Pressure (mm Hg)	
	Systolic	Diastolic
Normal	<120	<80
Prehypertension	120–139	Or 80–89
Stage 1 hypertension	140–159	Or 90–99
Stage 2 hypertension	≥160	≥100

○ **What are the most important risk factors for osteoarthritis?**

Female gender, family history, obesity, and a history of joint trauma.

○ **How do the symptoms of osteoarthritis differ from those of rheumatoid arthritis?**

Osteoarthritis is typically exacerbated by exercise and relieved by rest, whereas rheumatoid arthritis is associated with morning stiffness and improvement with activity.

○ **At what rate do women experience bone loss in the first 5 years after menopause?**

Bone mineral density decreases by approximately 3% per year during this time frame, then it returns to 1% per year.

○ **Define osteopenia and osteoporosis.**

Osteopenia is classified as having a bone mineral density between 1 and 2.5 standard deviations below the mean value for a reference population of young women.

Osteoporosis is defined as a bone mineral density of 2.5 or more standard deviations below the mean for the reference population.

○ **When does ACOG recommend screening for osteoporosis?**

All women starting at age 65. Starting at age 60 for women with an increased risk of osteoporotic fractures, no more frequently than every 2 years. Risk factors include, white race, history of a fracture, family history, poor nutrition, smoking, low BMI, early menopause, inadequate physical activity.

○ **What percentage of women are likely to have subclinical hypothyroidism?**

Up to 5%. The prevalence increases with age and is more common in white women than African Americans.

○ **What is the ACOG recommendation for screening for thyroid dysfunction?**

ACOG recommends checking a TSH every 5 years, beginning at age 50.

○ **A PPD of 5 mm or more is considered positive in which populations?**

HIV positive.
Those in close contact with a TB-positive person.
Those who have had TB in the past.
Those who do IV drugs and have unknown HIV status.

○ **What are the two most common reasons for a false-positive PPD?**

Infection with nontuberculosis mycobacteria and vaccination with BCG (bacillus Calmette-Guérin).

○ **If a patient has a positive PPD and she tells you that she had the BCG vaccine as a child, is any further work-up needed?**

Yes.

○ **What is the appropriate work-up for a first-time positive PPD?**

A chest x-ray should be performed and then based on the results, treatment initiated.

○ **In 1997, what percentage of American women was using complementary or alternative medicine?**

Forty nine percent. Most patients who use complementary and alternative therapies self-refer and do not tell their physicians.

○ **What is the body mass index (BMI) used for? What are the different categories?**

BMI is used as a screening tool to identify weight problems. The calculation is based on the patients' weight and height.

BMI	Category
<18.5	Underweight
18.5–24.9	Normal
25–29.9	Overweight
>30	Obese

○ **What percentage of females will pass away from CAD?**

33%.

○ **How many women annually will have an MI?**

500,000.

○ **What is the recommendation for physical activity for adults by the CDC and the American College of Sports Medicine?**

(1) Adults should engage in moderate intensity physical activities for at least 30 minutes on 5 or more days per week.

(2) Adults should engage in vigorous intensity physical activities 3 or more days per week for 20 minutes minimum per activity.

○ **When are therapeutic interventions recommended for blood pressure management?**

When elevations in blood pressure readings are obtained with 3 measurements performed at different times over the course of several weeks.

○ **What are the nonpharmacologic interventions for blood pressure management? How long should these interventions be pursued before they are deemed ineffective?**

The nonpharmacologic interventions include weight reduction, exercise, dietary sodium restriction, decreased alcohol intake, decreased fat consumption, smoking cessation, and stress reduction. If no success after 3 months, drug therapy is recommended.

○ **What tests other than fasting lipid panel are used to evaluate dyslipidemia?**

Other tests include fasting blood glucose, liver function, thyroid function, renal function, and urinalysis to rule out secondary causes of dyslipidemia.

○ **What values are considered normal for LDL, HDL, triglycerides, and total cholesterol?**

LDL	<100
HDL	>40
Triglycerides	<150
Total cholesterol	<200

CHAPTER 24 Functional and Dysfunctional Uterine Bleeding

Jeffrey Sellers, MD

○ **Define the normal menstrual cycle?**

The normal menstrual cycle is 28 days with a flow lasting 2 to 7 days. The variation in cycle length is set at 24 to 35 days.

○ **In a normal menstrual cycle, when does ovulation typically occur?**

Ovulation in a 28-day cycle occurs on day 14. The luteal phase of the cycle is normally 14 days. The estrogenic (proliferative) phase of the cycle can be variable.

○ **A woman normally has 32-day cycles. In this woman when does ovulation occur?**

In this clinical situation ovulation should occur on day 18. The luteal phase of the cycle should remain constant at 14 days.

○ **Name the hormones, and their source, that are involved in maintaining a normal menstrual cycle.**

From the ovary: Estrogen, progesterone, and Inhibin A.
   From the pituitary: Follicle stimulating hormone (FSH) and luteinizing hormone (LH). Prolactin and thyroid stimulating hormone are also vital in maintaining a normal menstrual cycle.
   From the hypothalamus: Gonadotropin-releasing hormone (GnRH).

○ **Describe the effect of estrogen on the endometrium.**

Estrogen causes growth of the endometrium. The endometrial glands lengthen and the glandular epithelium becomes pseudostratified. Mitotic activity is present in both the glands and the stroma.

○ **What are the earliest histologic changes in the endometrium following ovulation and when do they occur?**

Progesterone causes mitotic arrest. The earliest histologic change that can be identified is the development of subnuclear vacuoles. Both mitotic arrest and subnuclear vacuoles are present by postovulatory day 3 (day 17), assuming a normal 28-day cycle.

○ **By which postovulatory day do the endometrial glands appear exhausted as it relates to the secretory phase?**

By postovulatory 6 (day 20), assuming a normal 28-day cycle.

○   **On which postovulatory day does the endometrium demonstrate peak endometrial stromal edema?**

Postovulatory day 8 (day 22), assuming a normal 28-day cycle.

○   **On which postovulatory day does predecidual change first begin to appear and where does it first appear?**

Postovulatory day 9 (day 23). Predecidual change (periarteriolar cuffing) first appears around the spiral arterioles. Predecidual cells contain glycogen, assuming a normal 28-day cycle.

○   **When does implantation of the fertilized ovum typically occur?**

At approximately postovulatory day 9 (day 23), assuming a normal 28-day cycle.

○   **How big is the dominant follicle at the time of ovulation?**

Approximately 20 to 26 mm.

○   **Define menorrhagia.**

Menses at regular normal intervals with excessive flow and duration.

○   **Define menorrhagia quantitatively.**

Blood loss in excess of 80 mL.

○   **Define oligomenorrhea.**

Menses at intervals greater than 35 days.

○   **Define polymenorrhea.**

Menses at intervals less than 21 days.

○   **Define metrorrhagia.**

Menses at irregular intervals.

○   **Define menometrorrhagia.**

Menses with heavy, irregular bleeding.

○   **Define secondary amenorrhea.**

The absence of bleeding for at least three usual cycle lengths or 6 months in women who previously had menses.

○   **What percentage of patients present with chief complaint of abnormal vaginal bleeding?**

Approximately 12% of gynecology referrals are because of menorrhagia. Among women between ages 30 and 49, 5% consult physician for evaluation of menorrhagia.

○   **What percentage of women complaining of excessive or prolonged bleeding meets criteria for menorrhagia?**

40%.

○ **What is the percentage of women with menorrhagia that consider their periods as light or moderate?**

40%.

○ **What are the two direct (definitive) signs of ovulation?**

Pregnancy and visualization of follicle rupture either during laparoscopy or ultrasound.

○ **Broadly characterize the causes of abnormal uterine bleeding.**

Reproductive tract disease, systemic disease, trauma, pharmacologic alterations, anovulation, ovulation, etc.

○ **Define dysfunctional uterine bleeding (DUB).**

Bleeding that is not attributable to an underlying organic pathologic condition. DUB usually refers to anovulatory bleeding (90%).

○ **What are the components of the work up for abnormal uterine bleeding?**

A complete history, physical exam, laboratory studies, imaging studies, and tissue sampling.

○ **What is the first step in the evaluation of abnormal uterine bleeding following the history and physical examination in a woman?**

Hemodynamic status.

○ **What is the next step in the evaluation of abnormal uterine bleeding following the history and physical examination in a woman of reproductive age?**

A pregnancy test.

○ **What additional laboratory studies are important in the work up of abnormal uterine bleeding?**

CBC, PT/PTT, TSH, Prolactin levels, androgen levels, and testing for infection with Chlamydia and Gonorrhea.

○ **What is the next step in the evaluation of a woman abnormal uterine bleeding?**

Evaluation of the endometrial cavity by HSG, sonohysterography (SHG), or hysteroscopy.

○ **In a woman after age 30 with abnormal bleeding, what should be obtained next?**

Obtain a tissue biopsy. This may be in the form of endometrial biopsy or curettage.

○ **What is the advantage of curettage?**

In the woman with heavy bleeding, it may be therapeutic as well as diagnostic.

○ **What is the most important diagnosis to rule out in the postmenopausal woman?**

Cancer, primarily endometrial.

○ **Usual cause of abnormal genital bleeding in neonates?**

Withdrawal from maternal estrogens.

○ **What is the most common cause of vaginal bleeding in childhood?**

A foreign body.

○ **What is most common cause of abnormal bleeding in adolescence?**

Anovulation.

○ **What percentage of adolescents that require hospitalization for abnormal bleeding have an underlying coagulation disorder?**

Approximately 25%. The majority of these patients will have Von Willebrand's disease, problems with platelet count, or problems with platelet function.

○ **A 37-year-old woman, G2 P2 presents with a history of lengthening menses and acquired dysmenorrhea. This problem had been subtly going on for 2 years and now is a quality of life issue. Examination reveals a top normal size globular shaped uterus. What is the most likely diagnosis?**

Adenomyosis.

○ **What is the most common cause of postmenopausal bleeding?**

Atrophic endometrium and/or atrophic vaginitis.

○ **In what groups of patients other then postmenopausal women can you find vaginal bleeding secondary to atrophic vaginitis?**

Premenarchal girls, postpartum lactating women, and women on chronic progestins, like megace.

○ **What are the most common bleeding patterns seen in a woman with cervical cancer?**

Intermenstrual and postcoital bleeding.

○ **What is the size of the normal uterus?**

7.5 to 9.5 cm in length (cervix to fundus), 4.5 to 6.5 cm in width (from cornua to cornua), and 2.5 to 3.5 cm in anteroposterior diameter.

○ **What is the normal thickness of the myometrium?**

1 to 2 cm.

○ **What is the volume of a normal endometrial cavity in a woman of reproductive age?**

7 to 10 mL.

○ **When in the cycle should an endometrial biopsy be performed?**

At or beyond day 18, because if it shows secretory endometrium then it confirms that ovulation has occurred in that cycle.

○ **When should ultrasound be performed on premenopausal women for endometrium evaluation?**

Day 4 to 6, when endometrium is expected to be the thinnest.

○ **What is the normal endometrial thickness in women of reproductive age?**

Proliferative phase 4 to 8 mm; secretory phase 8 to 14 mm.

○ **Broadly characterize the major categories of dysfunctional uterine bleeding.**

Estrogen breakthrough bleeding, estrogen withdrawal bleeding, and progesterone breakthrough bleeding.

○ **What are causes of estrogen withdrawal bleeding?**

Bilateral oophorectomy, radiation of mature follicles, administration of estrogen to a previously oophorectomized woman followed by its withdrawal.

○ **What is the cause of midcycle spotting or light bleeding?**

The decline in estrogen that occurs immediately prior to the LH surge.

○ **How does estrogen affect breakthrough vaginal bleeding?**

Low doses of estrogen cause intermittent spotting that may be prolonged. High levels of estrogen lead to amenorrhea followed by acute, often profuse bleeding.

○ **What are the causes of progesterone withdrawal bleeding?**

Removal of the corpus luteum, medically or surgically. Pharmacologically, a similar event can be achieved by administration and discontinuation of progesterone or a synthetic progestin, provided the endometrium is estrogen primed.

○ **How can you narrow the differential diagnosis of uterine bleeding in patients of reproductive age?**

By establishing ovulatory status.

○ **How can you determine ovulatory status?**

Menstrual cycle charting, basal temperature monitoring, measurement of the serum progesterone concentration, monitoring urinary LH excretion, sonographic demonstration of periovulatory follicle.

○ **How can you determine ovulatory status based on menstrual history?**

If there are predictable cyclic menses, with duration of cycle 24 to 35 days, then most likely they are ovulatory. If the cycles vary in length by more than 10 days from one cycle to the next, then they are most likely anovulatory.

○ **If a single value of serum progesterone is low for the luteal phase, does it mean that the patient is not in the luteal phase?**

Not necessarily because it may be obtained between LH pulses. Although a single level above 6 ng/mL is usually indicative of normal luteal phase.

○ **What are the systemic illnesses that may cause anovulatory bleeding?**

Hypo and hyperthyroidism, chronic liver disease, chronic renal failure, Cushing's disease, PCOS, Prolactinoma, Empty sella syndrome, Sheehan's syndrome, adrenal and ovarian tumors, tumors infiltrating hypothalamus.

○   **What are the lifestyle elements that may cause anovulatory bleeding?**

Sudden weight loss, stress, and intense exercise.

○   **Decline in which hormone heralds the onset of menses?**

Normal menses occurs because of progesterone withdrawal.

○   **What is the life-span of a normal corpus luteum in the absence of pregnancy?**

Approximately 14 days.

○   **What is Halban's syndrome?**

It is the persistence of a corpus luteum. Patients commonly present with delayed menses, pelvic mass, and negative pregnancy test. Clinically, this is often confused with an ectopic pregnancy.

○   **How does one measure the strength of a progestational agent?**

Delay of menses.

○   **In women of reproductive age, what is the most common cause of estrogen excess bleeding?**

Chronic anovulation associated with polycystic ovaries.

○   **What are the usual causes of abnormal genital bleeding in premenarchal patients?**

Foreign body, trauma including sexual abuse, infection, urethral prolapse, sarcoma botryoides, ovarian tumor, precocious puberty.

○   **What are the usual causes of abnormal genital bleeding in patients early after menarche?**

Anovulation (hypothalamic immaturity), bleeding diathesis, stress (psychogenic, exercise induced), pregnancy, infection.

○   **What are the usual causes of abnormal genital bleeding in reproductive years?**

Anovulation, pregnancy, cancer, polyps, fibroids, adenomyosis, infection, endocrine dysfunction (PCOS, thyroid, pituitary adenoma), bleeding diathesis, and medication related.

○   **What are the usual causes of abnormal genital bleeding in perimenopausal women?**

Anovulation, polyps, fibroids, adenomyosis, and cancer.

○   **What are the usual causes of abnormal genital bleeding in postmenopausal women?**

Atrophy, cancer, and estrogen replacement therapy.

○   **What are the medications that can cause vaginal bleeding?**

Contraceptive medication (OCP, IUD, Depo-Provera), HRT, anticoagulants, corticosteroids, chemotherapy, dilantin, antipsychotic medication, and antibiotics (e.g., because of toxic epidermal necrolysis or Stevens-Johnson syndrome).

○ **What is the immediate objective of medical therapy in treating anovulatory bleeding?**

To stabilize the endometrium and control acute hemorrhage.

○ **How does progesterone work at the cellular level to control dysfunctional uterine bleeding when prescribed in pharmacologic doses?**

Progestins are powerful antiestrogens. They stimulate 17β hydroxysteroid dehydrogenase and sulfotransferase activity. This results in conversion of estradiol to estrone sulfate, which is rapidly excreted in the urine. Progestins also inhibit augmentation of estrogen receptors. Additionally, progestins suppress estrogen-mediated transcription of oncogenes.

○ **Failure of oral contraceptives to control bleeding when given twice daily for 5 to 7 days should prompt further evaluation. What are the most common diagnostic possibilities?**

Complications of pregnancy (incomplete abortion, ectopic pregnancy), endometrial polyps, endometrial neoplasia (including hyperplasia).

○ **A 14-year-old female presents with her first menses. Her bleeding is profuse and her hemoglobin is 4 g/dL. The pregnancy test is negative and to the best of your ability a bleeding disorder is excluded. What would be your pharmacologic approach to this patient?**

Conjugated estrogens 25 mg intravenously every 4 hours until bleeding stops or for four doses (12 hours). Progestin treatment is started concurrently.

○ **What is the best medical treatment of severe acute menorrhagia related to anovulation?**

High-dose estrogens. Intravenous conjugated equine estrogen (CEE) for up to 24 hours (25 mg IV/IM every 4 hours), followed with oral CEE (e.g., 2.5 mg four times a day) for 21 to 25 days, with medroxyprogesterone acetate (10 mg/d) for the last 10 days to induce bleeding. A Foley catheter can be placed to tamponade bleeding temporarily. Antiemetics are required in 40% of patients.

○ **Can severe acute menorrhagia related to anovulation be treated with progestins only?**

Yes, but it is less effective. Treatment involves medroxyprogesterone acetate (20–40 mg per day in divided doses), or megestrol acetate (40–120 mg per days), or norethindronate (5–10 mg per day) for 5 to 10 days. A 2 to 3 weeks regimen may be prescribed to allow for an increase in the hemoglobin concentration of anemic patients.

○ **What is the best medical treatment of severe acute menorrhagia secondary to atrophic bleeding?**

Ethinyl estradiol (10–20 mcg) for 2 to 3 weeks.

○ **A patient is taking a low-dose oral contraceptive pills. She experiences repetitive spotting during the first week of therapy. How would you treat this?**

Estrogen therapy for 7 days in addition to her oral contraceptive pill. This could be as conjugated estrogens 1.25 mg or estradiol 2.0 mg. This is preferable to changing pills. May reassure patient that this is normal and wait for three cycles, as most of such symptoms resolve by that time, if not then may change the pill.

○ **What the best pharmacologic approach to treat a woman with ovulatory cycles but heavy menses?**

A prostaglandin synthetase inhibitor, beginning with the onset of symptoms.

○   **What percentage decrease in blood loss can be expected with the use of a prostaglandin synthetase inhibitor?**

Approximately 40% to 50%.

○   **What are the options for treatment of chronic or less severe acute menorrhagia?**

OCPs, IUDs, NSAIDs, antifibrinolytics: tranexamic acid, danazol, D&C, hysteroscopic endometrial ablation (if completed child bearing).

○   **In what clinical situation is dysfunctional uterine bleeding best treated with a progestin containing IUD?**

Bleeding associated with chronic illnesses (such as renal failure).

○   **In what clinical situations is dysfunctional uterine bleeding best treated with a GnRH agonist?**

Renal failure, blood dyscrasia, or organ transplantation (especially liver transplantation).

○   **What percentage of women develop amenorrhea following endometrial ablation?**

Approximately 60%.

○   **What percentage of women will development improvement in their menstrual blood loss following endometrial ablation?**

Up to 90%.

○   **What percentage of patients after endometrial ablation require further procedures?**

Hysterectomy or repeat endometrial ablation is required in 20 to 40% of patients within 4 years.

○   **In what clinical situations should estrogen be the initial choice of treatment for abnormal uterine bleeding?**

(1) When the bleeding has been heavy for many days, (2) when endometrial sampling yields minimal tissue, (3) when the patient has been on progestins and the endometrium is atrophic, and (4) when follow-up is uncertain, because estrogen will temporarily stop all categories of DUB.

○   **What is the role of curettage in the treatment of DUB?**

It is effective in controlling acute hemorrhage when hormonal therapy fails.

○   **What are common clinical conditions present when medical therapy fails to control menorrhagia?**

Submucous fibroids, endometrial polyps, hyperplasia, or cancer.

○   **How can one increase sensitivity and specificity of transvaginal ultrasound in assessment of endometrial cavity?**

By performing saline infusion sonography with instillation of sterile saline into the endometrial cavity. Sensitivity increases from 75% to 93%, specificity from 76% to 94%.

○   **What is the probability of endometrial cancer in a postmenopausal woman with vaginal bleeding with endometrial thickness <4 mm?**

0.5%.

○   **What is the probability of endometrial cancer in postmenopausal woman with vaginal bleeding after a negative hysteroscopy ?**

0.4% to 0.5%.

○   **What is the probability of endometrial cancer in postmenopausal women with vaginal bleeding with endometrial thickness >10 mm?**

10% to 20%.

○   **What are the diseases that may mimic vaginal bleeding?**

Urethritis, bladder cancer, urinary tract infection, inflammatory bowel disease, and hemorrhoids.

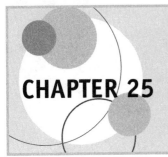

CHAPTER 25

Adenomyosis and Endometriosis

Michael Lempel, MD

○ **What is the prevalence of endometriosis?**

7% to 10% of reproductive age women.

25% to 35% of infertile women.

○ **The most common symptom of endometriosis is:**

Dysmenorrhea and pain throughout the menstrual cycle (25%–67% of women with endometriosis).

Dyspareunia is found in 25% and associated with uterosacral involvement.

○ **Other common symptoms and signs of endometriosis are:**

Intraperitoneal bleeding, pelvic adhesions, pelvic pain, infertility, cyclic bowel and bladder symptoms, and inflammation.

○ **What proportion of patients have uterosacral and cul-de-sac nodularity?**

One-third of all patients with endometriosis.

○ **The most common age of a diagnosis of endometriosis is:**

25 to 35 years.

○ **What is the best imaging technique for diagnosing endometriosis?**

Laparoscopy remains the optimal method, but MRI using the fat-saturation technique has a PPV of 95% and NPV of 50% with implants ≥4 mm.

○ **True or False: The black powder lesions seen here in the posterior cul-de sac should be biopsied to confirm the diagnosis of endometriosis?**

True. A biopsy is always recommended to confirm endometriosis on histology.

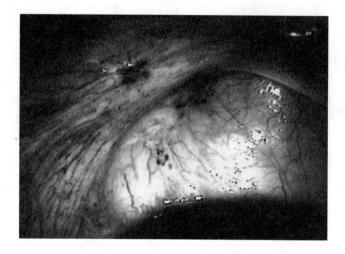

○ **What are the ultrasound findings consistent with endometriosis?**

Cystic structures with diffuse low-level internal echoes indicating a possible endometrioma.

○ **Does medical treatment of minimal-mild endometriosis increase fertility? How about surgical treatment?**

No. Surgical treatment may increase fertility rates therefore it is still recommended at time of laparoscopy.

○ **Does preoperative medical treatment assist in surgical treatment of endometriosis?**

Yes, it softens the endometrial implants for surgical removal.

○ **When does one achieve the highest pregnancy rates after surgical treatment?**

In the first year, success is inversely related to the severity of disease.

○ **What are the recurrence rates after surgical treatment and after medical treatment?**

For surgical tx: 10% in first year, 20% in 5 years.
For medical tx: 5% to 20% per year, 40% in 5 years.

○ **Is there any role for postoperative medical treatment?**

Yes, medical treatment after surgical treatment can delay return of symptoms with at least 6 months postoperative medical treatment.

○ **What are the options for postoperative medical treatment?**

GnRH agonist
Danazol
Oral contraceptives

○ **How do oral contraceptive pills treat endometriosis?**

They suppress FSH and LH secretion causing decreased estrogen production and reduced menstrual volume.

○ **Can tubal ligation be performed as a treatment for endometriosis?**

No. Some women even experience symptoms of endometriosis after hysterectomy.

○ **Can an intrauterine device (IUD) be used to treat endometriosis?**

Yes, the levonorgestrol IUD causes decidualization of the endomtrium and decreased menstrual flow.

○ **True or False: A CA-125 level can predict active endometriosis.**

True, but controvertial; CA-125 levels often correlate with the degree of disease; however, a normal level does not exclude the absence of disease.

○ **Name the three main theories for the pathogenesis of endometriosis.**

Coelomic metaplasia (Robert Meyer): tissue from prenatal development transforms into endometrial cells.
Transplantation theory: lymphatic, vascular, iatrogenic, retrograde menstruation (Sampson)
Induction theory: possible substance in body that results in cellular transformation/differentiation

○ **The familial nature of endometriosis has been reported in case reports and retrospective reviews. Simpson studied 123 patients with histologically demonstrated endometriosis: 5.9% of sisters and 8.1% of mothers were also affected. However, when the patient's husband's family history was looked at, only 1% of sisters and 0.8% of mothers had endometriosis. Propose a genetic mechanism for these findings.**

It can be polygenetic inheritance or a single mutant autosomal dominant or autosomal recessive gene, or lastly, a single mutant gene occurring in a small subset of patients with endometriosis. The most likely mode is polygenic and multifactorial.

○ **Name one characteristic of endometriosis that histomorphologically separates it from eutopic endometrium.**

Extensive stromal hemorrhage or dense stromal fibrosis.

○ **Chronic progesterone therapy has what specific effect on endometriosis?**

Initial decidualization of endometrial tissue with eventual atrophy.

○ **What is the currently accepted rate of transformation of endometriosis to malignancy?**

Less than 1%.

○ **Name at least three malignant neoplasms arising in endometriosis.**

Clear cell adenocarcinoma, adenoacanthoma, adenosquamous carcinoma, leiomyosarcoma, endometrial stromal sarcoma, mixed mullerian tumor, or carcinosarcoma.

○ **You have seen a suspicious lesion at laparoscopy and biopsied the lesion. The pathology report indicates endosalpingiosis. What does this mean?**

The characteristics of the cells and stroma of the epithelial cells and the stroma of the biopsy specimen indicate tubal-type epithelium. Involvement of the canal of Nuck with endometriosis indicates the presence of a hernial sack of hydrocele to provide communication with the peritoneal cavity.

○   **Endometriosis of the cervix is well known. It usually is a result of cervical trauma. In retrospective study, what percent of cases are associated with trauma?**

90%.

○   **With what tumor is endometriosis of the appendix associated with?**

Mucinous carcinoid.

○   **What is a catamenial pneumothorax?**

This is a rare condition that often involves endometriosis of the diaphragm, causing the lung to collapse during menses.

○   **List three causes of pelvic pain associated with endometriosis?**

(1) Inflammatory factors

(2) Scarring and retraction

(3) Compression and stretching

○   **Abnormal bleeding occurs in what percent of women? (Specify a range.)**

10% to 35%.

○   **State the macrophage hypothesis in endometriosis.**

The inflammatory response caused by endometriosis results in increased concentration of pelvic macrophages. This causes a decrease in fertility by phagocytosis of sperm and secretion of IL-1, which is shown to be toxic to mouse embryos.

○   **True or False: Spontaneous abortions are increased in women with endometriosis.**

False. There is no evidence that spontaneous abortion rate is altered in patients with this disease.

○   **True or False: Endometriosis is a risk factor for ectopic pregnancy?**

True

○   **List two characteristics that increase the risk of endometriosis.**

Cycle lengths less than 27 days and menstrual flow greater than 1 week.

○   **How do you choose medical treatment?**

By cost and side effect profile; no one medication has been shown to be more effective than any other

○   **Name some side effects of Danazol.**

Weight gain, fluid retention, fatigue, smaller breast size, acne, facial hair, atrophic vaginitis, hot flushes, muscle cramps, emotional lability, irreversible deepening of the voice, hepatocellular damage (check LFTS first), increase LDL, lower HDL, and in utero female pseudohermaphroditism

○ **True or False: In premenopausal women, Danazol lowers basal gonadotropin secretion.**

False. Danazol eliminates the midcycle LH and FSH surge, and inhibits steroidogensis in the corpus luteum creating a high androgen, low estrogen state and amenorrhea

○ **Name four currently used regiments in the treatment of endometriosis.**

Progestins, combination estrogen/progesterone pills (oral contraceptives), Danazol, and GnRH agonists. Recent reports also suggest hetrozole - (an aromatase inhibitor that presents androgen to estrogen conversion) may also be useful in treatment of endometriosis.

○ **What are the side effects of progestational agents?**

Weight gain, fluid retention, breakthrough bleeding, and depression.

○ **Name some side effects of GnRH agonists.**

Flare response, menopausal symptoms, and bone loss (need add back therapy after 6 months of treatment).

○ **Name two goals of surgery for endometriosis.**

Restoration of normal anatomy and elimination of pelvic pain; 90% of patients note some degree of pain relief with surgery.

○ **Total abdominal hysterectomy-bilateral salpingo-oophorectomy has generally been considered an excellent way to treat endometriosis definitively. If hormone replacement therapy is given, what is the expected rate of recurrence of endometriosis?**

8%.

○ **Endometriosis of the bladder has been reported in males. What treatment regimen are these men on?**

High-dose estrogen for prostate cancer.

○ **Presacral neurectomy is advocated for treating what condition associated with endometriosis?**

Dysmenorrhea; midline pain only (it is not a treatment for infertility)

○ **True or False: Provera at 30 mg/d was as effective as Danazol in treatment of endometriosis.**

True.

○ **The Guilliam suspension utilizes which anatomic structure of the uterus?**

The round ligament.

○ **How would you diagnose ovarian remnant syndrome?**

Check an FSH.

○ **To prevent adhesions after conservative surgery for endometriosis, name two parameters that must be satisfied.**

1. Impeccable hemostasis.

2. Lack of tissue necrosis.

○ **What is intercede?**

It is a physical barrier composed of oxidized regenerated cellulose.

○ **What is Sepra film?**

Sodium hialuronate-carboxy methyl cellulose absorbable adhesion barrier.

○ **What medication causes the estradiol level to be less than 20 pg/mL?**

Depo GnRH.

○ **Name a model that proposes a preexisting congenital or learned vulnerability that heighten the risk for chronic pain.**

The diathesis-stress model.

○ **Describe the diathesis-stress model.**

In the diathesis-stress model, a genetic vulnerability or predisposition (diathesis) interacts with the environment and life events (stressors) to trigger behaviors or psychological disorders.

○ **What class of medications have now supplanted narcotics as a treatment of chronic pelvic pain?**

Heterocyclic antidepressants.

○ **Based on a recent review of 500 consecutive cases by Shaw, what pelvic structure has a higher incidence of implants than the ovary?**

Uterosacral ligaments.

○ **As a woman with endometriosis ages, her endometriotic lesions change from clear papules to_____.**

Black.

○ **Who was the first person to describe adenomyosis in the medical literature?**

Rokitansky, in 1860.

○ **What is the definition of adenomyosis?**

The presence of endometrial glands and stoma within the myometrium with compensatory hypertrophy of the myometrium (most articles today used a depth of 3 mm, or 1 low-powered field, below the basal layer of endometrium as the required depth of invasion) It has an incidence of 31% to 61%.

○ **True or False: Adenomyosis appears equally in parous and nulliparous women.**

False, it has been correlated with increasing parity.

○ **What are the four theories of causality of adenomyosis?**

Heredity, trauma, hyperestrogenemia, and viral transmission.

○ **Name the most common symptom in patients with adenomyosis.**

Abnormal uterine bleeding, secondary dysmenorrhea, enlarged and tender uterus (but up to 35% may be asymptomatic)

○ **Name the imaging technology most likely to diagnosis adenomyosis.**

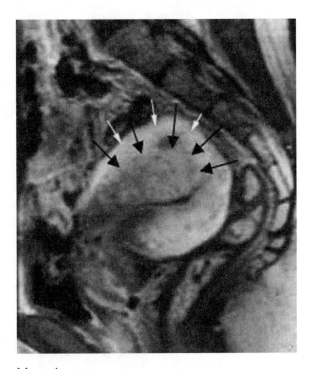

Magnetic resonance.

○ **What other condition is commonly associated with adenomyosis?**

Leiomyomata, up to 57% of the time.
Also frequently occurs in association with endometrial adenocarcinoma.

○ **What is the treatment for adenomyosis?**

Hysterectomy remains the first choice; Bromocriptine and RU486 have been shown to suppress adenomyosis.

○ **True or False: Endometrioid carcinoma is of endometriosis origin.**

False. This designation is merely a description of the microscopic findings and have nothing to do with the etiology of the carcinoma.

○   **What are the ultrasound characteristics of adenomyosis?**

- Ill-defined hypoechoic areas.
- Hetrogeneous myometrial echotexture.
- Small anechioc lakes.
- Asymetrical uterine enlargement.
- Indistinct endometrial-myometrial border.
- Subendometrial halo thickening.

CHAPTER 26

Benign Disorders of the Upper Genital Tract

Gretchen Glaser, MD

○ **What is the average weight of the mature woman's uterus?**

30 to 40 g.

○ **What is the normal length of the uterine cavity?**

3.5 cm.

○ **Approximately what percentage of uteri will be retroverted on exam?**

About one-third. It is important to emphasize that this is a normal variant as many "old wives' tales" exist regarding a "tipped" uterus.

○ **What is a cystocele?**

The downward displacement of the bladder.

○ **What is a cystourethrocele?**

A cystocele that includes the urethra as part of the prolapsing organ complex.

○ **What is uterine prolapse?**

The descent of the uterus and cervix down the vaginal canal toward the vaginal introitus.

○ **What is a rectocele?**

The protrusion of the rectum into the posterior vaginal lumen.

○ **What is an enterocele?**

The herniation of small bowel in the vaginal lumen.

○ **What is the Pelvic Organ Prolapse Quantitative (POP-Q)?**

An objective, standardized system for describing pelvic support in women. It allows for consistency between examiners and is the most commonly used pelvic support scoring system.

○   **How should physical exam be performed when using the POP-Q system?**

The patient should be standing and performing a Valsalva maneuver to elicit maximum prolapse.

○   **What is the vaginal reference point for POP-Q scoring?**

Hymen.

The following questions relate to POP-Q.

○   **Define point Aa.**

A point located in the midline of the anterior vaginal wall 3 cm proximal to the external urethral meatus, The position of point Aa relative to the hymen can range from −3 to +3 cm.

○   **Define point Ba.**

Ba represents the most distal position of any part of the upper anterior vaginal wall from the vaginal cuff or anterior vaginal fornix to point Aa. By definition, point Ba is at −3 cm in the absence of prolapse.

○   **Define point C.**

C represents either the most distal (i.e., most dependent) edge of the cervix or the leading edge of the vaginal cuff after total hysterectomy.

○   **Define point D.**

Point D represents the location of the posterior fornix (or pouch of Douglas) in a woman who still has a cervix. Point D is omitted in the absence of the cervix.

○   **Define point Bp.**

Point Bp is the most distal position of any part of the upper posterior vaginal wall from the vaginal cuff or posterior vaginal fornix to point Ap. By definition, point Bp is at −3 cm in the absence of prolapse.

○   **Define point Ap.**

A point located in the midline of the posterior vaginal wall 3 cm proximal to the hymen. By definition, the range of position of point Ap relative to the hymen is −3 (normal) to +3 cm (complete prolapse).

○   **What other landmarks are used in the POP-Q 3 × 3 grid?**

Genital hiatus, gh: measured from the middle of the external urethral meatus to the posterior midline hymen.

Perineal body, pb: measured from the posterior margin of the genital hiatus to the midanal opening.

Total vaginal length (TVL) is the greatest depth of the vagina in centimeters when point C or D is reduced to its full normal position.

○   **How is pelvic organ prolapse staged according to the ordinal staging system?**

Stage 0: No prolapse is demonstrated. Points Aa, Ap, Ba, and Bp are all at −3 cm and either point C or D is between −TVL (total vaginal length) cm and −(TVL − 2) cm.

Stage I: The criteria for stage 0 are not met, but the most distal portion of the prolapse is >1 cm above the level of the hymen.

Stage II: The most distal portion of the prolapse is less or equal to 1 cm proximal to or distal to the plane of the hymen.

Stage III: The most distal portion of the prolapse is >1 cm below the plane of the hymen but protrudes no further than 2 cm less than the total vaginal length in centimeters.

Stage IV: Essentially, complete eversion of the total length of the lower genital tract is demonstrated. The distal portion of the prolapse protrudes to at least +(TVL − 2) cm In most instances, the leading edge of stage IV prolapse will be the cervix or vaginal cuff scar.

○ **How common is pelvic organ prolapse?**

The Women's Health Initiative found that in women with a uterus, 14% had uterine prolapse, 34% had a cystocele, and 19% had a rectocele. In women who had undergone hysterectomy, 33% had a cystocele and 18% had a rectocele.

○ **What factors are strongly associated with an increased risk of pelvic organ prolapse?**

Increased parity and obesity. Race also seems to play a role, as African American women have the lowest rates of pelvic organ prolapse, while Hispanic women have the highest rates.

○ **What is the course of the ascending limb of the uterine artery?**

It courses below the fallopian tube and eventually anastomoses with the ovarian artery.

○ **What are Mackenrodt's ligaments?**

Also known as the cardinal ligaments, these are transverse fibrous bands which attach to the uterine cervix and to the vault of the lateral vaginal fornix, serving to stabilize the cervix.

○ **What three structures form the boundaries of the broad ligament?**

(1) The fold of peritoneum over the fallopian tube, (2) the infundibulopelvic vessels, and (3) the hilus of the artery.

○ **What are the three layers of the endometrium?**

(1) The pars basalis, (2) the zona spongiosa, and (3) the superficial zona compacta.

○ **What vascular event triggers shedding of the endometrium?**

Spasm of the spiral arteries resulting in ischemia of the tissue and sloughing.

○ **What is the embryologic origin of the fallopian tube?**

Paramesonephric duct.

○ **What is the average length of the fallopian tube?**

10 to 12 cm.

○ **What is the largest and longest portion of the fallopian tube?**

The ampulla.

○ **What is the site of most ectopic *pregnancies*?**

The ampulla.

○ **Where do primitive germ cells originate?**

They originate in the dorsal part of the hindgut and then migrate to the gonad.

○ **What is the normal weight of the mature ovary?**

3 to 8 g.

○ **What is the location of the ovarian fossa?**

Below the external iliac vessel and in front of the ureter.

○ **What *cell type* covers the ovary?**

Germinal epithelium.

○ **What two ligaments support the ovary?**

The suspensory ligament at the tubal pole and the utero-ovarian ligament at the opposite pole.

○ **What is the name of the vestige of the mesonephric (wolffian) tubule in the female?**

The epoophoron, which is an important potential source of cyst formation.

○ **What is the name of the vestige of the mesonephric duct in the female?**

The Gartner's duct, which can course along the uterus, cervix, and vagina.

○ **What does the primordial follicle consist of?**

The primordial follicle consists of the oocyte with a layer of follicular cells surrounding it.

○ **What is the cumulus oophorus?**

A cluster of granulosa cells around the oocyte.

○ **What action creates the corpus hemorrhagicum, and into what structure does it evolve?**

The formation of a clot at the site of follicular rupture; as the granulosa cells grow into this clot it becomes the corpus luteum.

○ **What functional ovarian cyst is most commonly associated with a hydatidiform mole?**

The theca lutein cyst is associated with up to 50% of molar gestations and 10% of choriocarcinomas. They are usually bilateral and produce moderate to massive enlargement of the ovaries. Theca lutein cysts may also be associated with ovulation induction or pregnancies where large placentas are produced (diabetes, twins and Rh sensitization).

○ **What is the luteoma of pregnancy?**

A benign hyperplastic reaction of ovarian theca lutein cells, which may cause virilization in the mother or female fetus, although most cases are asymptomatic.

○ **A 10-year-old girl presents with an adnexal mass. What is the most common etiology?**

Mature cystic teratomas (also known as dermoid cysts) develop from totipotential cells and are composed of well-differentiated ectodermal, endodermal, and mesodermal elements. They account for greater than 50% of adnexal masses in the prepubertal period.

○ **A 6-year-old girl presents for evaluation of premature thelarche. Her workup reveals Tanner stage 4 breast development, numerous café au lait spots and ovarian cysts. What is her most likely diagnosis?**

McCune-Albright syndrome is associated with an ovarian etiology of excess hormone production and is characterized by polyostotic fibrous dysplasia and café au lait spots. Patients have a genetic mutation in the G protein, which results in polyglandular lesions involving the thyroid, pituitary, and gonads.

○ **What percentage of teratomas are bilateral?**

Approximately 10% to 15%. The contralateral ovary should be inspected carefully at the time of surgery by visualization and palpation. The presence of a mature unilateral teratoma does not necessitate a wedge resection or bivalving of the contralateral ovary.

○ **What is the karyotype of a mature teratoma?**

The karyotype is 46 XX and arises from a single germ cell after the first meiotic division.

○ **What are the most common complication of teratomas?**

Torsion occurs in nearly 15% of cases and is more common in younger women. Other complications include rupture, infection, hemorrhage, and malignant degeneration.

○ **What is the risk of malignant transformation in a mature teratoma?**

Malignant transformation occurs in less than 2% of mature teratomas and more than 75% of the time this is in patients older than 40 years. Squamous cell carcinoma arising in ectodermal layers accounts for 80% of malignant transformations.

○ **What is struma ovarii?**

An ovarian mass (usually a teratoma) in which thyroid tissue is a major component. Thyroid tissue occurs in approximately 10% of teratomas. Patients usually present with a pelvic mass, and less than 5% of women with struma ovarii develop thyrotoxicosis. Struma ovarii occurs most often in women aging 40 to 60.

○ **What are the Rotterdam criteria for diagnosing PCOS?**

Two out of three of the following:

- Oligo- and/or anovulation
- Clinical and/or biochemical signs of hyperandrogenism
- Polycystic ovaries by ultrasound

    Other etiologies must also be excluded.

○ **What percentage of patients with anovulation associated with PCOS do not have the expected reversal of the LH:FSH ratio?**

Between 20% and 40% of patients with PCOS will not have the expected reversal of the LH:FSH ratio. For this reason it is not recommended to routinely measure FSH and LH levels in anovulatory patients and make the diagnosis on clinical presentation alone.

○ **What is the most common benign, solid ovarian tumor?**

The fibroma is the most common, with a malignant potential of under 1%. These are slow-growing tumors with less than a 10% occurrence of bilaterality. On cut section a homogeneous white or yellowish white solid tissue with a trabeculated appearance is seen.

○ **What is Meigs' syndrome?**

The clinical triad of an ovarian fibroma, ascites, and hydrothorax. These clinical features are not specific to fibromas, and a similar clinical picture can be found with many other ovarian tumors. *The ascites and hydrothorax are most likely caused by substances such as vascular endothelial growth factor (VEGF), which increases vessel permeability.* Both the ascites and hydrothorax resolve after removal of the tumor.

○ **A benign ovarian tumor is removed from a 50 year old. The pathology report makes note of pale epithelial cells with a "coffee bean" nucleus. What is the diagnosis?**

Brenner tumors are rare transitional cell ovarian tumors that usually occur in women from 40 to 60 years of age. They are rarely bilateral and less than 2% undergo malignant degeneration.

○ **A 43-year-old women presents 5 years following a TAH/BSO for benign disease with a palpable pelvic mass and cyclical pelvic pain. A FSH level is in the premenopausal range. What is the most likely diagnosis?**

The ovarian remnant syndrome occurs in patients who have undergone bilateral oophorectomy usually complicated by endometriosis or pelvic inflammatory disease. This syndrome occurs when failure to skeletonize the infundibulopelvic ligament or incorrect clamp placement results in retention of a piece of ovarian tissue. Many patients present with cyclic pain and a mass. Sonography may aid in the diagnosis, as will FSH levels. CT/MRI may be useful in defining the relation of the ovarian remnant to surrounding structures.

○ **What is the risk of malignant degeneration in a leiomyoma?**

Malignant degeneration in a preexisting leiomyoma is extremely rare, and occurs in less than 0.5%.

○ **What is leiomyomatosis peritonealis disseminata?**

A rare condition in which benign leiomyomatous nodules are spread out over the pelvic and abdominal peritoneum, simulating disseminated carcinoma. This usually occurs in young women and is associated with a recent pregnancy, estrogen secreting granulosa tumor, or oral contraceptive use.

○ **What are the clinical findings of leiomyoma?**

Abnormal uterine bleeding

Pelvic pain

Pressure effects (constipation, incontinence)

Infertility

Spontaneous abortions

○ **Leiomyomas undergo what type of benign degeneration?**

Atrophic, hyaline, cystic, calcification, septic, and carneous (red).

○ **What is the natural history of leiomyomas during pregnancy?**

Nearly three-fourth of all leiomyomas do not change size significantly during pregnancy; 5% to 10% undergo carneous or red degeneration, and may cause severe pain and peritoneal irritation. The larger the leiomyoma the greater the risk of premature labor.

○ **What are the options for medical treatment of uterine myomas?**

GnRH agonist with add-back therapy (i.e., addition of estrogen-progestin therapy)

GnRH antagonist

Mifepriston (RU-486)

Danozol

Raloxifene

Levonorgestrel-releasing intrauterine device

○ **What is the incidence of leiomyomas that are clinically apparent?**

25% to 50% of women have clinically apparent leiomyomas.

○ **When using GnRH agonists to "shrink" leiomyomas, when does the maximum effect occur?**

Nonpulsatile GnRH agonist therapy has been shown to decrease leiomyoma size by 30% to 50% with the maximal effect noted in 2 to 3 months.

○ **For the symptomatic treatment of uterine leiomyomas, what is the rate of resolution of symptoms following abdominal myomectomy?**

Overall 81% with a range of 40% to 93%.

○ **What is the risk of reoperation following abdominal myomectomy?**

11% for a single myoma.

26% for multiple myomas.

18% overall risk of reoperation following abdominal myomectomy.

○ **What is the risk of undergoing unexpected hysterectomy at the time of abdominal myomectomy?**

<1% for the experienced surgeon, higher rates appear for the inexperienced surgeon.

○ **What are side effects of uterine artery embolization?**

Pelvic infection

Premature menopause

Vaginal expulsion of necrotic fibroids

Severe pelvic pain requiring analgesia

○ **Who is a candidate for uterine artery embolization?**

Patients whose symptoms are directly related to fibroids

Patients who have been ruled out for malignancy

Absence of endometrial hyperplasia or neoplasm on pippelle for patients with intermenstrual bleeding

○　**What are contraindications to UAE?**

Pregnancy, active pelvic infection, active vasculitis, history of pelvic irradiation, evidence of pelvic malignancy, life threatening contrast allergy, uncontrollable coagulopathies, and severe renal insufficiency.

○　**What percentage of patients undergoing UAE will pass fibroid sloughing through the vagina?**

5%.

○　**What percentage of patients undergoing UAE begin menopause following the procedure?**

5%.

○　**What is the success rate of UAE?**

85% to 94%.

○　**A 23-year-old women presents for a primary infertility workup and is found to have a septate uterus. What treatments can be offered and what are their success rates?**

A septate uterus is associated with pregnancy wastage. Only 15% of patients without treatment achieve a term pregnancy. Most septums can be excised via hysteroscopy. Occasionally a very large septum may necessitate a Jones (wedge) metroplasty. Term pregnancy rates of 75% are possible following repair.

○　**A 30-year-old women presents 6 weeks postpartum from a vaginal delivery with mild uterine tenderness, heavy bleeding, and an 8-week size, boggy uterus. A serum pregnancy test is negative. What is the most likely diagnosis?**

Failure of the uterus to return to its normal size postpartum is referred to as "subinvolution." Microscopy of the placental site reveals retention of trophoblastic cells, enlarged vessels, and necrotic decidua. This may serve as a nidus for infection as well as cause delayed postpartum bleeding.

○　**What is the incidence of benign endometrial polyps?**

The reported incidence of polyps is nearly 25% of all uteri. They frequently present with abnormal uterine bleeding. This diagnosis should be considered especially when bleeding persists following D+C because the curette may miss small polyps.

○　**An endometrial biopsy is performed on a 36-year-old anovulatory, fertility patient and shows "tubal metaplasia." What does this mean?**

Ciliated cells are usually not seen in endometrial glands. The presence of a significant number of ciliated glandular cells is referred to as tubal metaplasia or ciliated cell change because of the resemblance to epithelium of the fallopian tube. This is a benign finding and reflects a mild degree of estrogenic stimulation. It may accompany endometrial hyperplasia.

○　**What is the first histologic sign on an endometrial biopsy that ovulation has occurred?**

The first sign of the secretory phase is the appearance of subnuclear intracytoplasmic glycogen vacuoles in the glandular epithelium. This is soon followed by active secretion into the endometrial cavity with a peak level reached about 7 days after ovulation, coinciding with the time of blastocyst implantation.

○ **What is the primary histologic feature of the endometrium at the time that implantation should occur?**

On days 21 to 22 of a normal cycle the predominant feature is stromal edema. This may be caused by an increased vascular permeability secondary to greater prostaglandin production.

○ **Which layer of the endometrium is responsible for the greatest increase in height during the menstrual cycle?**

The functionalis layer is primarily responsible for the increased height of the endometrium during the proliferative phase. After ovulation the height is generally fixed at approximately 6 mm by the growth restraining effects of progesterone.

○ **What is the risk of progression to malignancy with complex atypical hyperplasia of the endometrium?**

Approximately 25% of these cases progress to carcinoma without treatment. Only 2% of endometrial hyperplasia without atypia progresses this way.

○ **What percent of adolescents with heavy dysfunctional uterine bleeding will have a coagulation defect?**

Although the most common cause is anovulation, as many as 20% of adolescents will have a coagulation defect, the most common being von Willebrand's disease. Bleeding is usually a heavy flow with regular, cyclic menses. This is the same pattern seen in patients treated with anticoagulants.

○ **How much do oral contraceptive pills reduce menstrual flow?**

In normal uteri, OCPs reduce flow by 50% to 60% by limiting maximal endometrial growth and allowing orderly menses.

○ **What is adenomyosis?**

Adenomyosis is the presence of endometrial glands and stroma within the myometrium. It occurs most commonly in perimenopausal women and is present in approximately 15% of uteri. Some pathologists only use this term when the lower border of the endometrium and the adenomyosis are separated by at least one-half of a low-power field (about 2.5 mm).

○ **How is the diagnosis of adenomyosis made?**

Adenomyosis is primarily diagnosed postoperatively, upon histologic review of the uterus. Clinical suspicion is increased when a patient in her fourth or fifth decade presents with worsening dysmenorrhea and menorrhagia in the presence of a symmetrically enlarged, firm, and tender uterus. MRI can make this diagnosis preoperatively with a high degree of accuracy. Curettage does not help in diagnosis or treatment.

○ **What is the embryological derivative of the hydatid cyst of Morgagni?**

This is the most common paramesonephric (mullerian) cyst. Other paratubal cysts can arise from mesonephric (wolffian) structures or mesothelial inclusions.

○ **What is Salpingitis Isthmica Nodasa?**

These are outpouchings or diverticula of tubal epithelium in the isthmic region. Involvement is often bilateral and is associated with ectopic gestation and infertility. The etiology is unknown, although some evidence exists for a noninflammatory adenomyosis-like origin.

○ **Following tubal sterilization procedures, what is the rate of hysterosalpingogram documented "leak"?**

Hysterosalpingogram "leak rates" may reach 25% after Pomeroy or any of the other operations but the actual fertility "failure rate" is much lower. Additional surgery on a fallopian tube found to leak dye does not guarantee permanent sterilization. Injection of dye under hydraulic pressure through the uterus may open a previously occluded fallopian tube.

○ **What are Nabothian cysts?**

Nabothian cysts are retention cysts of endocervical columnar cells where a cleft has been covered by squamous metaplasia.

○ **What is the size of a Nabothian cyst?**

It can vary from 3 mm to 3 cm.

○ **What are the symptoms of Nabothian cysts?**

Nabothian cysts are asymptomatic.

○ **What is hematometra?**

Hematometra is a uterus distended with blood secondary to partial or complete obstruction of the lower genital tract.

○ **What are the most common causes of hematometra?**

Imperforate hymen and transverse vaginal septum.

○ **What are acquired causes of lower tract stenosis?**

Senile atrophy of the endocervical canal, cervical stenosis associated with surgery, radiation, cryocautery or electrocautery, malignant disease of the endocervical canal.

○ **What are the symptoms of hematometra?**

Primary and secondary amenorrhea, cyclic lower abdominal pain.

CHAPTER 27
Dysmenorrhea and Premenstrual Syndrome

Miki Chiguchi, MD

○ **Define primary dysmenorrhea.**

Menstrual pain without pelvic pathology.

○ **What percentage of women are affected by dysmenorrhea?**

60%, of which 10% may be incapacitated for 1 to 3 days each month. Most common reason women miss work.

○ **What is the cause of primary dysmenorrhea?**

Increased endometrial prostaglandin production. Prostaglandin levels increase threefold from the follicular to the luteal phase and further during menstruation.

○ **In what phase of the endometrium are these compounds increased?**

The secretory endometrium.

○ **The fall of what hormone in the late luteal phase triggers the pathway that increases prostaglandin production?**

Progesterone.

○ **Name the compound that is the substrate for the release of prostaglandin?**

Arachidonic acid.

○ **Name the pathway through which prostaglandins are released.**

Cyclooxygenase pathway.

○ **What compound is responsible for dysmenorrhea?**

PGF.

○ **Name another pathway that is not blocked by NSAIDs and produce leukotrienes?**

The lipoxygenase pathway.

○   **In primary dysmenorrhea, when is the typical onset in relation to the menstrual cycle?**

The pain usually begins a few hours prior to or just after the onset of menses. The pain may last for 48 to 72 hours.

○   **Describe the nature of the pain.**

It is colicky, with suprapubic cramping that may or may not be accompanied by back pain, nausea, vomiting, and diarrhea.

○   **How is it diagnosed?**

It is generally a diagnosis of exclusion, once underlying pathology has been excluded.

○   **What is the treatment of choice?**

Prostaglandin synthase inhibitors (i.e., nonsteroidal anti-inflammatory agents).

○   **How should they be taken?**

Take the inhibitors just prior to or at the onset of pain and then continuously every 6 to 8 hours to prevent reformation of prostaglandin by-products.

○   **In what percentage of cases are prostaglandin inhibitors effective treatment?**

80%.

○   **Name a form of treatment that acts by decreasing endometrial proliferation, thus decreasing the production of prostaglandins?**

Birth control pills.

○   **What percentage of women with primary dysmenorrhea will have relief with birth control pills?**

90%.

○   **What other pharmacological agents may improve dysmenorrhea?**

Glyceryl trinitrate, magnesium, calcium antagonists, vitamin B, vitamin E, herbs.

○   **What other nonpharmacologic approaches may improve dysmenorrhea?**

Rest, heating pad to lower abdomen and back, regular nutritious diet, exercise, transcutaneous electrical nerve stimulation (TENS), acupuncture/acupressure, and uterosacral nerve ablation/resection.

○   **Define secondary dysmenorrhea.**

Menstrual pain with underlying pelvic pathology.

○   **In relation to the menstrual cycle, when does the pain of secondary dysmenorrhea begin?**

1 to 2 weeks prior to menses. It will generally continue until a few days after the cessation of bleeding.

○ **Name the most common cause of secondary dysmenorrhea?**

Endometriosis. This is followed by adenomyosis, infection (i.e., intrauterine device), and adhesions.

○ **Name three causes of secondary dysmenorrhea that are a result of blockage of the outflow tract.**

Imperforate hymen, transverse vaginal septum, and cervical stenosis.

○ **Name five causes of secondary dysmenorrhea that are uterine related.**

Endometrial polyps, uterine leiomyoma, adenomyosis, Asherman's syndrome, pelvic congestion, and uterine anomalies.

○ **What is pelvic congestion syndrome?**

It is one of the etiologies of secondary dysmenorrhea and results from congestion of the uterus and engorgement of varicosities of broad ligaments.

○ **What is the term for the cyclic appearance of a large constellation of symptoms (more than 100) just prior to menses followed by a period of time entirely free of symptoms?**

Premenstrual syndrome or PMS.

○ **Who first defined premenstrual syndrome and when?**

R.T. Frank, MD, Chief of Obstetrics and Gynecology at Mt. Sinai Hospital in NYC, in 1931.

○ **Name the most common symptoms of PMS.**

Bloating, anxiety or tension, breast tenderness, depression, fatigue, irritability, and appetite changes.

○ **How is the diagnosis of PMS made?**

It is a clinical diagnosis often based on a cycle diary. However, the National Institute of Mental Health has suggested that PMS requires documentation of at least a 30% increase in the severity of symptoms within 5 days prior to menses, and a symptom-free period starting sometime during the menses.

○ **What percentage of women suffers from PMS?**

It is actually difficult to ascertain, but up to 80% of women develop emotional and physical changes related to their cycles during the reproductive years.

○ **How is the cognitive function of women with PMS changed during the luteal phase?**

Despite the feelings of inadequacy, women with PMS show no deficit in memory, attention, or concentration.

○ **Name six nonpharmacologic treatments that should be initial treatment for PMS?**

Elimination of caffeine

Smoking cessation

Regular exercise

Adequate sleep

Decreased stress

Regular, nutritious diet

○ **What dietary supplement has been associated with 48% reduction in symptom scores?**

Calcium (1200 mg daily).

○ **Name the differential diagnoses of premenstrual dysphoric disorder (PMDD).**

Underlying psychiatric disorder, thyroid abnormalities, migraine, diabetes, asthma, epilepsy, irritable bowel syndrome, and autoimmune disorders.

○ **What is PMDD?**

PMDD is considered a psychiatric disorder; where women predominantly have emotional symptoms that are serious enough to disrupt their personal relationships and interfere with their daily lives.

○ **Approximately what percentage of women suffer from PMDD?**

2% to 8%.

○ **What is the treatment for PMDD?**

Selective serotonin uptake inhibitors (SSRIs) are most effective in low doses taken during the luteal phase of the menstrual cycle.

○ **Which patient group with PMDD may be recommended continuous SSRI therapy?**

Patients who have comorbid depressive or anxiety disorders, and who are not adherent to dosing schedule or not able to tolerate intermittent therapy.

○ **What other medications may relieve PMS symptoms?**

Oral contraceptives, diuretics, and danazol.

CHAPTER 28 Ectopic Pregnancy

Radmila Kazanegra, MD

○ **What has happened to the rate of ectopic pregnancies in the United States during the past 20 years?**

The rate went from 4.5/1000 to 20/1000 pregnancies during 1970 to 1992.

○ **What percentage of conceptions are ectopic pregnancies?**

About 2 in 100 women have an ectopic pregnancy (2%).

○ **Are ectopic pregnancies more common in multigravid or nulligravid women?**

Multigravid. Only 10% to 15% of ectopic pregnancies are found in nulligravid women.

○ **What has happened to ectopic mortality since 1970?**

The rate of death has dropped sevenfold from 3.5/1000 to 0.5/1000 cases. Ectopic pregnancy remains the most common cause of maternal death in the first trimester and accounts for 4% to 10% of all pregnancy-related deaths.

○ **What is the most common cause of death in women with ectopic pregnancies?**

Acute blood loss accounts for more than 85% of deaths.

○ **What is the most common misdiagnosis for fetal ectopic pregnancy?**

Gastrointestinal disorder is the most common misdiagnosis, followed by intrauterine pregnancy and pelvic inflammatory disease.

○ **What can increase the likelihood of early diagnosis of ectopic pregnancy?**

Identification of risk factors, high index of suspicion, and transvaginal ultrasound.

○ **What is the most common etiology of ectopic pregnancy?**

About half of ectopic pregnancies can be linked to a history of pelvic inflammatory disease.

○   **Do chromosomal abnormalities increase the risk of ectopic pregnancy?**

Pregnancy associated with chromosomal abnormality does not increase the risk of having an ectopic pregnancy.

○   **What is the rate of ectopic pregnancy in women with a history of pelvic inflammatory disease, as compared to the general population?**

A fivefold increase in ectopic pregnancy from 16.8/1000, is seen in women with a history of PID.

○   **List the high risk factors for ectopic pregnancy.**

Previous ectopic pregnancy
Previous tubal surgery
Tubal ligation
Tubal pathology
In utero DES exposure
Current IUD use

○   **List the moderate risk factors for ectopic pregnancy.**

Infertility
Previous cervicitis (gonorrhea, chlamydia)
History of pelvic inflammatory disease
Multiple sexual partners
Smoking

○   **List the low-risk factors for ectopic pregnancy.**

Previous pelvic/abdominal surgery
Vaginal douching
Early age of intercourse (<18 years)

○   **What percentage of pregnancies after tubal ligation are ectopic pregnancies?**

The incidence depends on the type of tubal ligation; up to 50% of pregnancies after laparoscopic fulguration are ectopic pregnancies.

○   **What percentage of women with a previous ectopic pregnancy will conceive again?**

About 60% of women with a history of an ectopic pregnancy will conceive again; 15% will be another ectopic pregnancy. This may be dependent on age, history, prior infertility, and ectopic management.

○   **What is the best predictor of a successful intrauterine pregnancy in a woman with a history of ectopic pregnancy?**

The best predictor of another pregnancy is the condition of the contralateral tube.

○   **Is the rate of ectopic pregnancy higher or lower in women with an IUD?**

The rate of any pregnancy is much lower with an IUD, including ectopic pregnancies. IUDs, however, are more effective at preventing intrauterine pregnancy, making an ectopic pregnancy more likely (about 5%), if an IUD is in place. This varies with a copper device having a very low rate, while a progesterone IUD increases the risk caused by lowered tubal motility.

○ **Are ectopic pregnancies more or less likely during in vitro fertilization?**

Ectopic pregnancies are more likely, accounting for 3% of IVF pregnancies, especially with tubal disease and very high hormone levels.

○ **Does therapeutic abortion increase the risk of an ectopic pregnancy in the future?**

When controlling for other variables, studies have found no association between elective abortion and subsequent ectopic pregnancy.

○ **What is the most likely site of an ectopic pregnancy within the tube?**

More than 80% of tubal pregnancies are ampullary; the next most common site is isthmic.

○ **Besides the tube, what is most common location for an ectopic pregnancy?**

Although 98% of ectopics are found in the tube, 1.4% are in the abdomen. Less common are ectopics in the uterine cornua, cervix, and ovary.

○ **What is the incidence of ovarian pregnancy?**

Ovarian pregnancy occurs in 1 per 7000 pregnancies and is becoming more common.

○ **What are the risk factors for ovarian pregnancy?**

It is a random event. History of pelvic inflammatory disease or the use of an intrauterine contraceptive device does not increase the risk of ovarian pregnancy.

○ **Does a history of ovarian pregnancy increase the risk for recurrent ectopic pregnancy or infertility?**

There is no such association established.

○ **What is the source of an abdominal pregnancy?**

It is thought that most abdominal pregnancies were tubal abortions.

○ **What is the appropriate treatment for an abdominal pregnancy?**

Delivery of the fetus at the time of diagnosis with retention of the placenta if attached to mesentery or bowel.

○ **What is an interstitial pregnancy?**

A pregnancy implanted at the proximal segment, interstitial portion of the fallopian tube, which is embedded within the muscular wall of the uterus.

○ **What is the incidence of interstitial pregnancy?**

2% of all ectopic pregnancies.

○ **What are the risk factors for interstitial pregnancy?**

Risk factors are the same as for other tubal pregnancies. However, ipsilateral salpingectomy is a risk factor specific for interstitial pregnancy.

○ **What is a hysterotomy scar pregnancy?**

A pregnancy implanted at the previous hysterotomy (cesarean) scar.

○ **What is the incidence of hysterotomy scar pregnancy?**

6% of ectopic pregnancies among women with a prior cesarean delivery, 2% of all ectopic pregnancies.

○ **Is the incidence of hysterotomy scar pregnancies related to number of previous cesarean deliveries?**

No. Implantation occurs because the embryo migrates through a defect within the scar.

○ **How frequent are heterotopic pregnancies?**

About 1/4000 to 1/8000 pregnancies. The incidence increases to about 1/100 with assisted reproductive technologies.

○ **In a heterotopic pregnancy, how often will the intrauterine pregnancy survive after surgery for the ectopic pregnancy?**

About two-thirds of the intrauterine pregnancies survive following salpingectomy.

○ **How deep does the trophoblast invade into the tube?**

As there is no decidua to limit trophoblast growth, the pregnancy frequently grows through the muscularis of the tube.

○ **What percentage of women with ectopic pregnancy reports, "passing tissue"?**

5% to 10% of women with ectopic pregnancy report passing tissue; women with ectopic pregnancy can pass the decidual cast, which can be misinterpreted as a spontaneous abortion.

○ **What are some of the symptoms associated with tubal rupture and hemoperitoneum?**

Worsening pain, shoulder pain (as a result of diaphragmatic irritation), and dizziness/syncope.

○ **In addition to pain, what is the most common presenting symptom for women with an ectopic pregnancy?**

The second most common symptom is amenorrhea/missed menses.

○ **What is the most common location of pain with an ectopic pregnancy?**

Most commonly the pain is generalized over the abdomen. When localized, the most common site is unilateral lower quadrant. Shoulder pain is also common.

○ **What sign can distinguish an ectopic pregnancy from pelvic inflammatory disease?**

Fever is rare with ectopic pregnancy (<2% of women).

○ **How often is an adnexal mass found in women with an ectopic pregnancy?**

Fifty percent of women with an ectopic pregnancy have an adnexal mass.

○ **How often is an ectopic pregnancy diagnosed the first time the patient presents?**

About half of the patients are incorrectly diagnosed at least once prior to identification of the ectopic pregnancy.

○ **What are the most commonly used tools for establishing a diagnosis of ectopic pregnancy?**

hCG levels and pelvic ultrasound are the most common tools for diagnosing ectopic pregnancy. In 85% of women with ectopic pregnancy, the hCG level is lower than expected. hCG levels should increase at least 66% every 48 hours. There is a 90% chance that a rise less than this indicates an abnormal pregnancy (ectopic or spontaneous abortion), although 15% of normal pregnancies rises slower.

○ **What three patterns of hCG rise can be seen with an ectopic pregnancy?**

The hCG patterns associated with an ectopic pregnancy can be an abnormal rise (see previous question), a falling level, or a shift to the right (normal rise occurring later than expected based on menstrual dates).

○ **When culdocentesis is done to diagnose an ectopic pregnancy, what finding is considered diagnostic?**

Nonclotting blood with a hematocrit more than 15% is diagnostic.

○ **How often does a positive culdocentesis indicate an ectopic pregnancy?**

About 85% of positive tests are associated with an ectopic pregnancy; a bleeding corpus luteum can give a false-positive result.

○ **What progesterone level predicts a normal intrauterine pregnancy?**

A progesterone value greater than 25 ng/mL suggests a normal pregnancy. There is no single level that will definitely confirm a normal pregnancy or rule out an ectopic.

○ **What progesterone level predicts an abnormal pregnancy?**

A progesterone level less than 5 ng/mL suggests an abnormal pregnancy; this does not distinguish between a spontaneous abortion and an ectopic pregnancy.

○ **At what hCG level would an intrauterine pregnancy be seen by transabdominal pelvic ultrasound?**

An hCG level greater than 6500 mIU/mL should show a gestational sac. The yolk sac and fetal pole may not be seen at this level.

○ **At what hCG level would an intrauterine pregnancy be seen by transvaginal ultrasound?**

The discriminatory zone for detecting an intrauterine pregnancy by transvaginal ultrasound is an hCG level greater than 1500 mIU/mL.

○ **Which of the two following findings is the most common sign of an ectopic pregnancy by transvaginal ultrasound: adnexal mass or absence of an intrauterine pregnancy?**

An adnexal mass or gestational sac in the adnexa is a less reliable finding and is not always seen in early ectopic pregnancies. The absence of an intrauterine pregnancy at an hCG level >1500 mIU/mL is highly predictive of an ectopic pregnancy.

○ **If the hCG level is less than 3000 mIU/mL and rising abnormally, what diagnostic test(s) can be used to confirm the diagnosis of ectopic pregnancy?**

If the woman is not symptomatic, the options are: Continue to follow the hCG level until it reaches the diagnostic level and repeat the transvaginal ultrasound or perform a diagnostic dilation and curettage (D & C) to rule out an abnormal intrauterine pregnancy. If symptomatic, diagnostic laparoscopy can be performed.

○ **Does the presence of a thick endometrial stripe indicate an intrauterine pregnancy?**

The endometrium can be thickened as a result of the hormonal stimulation associated with either an ectopic or intrauterine pregnancy, so this is not a consistent sign of a normal pregnancy.

○ **Does the presence of a gestational sac always rule out an ectopic?**

Up to 15% of women with an ectopic pregnancy can have a "pseudosac" or fluid area (representing blood and mucus) within the cavity. Therefore, it is critical with women at high risk for an ectopic pregnancy to confirm an intrauterine pregnancy with a follow-up ultrasound. This ultrasound will identify the yolk sac ("double ring sign") or fetal pole within the gestational sac.

○ **Is Doppler flow ultrasonography useful in the diagnosis of ectopic pregnancy?**

Studies suggest that Doppler flow may be useful in identifying the presence and location of a cervical ectopic pregnancy.

○ **What series of test(s) are considered to be the best predictors of early ectopic pregnancies?**

The combination of serial hCG levels and transvaginal ultrasound gives the best positive (and negative) predictive value for diagnosing ectopic pregnancies.

○ **In a symptomatic patient, when ultrasound is not available, what tests give the best positive predictive value of an ectopic pregnancy?**

The combination of a positive hCG and a positive culdocentesis is an excellent predictor of ectopic pregnancy.

○ **Does a positive culdocentesis indicate a ruptured ectopic pregnancy?**

Although a positive culdocentesis is a strong predictor of an ectopic pregnancy, the tube may not be ruptured. Bleeding within the fallopian tube will frequently lead to a hemoperitoneum even when the tube is not ruptured. Similarly, cul de sac fluid can be found in 60% of nonruptured ectopics on ultrasound.

○ **Does color Doppler ultrasonography have advantages over gray-scale scans?**

Yes, there is an increased diagnostic sensitivity for both ectopic and failed intrauterine pregnancies.

○ **At what gestational age does tubal rupture most commonly occur?**

Rupture of an ampullary ectopic typically occurs at 8 to 12 weeks, allowing adequate time for early diagnosis and treatment prior to rupture in most cases. Isthmic ectopics may rupture earlier at 6 to 8 weeks.

○ **What type of ectopic pregnancy has the highest mortality rate?**

Although a rare site of an ectopic pregnancy, the highest mortality rate occurs with cornual pregnancies.

○ **Should women with ectopic pregnancies be given RhoGAM?**

Most authors recommend administration of miniRhoGAM (50 μg) with any failed pregnancy up to 12 weeks (with full dose Rhogam after 12 weeks).

○ **What are the indications for laparotomy for treatment of ectopic pregnancy?**

Common indications for laparotomy include an unstable patient, large hemoperitoneum, cornual pregnancy, and lack of appropriate surgical tools for laparoscopy. Some authors would also include a large ectopic (>6 cm) and fetal heart tones in the adnexa as indications for laparotomy.

○ **What are the indications for conservative surgical therapy (conservation of the fallopian tube)?**

The tube can be conserved if the tube has minimal damage and the woman desires further fertility.

○ **List the possible techniques for conservative tubal surgery.**

Possible conservative techniques include salpingostomy, fimbrial evacuation, and segmental resection (with future reanastomosis of the tube).

○ **Which of the techniques listed in the previous question increase the risk of a future ectopic pregnancy?**

Fimbrial evacuation, with milking of the ectopic from the distal end of the tube, increases the risk of another ectopic pregnancy.

○ **When should salpingectomy be performed?**

With a severely damaged tube, recurrent ectopic in that tube, uncontrolled hemorrhage or a desire for sterility especially after previous tubal ligation.

○ **What is the advantage of linear salpingostomy for a woman desiring future fertility?**

The rate of subsequent ectopic pregnancy is not increased when compared to salpingectomy, and the chance of future delivery is increased.

○ **If a salpingectomy is performed, what is the best predictor of future fertility?**

The best predictor is the degree of adhesive disease and the quality of the contralateral tube as well as a history of past fertility.

○ **What is the advantage of closing the salpingostomy site on the fallopian tube?**

There is no advantage to suturing the salpingostomy site.

○ **What follow up is required for women undergoing linear salpingostomy?**

Serial hCG levels are necessary to rule out persistent trophoblastic tissue.

○ **What is the risk of persistent ectopic pregnancy with linear salpingostomy?**

About 5% to 10% of ectopic pregnancies treated by linear salpingostomy will have retained trophoblastic tissue and require further therapy.

○ **How is a persistent ectopic pregnancy treated?**

This can be treated with medical therapy or removal of the affected tube. Expectant management can be considered, if the hCG levels are falling.

○ **When observing the tube at surgery, what is the most likely site of the ectopic pregnancy?**

The most likely site of implantation is proximal to the most dilated portion of the tube.

○ **What is the advantage of laparoscopy vs laparotomy for treatment of an ectopic pregnancy?**

The primary advantages are: Decreased hospital stay, decreased recovery, and decreased costs (more than 20 million dollars/year, if laparoscopy is performed primarily).

○ **What is the most common clinical presentation of cervical pregnancy?**

Profuse painless vaginal bleeding.

○ **What is the incidence of cervical pregnancy?**

1/9000.

○ **What is the treatment for hemodynamically stable patients diagnosed with cervical pregnancy?**

Multidose systemic methotrexate (MTX) with intra-amniotic and/or intrafetal injection of local potassium chloride (KCL), if fetal cardiac activity is present.

○ **What is the treatment for a patient with hemorrhage diagnosed with cervical pregnancy?**

Hysterectomy; if there is uncontrolled hemorrhage (avoid, if possible, in cases of desired further childbearing). Dilation and evacuation with preoperative measures (such as transvaginal ligation of the cervical branches of the uterine arteries, Shirodkar cerclage, angiographic uterine artery embolization, or intracervical vasopressin injection) to reduce incidence of severe hemorrhage.

○ **What additional measures can be used to control the profuse bleeding in patient diagnosed with cervical pregnancy?**

- Foley catheter with a 30 mL balloon into the dilated cervix, with the tip extending into the uterine cavity for 24 to 48 hours in combination with a purse-string suture around the external cervical os to prevent expulsion of the balloon.
- Placement of hemostatic sutures, locally in the cervix.
- Angiographic embolization.
- Bilateral internal iliac artery ligation.
- Bilateral uterine artery ligation.

○ **What is the mode of action of methotrexate?**

Methotrexate is a folic acid antagonist.

○ **The original methotrexate treatment regimens included multiple doses of methotrexate and alternate "rescue" treatments. What was given for "rescue"?**

Leucovorin also known as folinic acid.

○ **What short-term side effect can be seen with the dose of methotrexate used for ectopic pregnancy?**

Nausea, vomiting, stomatitis, mouth ulcerations, diarrhea, and fatigue have been reported. Thrombocytopenia, liver abnormalities, and neutropenia are rare.

○ **What is the risk of early ovarian failure with methotrexate use?**

There does not appear to be an increased risk of ovarian failure with this chemotherapeutic agent.

○ **Single dose methotrexate therapy (typically 50 mg/m² of body surface area) has what primary advantage over multiple treatment regimens?**

Fewer side effects are seen with single dose treatment. The success rate is similar.

○ **What patients are reasonable candidates for medical treatment of an ectopic pregnancy?**

Early diagnosis of ectopic pregnancy in an asymptomatic patient, without a large adnexal mass allows the choice of medical therapy.

○ **What lab values should be checked prior to giving methotrexate?**

Baseline hCG levels, liver function tests, platelet count, and white blood cell count should be checked before and after treatment. After treatment, hCG levels should be followed to zero.

○ **What criteria are used for assuring the success of methotrexate?**

With a single dose therapy, the hCG levels should fall by 15% betweendays 4 and 7 after therapy and continue to fall weekly until undetectable.

○ **How common is pelvic pain following methotrexate therapy?**

Up to 30% of women will experience pain within 2 weeks of treatment.

○ **Does pelvic pain after methotrexate require surgery?**

Although these patients should be followed closely with ultrasound and CBCs, the pain often resolves without surgery.

○ **When is second dose of methotrexate required?**

If the hCG level does not fall at 1 week, a second dose is required.

○ **What percentage of women require a second dose of therapy?**

About 6% of women getting single-dose therapy require a second dose.

○ **What percentage of women are successfully treated with methotrexate?**

Studies suggest that between 85% and 95% of women are successfully treated with medical therapy.

○ **How does ectopic rate compare with medical vs surgical therapy?**

The rate of repeated ectopic pregnancy following medical therapy compares favorably with surgical therapy (8% vs 15%).

○   **What percentage of patients treated with methotrexate rupture?**

10%, depending on location and initial hCG titer.

○   **What percentage of ectopic pregnancies will spontaneously resolve?**

It has been estimated that up to 60% or more of ectopic pregnancies will resolve without therapy.

○   **What is the best predictor of spontaneous resolution of an ectopic pregnancy?**

The best predictor is an hCG level <1000 mIU/mL at the time of diagnosis (up to 85% resolve spontaneously).

○   **If the hCG levels are falling, is surgery or medical therapy required in a patient with an ectopic pregnancy?**

Treatment is only required if the patient is symptomatic or the hCG levels do not continue to fall. Active treatment is indicted if compliance is a concern.

○   **What materials have successfully treated ectopic pregnancy when injected into the fallopian tube?**

Prostaglandins, glucose solutions, salt solutions, and methotrexate have been used for injecting directly into the ectopic pregnancy. This procedure may have a higher failure rate and is technically difficult, and thus, less commonly used. The best success is with injected methotrexate.

○   **What counseling should be provided to a woman with an ectopic pregnancy?**

Women need to be aware of the decreased fecundity associated with a history of an ectopic pregnancy, as well as the increased risk of another ectopic pregnancy. As with any pregnancy loss, supportive counseling should be offered.

○   **How should a woman with a history of an ectopic pregnancy be followed in a subsequent pregnancy?**

Early monitoring of the pregnancy with hCG levels and transvaginal ultrasound.

CHAPTER 29 Genital Tract Infections and Pelvic Inflammatory Disease

Maria A. Giraldo-Isaza, MD

○ **What are some medical sequelae of Pelvic Inflammatory Disease (PID)?**

Increased rate of ectopic pregnancy, chronic and acute pelvic pain, and infertility.

○ **What are some common organisms causing PID?**

The infection is usually polymicrobial, commonly included are *Chlamydia trachomatis*, *Neisseria gonorrhea*, CMV, endogenous aerobic and anaerobic bacteria, and rarely genital *Mycoplasma species*.

○ **N. gonorrhea and C. trachomatis coexist in the same individual in what percentage of the time?**

25% to 50% of the time.

○ **What percentage of women with asymptomatic gonococcal cervical infection will develop acute salpingitis?**

15%.

○ **What is the incidence of infertility with one episode of PID?**

10% and 25% with second episode, and 40% to 60% with a third episode.

○ **What is Fitz-Hugh-Curtis Syndrome?**

Syndrome characterized by perihepatic inflammation that occurs in 5% to 10% of patients with PID, likely from transperitoneal or vascular route of *N. gonorrhea* or *C. trachomatis*.

○ **What is the most common nonviral sexually transmitted disease?**

Chlamydia trachomatis. It is more common than *Neisseria* by as much as 10 to 1 in some studies.

○ **What are the risk factors for sexually transmitted disease?**

Age at first intercourse, number of sexual partners, and lack of contraception.

○ **What is the alternative to doxycycline for treatment of *Chlamydia*?**

Azithromycin.

○ **What is the incidence of adnexal abscesses in patients with acute PID?**

Approximately 10%.

○ **What are some options for drainage of tubo-ovarian complexes?**

Laparoscopy, interventional radiology, colpotomy, or laparotomy.

○ **Which organisms should be covered when considering antibiotic treatment for tubo-ovarian abscess?**

Anaerobic organisms, which are predominantly present between 60% and 100% of cases.

○ **What is the infection most commonly associated with patients using an IUD?**

Actinomyces.

○ **What is the classic histologic finding of *Actinomyces israelii*?**

The classic "sulfur granules" are observed along with gram-positive filaments.

○ **What are the predominant presentations of pelvic tuberculosis?**

Infertility and abnormal uterine bleeding.

○ **What is the classic finding in chronic endometritis?**

The presence of plasma cells on endometrial biopsy.

○ **What are the three most prevalent primary viral infections of the vulva?**

Herpes genitalis, condyloma acuminatum, and molluscum contagiosum.

○ **What are some treatments of choice for symptomatic Bartholin duct cyst or abscess?**

Insertion of the Word catheter or marsupialization of the Bartholin duct cyst.

○ **What is the organism responsible for syphilis?**

The spirochete *Treponema pallidum.*

○ **In pregnant patients with penicillin allergies, what is the treatment for syphilis?**

Desensitization protocol and then treat with penicillin.

○ **What are the confirmatory tests for syphilis?**

The fluorescent treponemal antibody absorption (FTA-ABS) or microhemagglutination assay for antibodies to *T. Pallidum* (MHA-TP). The VDRL (Venereal Disease Research Laboratories) or RPR (rapid plasma reagin) are nonspecific and are only used for screening.

○   **What is the classic skin lesion of primary syphilis?**

It is the chancre—a firm, painless ulcer that develops at a mucus or cutaneous site of entry of the spirochete.

○   **When does a serologic test for syphilis become positive after exposure?**

Generally, 4 to 6 weeks after exposure.

○   **What percentage of women with primary herpes experience systemic symptoms?**

70%. Primary herpes is much more severe than recurrent infection.

○   **How long can viral shedding occur after herpetic vulvar lesions appear?**

Up to 2 to 3 weeks.

○   **What is the benefit of acyclovir in the treatment of genital herpes?**

It reduces the duration of ulcerative lesions and the median duration of viral shedding, and decreases the recurrence rate when given prophylactically.

○   **What is the pathognomonic microscopic finding of Granuloma inguinale?**

Donovan bodies, which are clusters of dark staining, bipolar-appearing bacteria in large mononuclear cells.

○   **What is lymphogranuloma venereum (LGV)?**

A chronic infection of lymphatic tissue produced by Chlamydia trachomatis, serotypes L1, L2, or L3.

○   **What is the classic clinical sign of LGV?**

A "groove sign", a linear depression between the inguinal and femoral groups of inflamed nodes.

○   **What is the treatment for LGV?**

Oral tetracycline or erythromycin (500 mg every 6 hours) for 21 days.

○   **What causes molluscum contagiosum?**

Poxvirus. It is acquired both through sexual and nonsexual contact.

○   **What is the difference between the ulcer of chancroid and syphilis?**

The lesion of chancroid is always painful and tender; whereas, the chancre of syphilis is usually asymptomatic.

○   **What is chancroid caused by?**

Haemophilus ducreyi, a nonmotile, anaerobic, small gram-negative rod.

○   **What is the treatment for pediculosis pubis?**

Topical application of lindane (Kwell) or 5% permethrin dermal cream (Nix). The organism responsible is the crab louse *Phthirus pubis.*

○   **How is scabies diagnosed?**

It is diagnosed by scraping of the papules, vesicles, or burrows and looking for the mite *Sarcoptes scabiei* under the microscope.

○   **What is the classic finding on wet smear of bacterial vaginosis?**

Clue cells, which are vaginal epithelial cells with clusters of bacteria covering their surfaces.

○   **What is the treatment of choice for bacterial vaginosis?**

Metronidazole. Alternatives included clindamycin or augmentin.

○   **The appearance of a "strawberry cervix" is a classic sign of what infection?**

Trichomonas vaginalis.

○   **What is the treatment for candidal vaginitis?**

Topical application of one of the synthetic imidazoles, terconazole, butonconazole, or oral fluconazole.

○   **What is the most practical method of diagnosing candidal vaginitis?**

Apply of KOH on a wet smear and look for presence of mycelial and blastospore forms.

○   **What human papillomavirus serotypes usually cause genital warts?**

Types 6 and 11.

○   **What percentage of individuals infected with the human papillomavirus develop genital warts?**

3%.

○   **What are some treatment options for vulvar condyloma?**

Provider applied: Trichloroacetic acid, podophyllin, cryosurgery, laser ablation, or 5-fluorouracil cream. Patient applied: Imiquimod or podophyllin (Condylox gel or liquid).

○   **What are the criteria for hospitalization of patients with PID?**

A patient should be hospitalized when: a surgical emergency cannot be excluded, the patient is pregnant, the patient does not respond to oral antibiotic therapy, the patient is unable to follow or tolerate oral therapy, the patient suffers from tubo-ovarian abscess, and the patient has severe illness, nausea, vomiting or high fever.

○   **What is the treatment of choice for the condition shown below?**

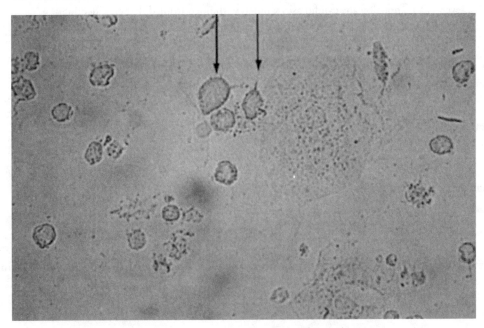

Reused, with permission, from Hansfield HH. Atlas of Sexuallty Transmitted Diseases. New York: McGraw-Hill, 1992.

Metronidazole 2 g orally, single dose or tinidazole 2 g orally, single dose is the treatment of choice for trichomoniasis.

○   **Which are the most specific criteria for the diagnosis of PID?**

Endometrial biopsy with histological evidence of endometritis, transvaginal ultrasound, or MRI showing thickened fluid-filled tubes with or without free pelvic fluid or tubo-ovarian abscess, or Doppler suggesting pelvic infection and laparoscopic findings of PID.

○   **Is a test of cure for chlamydia routinely recommended?**

No, unless the patient is pregnant, therapeutic compliance is in question, symptoms persist, or reinfection is suspected. If indicated, should be done 3- to 4 weeks after treatment is completed.

○   **Which are the clinical criteria for bacterial vaginosis, and how many do you need to make the diagnosis?**

The diagnosis is made if at least three of the following criteria are present:

(1) Homogeneous, thin, white discharge that coats the vaginal walls

(2) Clue cells on microscopic exam

(3) Vaginal pH >4.5

(4) Whiff test positive

○   **What is the definition of recurrent vulvo vaginal candidiasis (VVC)?**

Four or more episodes in 1 year.

○   **What is the first-line maintenance regimen for recurrent vulvovaginal candidiasis?**

Oral fluconazole, weekly for 6 months (100- to 150- or 200-mg weekly).

○ **Characteristics of complicated vulvovaginal candidiasis include?**

Recurrent VVC, severe VVC, nonalbicans candidiasis, women with uncontrolled diabetes, debilitation, immunosuppression, or pregnancy.

○ **When should the partner be treated when you made the diagnosis of chancroid?**

The partner should be treated if sexual contact occurs within the last 10 days preceding the symptoms.

○ **What is the most sensitive test for diagnosis of HSV?**

PCR.

○ **What is the current recommendation for screening of chlamydia?**

Annual screening should be performed in all sexually active women aged 25 years and younger, and other asymptomatic women at increased risk for infection.

○ **True or False: Suppressive therapy reduces the frequency of genital herpes recurrences by 70% to 80% in patients with more than six recurrences per year.**

True.

○ **What is the recommended regimen for granuloma inguinale?**

Doxycycline 100 mg bid for at least 3 weeks and until all lesions are completely healed.

○ **When should the sexual partner be treated, if you diagnose a patient with granuloma inguinale?**

Within 60 days before the symptoms.

CHAPTER 30

Benign Vulvar and Vaginal Lesions

Denise Hartman, MD

○ **What is the most common gynecologic problem of childhood?**

Vulvovaginitis.

○ **What are the two most common infectious causes of vulvovaginitis in children?**

Pinworms (*Enterobius vermicularis*) and *Candida*.

○ **What is the most common benign condition affecting the external genitalia?**

Contact dermatitis.

○ **What is vestibular adenitis?**

Chronic inflammation of the lesser vestibular glands lying just external to the hymenal ring; can get small, extremely painful ulcerations of the vestibular mucosa.

○ **What are the diagnostic criteria for vestibular adenitis?**

Characterized by dyspareunia, severe point tenderness by swab test, and vestibular erythema of varying degrees.

○ **How is vestibular adenitis best treated?**

Education, as this can be a chronic condition; alpha-interferon may be tried; surgical excision of the vestibular glands is a last resort but cures 60% to 80% of patients.

○ **What benign skin lesions commonly appear as white areas on the vulva and vagina?**

Vulvar dystrophies and vitiligo.

○ **What are the vulvar dystrophies as classified by the International Society for the Study of Vulvar Disease (ISSVD)?**

Lichen sclerosus, squamous cell hyperplasia, squamous cell carcinoma in situ, Paget's disease of the vulva, and other dermatoses.

○ **What features may histologically characterize the vulvar dystrophies?**

Excessive keratin (hyperkeratosis), relative avascularity, deep pigmentation, irregular thickening of the malpighian ridges (acanthosis), and inflammation.

○ **Why does hyperkeratosis occur?**

Because of disordered epithelial growth and nutrition, which can be a result of chronic irritation, chronic inflammation, cancer, or precancer.

○ **What is the treatment of squamous cell hyperplasia without atypia?**

Episodic mid- to high-potency topical corticosteroids.

○ **What is lichen sclerosus characterized by, histologically?**

Hyperkeratosis, thinning of the epidermis with acanthosis, and elongation of the rete pegs; upper dermis is hyalinized with a band of lymphocytes below this region.

○ **What is the appearance of vulvar lichen sclerosus?**

Thin, white, wrinkled skin, localized to the labia majora and/or minora. Although whitening may extend over the perineum and around the anus in a keyhole fashion; fissuring is frequently seen perianally, in intralabial folds, or around the clitoris; introitus may have yellow, waxy appearance.

○ **How is lichen sclerosus treated in a child?**

It usually regresses, but tiny amounts of clobetasol (topical corticosteroid) for a longer period of time appears successful in young girls and maintenance therapy not always required; topical corticosteroids can arrest the process and the symptoms.

○ **How is lichen sclerosus treated in the adult?**

High potency topical steroid, usually clobetasol 0.05% ointment or cream. The treatment is tapered over 4 to 6 weeks from initial BID/TID applications to a maintenance application of one- to three times weekly. This is a chronic condition that usually requires indefinite therapy.

○ **What is the new term for vulvodynia, according to the ISSVD?**

Generalized vulvar dysesthesia.

○ **What is generalized vulvar dysesthesia?**

Unexplained vulvar discomfort, usually described as burning pain occurring in the absence of a specific, relevant infection, inflammatory, or neoplastic condition. Generalized vulvar dysesthesia is thought to be of neuropathic etiology, and the most successful therapies are directed at treating the underlying neuropathy.

○ **What is the new term for vestibulitis according to the ISSVD?**

Localized vulvodynia. Unexplained localized tenderness and burning pain of the minor vestibular glands, in the absence of a specific, relevant infection, inflammatory or neoplastic condition. This is also considered a neuropathic condition, a diagnosis of exclusion.

○ **What are the most effective treatments for the generalized and localized vulvodynias?**

Systemic treatments aimed at treating neuropathies: Antidepressants (usually imipramine or desipramine) and/or gabapentin. In localized vulvodynia, vestibulectomy is curative in 60% to 80% of patients.

○ **What is intertrigo?**

Inflammatory condition of two closely opposed skin surfaces.

○ **In which patients is intertrigo of the vulva commonly found?**

Obese or diabetic women.

○ **What is the common distribution of intertrigo?**

Axilla, inframammary folds, groin, perineum, intergluteal folds, toe webs, interlabial, and intercrural folds.

○ **What causes labial agglutination?**

Chronic vulvar inflammation from any cause.

○ **What is the treatment for labial agglutination?**

If it is asymptomatic, no treatment is needed and often a girl's natural estrogen at the time of puberty will resolve the agglutination; if symptomatic, 2 to 4 weeks of topical estrogen may be used with manual separation.

○ **What symptom of labial agglutination requires prompt treatment for the agglutination?**

Inability to urinate.

○ **What is the most common cause of papillary lesions on the vulva?**

HPV.

○ **What characteristic of HPV explains the high rate of clinical relapse of treated warts?**

Viral latency.

○ **Which types of HPV are most commonly associated with malignancy?**

16 and 18.

○ **What cytotoxic agents are used in the treatment of HPV of the vulva?**

Podophyllin (mitotic poison), TCA (caustic agent), 5-FU (antimetabolite), imiquimod (immune modulator), alpha-interferon (immune modulator), and adefovir (nucleoside analog).

○ **What other techniques may be used in the treatment of HPV?**

Liquid nitrogen, electrocauterization, surgical excision, carbon dioxide laser, and CUSA (cavitary ultrasonic ablation).

○ **What is the duration of treatment of condyloma with 5-FU for vulvar and vaginal lesions?**

Two treatments of 5 to 7 days of consecutive nightly applications.

O **Which treatment for vaginal condylomas is contraindicated in pregnancy?**

Podophyllin.

O **What are the risk factors associated with vaginal condylomas and vaginal delivery?**

Trauma and heavy bleeding during delivery and infrequently, laryngeal papillomas in the newborn.

O **What is the most common cystic lesion of the vulva?**

Epidermal inclusion cyst.

O **What is an epidermal inclusion cyst?**

A cyst in which the cyst wall contains normal epidermis that produces keratin; most commonly these cysts arise from pilosebaceous ducts that have become occluded. A less common cause is traumatically buried skin fragments.

O **What is the treatment of inclusion cysts?**

They need no treatment unless infected or for cosmetic reasons. If infected, they can be incised and drained after antibiotic treatment is instituted.

O **What is the most common site of an inclusion cyst?**

The site of a previous laceration or episiotomy scar in the vagina or in the labia majora, especially the anterior half.

O **What is a syringoma?**

A benign adenoma of the eccrine sweat gland, found most often around the eyelids and less commonly on the vulva, chest, or abdomen.

O **How are Bartholin's duct abscesses treated?**

A small stab wound is made in the abscess and a Word catheter is inserted and left in place for 4 to 6 weeks to allow epithelialization of a tract and permanent opening of the gland.

O **How are recurrent Bartholin's duct cysts treated?**

Marsupialization.

O **How are Bartholin's duct cysts treated differently in postmenopausal women?**

Malignancy must be ruled out, all or part of the Bartholin's duct cyst should be removed for histologic evaluation.

O **What are the vulvovaginal cysts of embryonic origin?**

Mesonephric cysts, paramesonephric cysts, and urogenital sinus mucus cysts.

O **What is a Skene's duct cyst?**

Cystic dilatation of an occluded paraurethral duct, usually associated with infection in the duct.

○ **What is a complication of Skene's duct cysts?**

Urinary obstruction because of enlargement.

○ **The Gartner duct arises from what structure?**

Vestigial remnant of the vaginal portion of the mesonephric duct (wolffian duct).

○ **How do Gartner's duct cysts usually appear?**

Multiple tiny cystic dilations, most commonly, or rarely as a large single cyst in the anterolateral vaginal wall.

○ **Where does endometriosis most commonly appear in the vagina?**

Posterior fornix, as a result of penetration from the cul-de-sac.

○ **What is vaginal adenosis and what is it associated with?**

Presence of epithelial lined glands or their secretory products within the vagina and is associated with in utero exposure to DES.

○ **What are the exam findings of atrophic vaginitis?**

Vaginal mucosa is thin and pale with lack of normal rugae and often with visible blood vessels or petechial hemorrhages.

○ **What does a wet mount show with atrophic vaginitis?**

Small rounded parabasal epithelial cells with an increased number of PMNs.

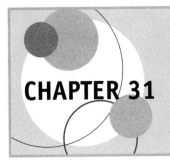

CHAPTER 31 Hysterectomy

Chase M. White, MD

○ **How many hysterectomies are done each year in the US?**

Approximately 600,000 hysterectomies are performed annually in the United States, making hysterectomy the second most-commonly performed operation for women of reproductive age, after caesarean section.

○ **What is the age distribution for women undergoing hysterectomy in the US?**

One study showed that two-thirds of all hysterectomies performed between 1994 and 1999 were for women aged 35 to 54.

○ **What are the most common indications for hysterectomy?**

From 1994 to 1999, 3,200,000 hysterectomies were performed in the US:

- 43.0% were done for leiomyomata.
- 19.9% for endometriosis.
- 18.8% for prolapse.
- 14.4% other indications (including malignancy).
- 3.8% for endometrial hyperplasia.

○ **What is the correct terminology regarding hysterectomy?**

(1) Simple hysterectomy means removal of the uterus.

(2) Subtotal hysterectomy leaves the uterine cervix in place.

(3) Total hysterectomy is the removal of the uterus as well as the cervix.

○ **Describe the various surgical approaches to hysterectomy.**

(1) Abdominal hysterectomy is performed through an abdominal incision.

(2) Vaginal hysterectomy is performed through the vagina.

(3) Laparoscopic hysterectomy is performed with the laparoscope.

(4) Laparoscope-assisted vaginal hysterectomy is a hysterectomy performed primarily via the vaginal approach, with the laparoscope used to take down pelvic adhesions and/or structures. This can also be done laparoscopically using the Da Vinci Robotic Surgical System.

(5) Radical hysterectomy is the removal of the uterus, the upper 25% of the vagina, all of the uterovesical and uterosacral ligaments, and the entire parametrium on either side, as well as pelvic lymph node dissection.

○   **What is the mortality associated with hysterectomy?**

12 deaths per 10,000 procedures, for all surgical indications.

○   **When is hysterectomy indicated in the management of dysfunctional uterine bleeding?**

Hysterectomy may be indicated for women with DUB who have completed their childbearing, particularly if the bleeding is severe and/or recurrent, and unresponsive to hormonal therapy and endometrial curettage.

○   **When is hysterectomy indicated for adenomyosis?**

Symptomatic patients who do not experience relief with D+C and hormonal therapy, and who have completed their childbearing, can be offered hysterectomy.

○   **When is hysterectomy indicated in treating uterine prolapse?**

When the symptoms are, especially in the patient's view, severe enough to justify the risks of surgery. Hysterectomy does not necessarily need to be done as part of an operation to correct stress incontinence. A retropubic urethropexy may be done with the uterus left in place.

○   **When is hysterectomy indicated in the treatment of leiomyomata uteri?**

If the patient has no symptoms, treatment can often be expectant. In women who have completed their childbearing and who have symptoms related to myomas, hysterectomy represents the definitive cure.

○   **When doing a hysterectomy for leiomyomata, what is the chance of discovering a leiomyosarcoma?**

Approximately 0.2% to 0.3%.

○   **What are the indications for cesarean hysterectomy?**
- Uterine rupture.
- An unrepairable uterine scar.
- Laceration of major uterine vessels.
- Placenta previa or accreta, unreducible uterine inversion.
- Placental abruption.
- Uterine atony unresponsive to conservative management.
- Severe cervical dysplasia or early cervical cancer may prompt a planned cesarean hysterectomy.

○   **What are the major causes of morbidity associated with cesarean hysterectomy?**

Febrile morbidity and injury to the urinary tract are more common than in the nonpregnant patient, and blood loss is usually much greater because of the hypertrophy of the uterus and the vessels. Elective cesarean hysterectomy is known to carry an average blood loss of 1,500 mL and should therefore not routinely be done for sterilization or for trivial indications.

○ **What other obstetrical problems may require hysterectomy?**

Occasionally, septic abortion fails to respond to medical management and must be treated with hysterectomy. Abdominal, cervical, and interstitial pregnancies may also result in hysterectomy.

○ **When is hysterectomy indicated in PID?**

Approximately 20% of patients with tubo-ovarian abscess will fail to respond to antibiotics and/or colpotomy drainage. These women are usually treated with TAH-BSO. Ruptured tubo-ovarian abscess may also be treated with TAH-BSO. Hysterectomy may also be recommended for patients with chronic PID who have completed childbearing or who are not interested in assisted reproductive technologies.

○ **When is hysterectomy indicated for cervical intraepithelial neoplasia?**

If there is persistent CIN 2 or 3 on follow-up after LEEP or conization, then reexcision is indicated. If reexcision is found to be technically impractical or if the woman has definitively completed childbearing, then hysterectomy is an option, but conization should be performed for frozen section prior to the hysterectomy to look for invasive cancer. If cancer is found by frozen section, radical hysterectomy may be appropriate; if no cancer is found, then simple hysterectomy is appropriate.

○ **When is hysterectomy indicated in the management of endometrial hyperplasia?**

Adenomatous hyperplasia with cytologic atypia is considered a precancerous lesion, and should be treated with hysterectomy except under very special circumstances. Less severe forms of hyperplasia, without cytologic atypia, can be managed medically. Hysterectomy for hyperplasia may be done vaginally or abdominally.

○ **What type of hysterectomy is done for adenocarcinoma of the endometrium?**

Systematic surgical staging for endometrial cancer requires total abdominal hysterectomy (TAH) with bilateral salpingo-oophorectomy (BSO), peritoneal washings, and bilateral pelvic and para-aortic lymphadenectomy.

○ **What procedures are used in the treatment of uterine sarcoma?**

TAH, BSO, pelvic washings, and pelvic and para-aortic lymphadenectomy make up the appropriate surgical treatment and staging of uterine sarcoma. Postoperative radiation and chemotherapy may be of benefit, but this is an evolving area.

○ **When is hysterectomy used in the treatment of gestational trophoblastic disease?**

In women who have completed their childbearing, hysterectomy performed during the first cycle of chemotherapy can reduce the total amount of chemotherapy required to achieve complete remission. Recurrence rates after successful treatment in these cases (with or without hysterectomy) are less than 5%.

Early hysterectomy is of no benefit in women with high-risk metastatic GTD with any of the following:

- hCG >40k
- brain or liver metastases
- antecedent term pregnancy
- >4 months since last pregnancy, or prior chemotherapy

○ **Is hysterectomy always part of the surgical management of ovarian cancer?**

Systematic surgical staging and debulking is required for ovarian cancer. The staging procedure includes TAH, BSO, pelvic washings and cytology, inspection of all peritoneal surfaces with debulking of any visible tumor, bilateral pelvic and para-aortic lymphadenectomy, omentectomy, and peritoneal biopsies. In younger women desiring fertility who at the time of operation are found to have ovarian cancer that is low grade and confined to one ovary, the staging procedure may be modified to leave the uterus and uninvolved ovary in place.

○ **What work-up should be done before recommending hysterectomy for chronic pelvic pain?**

Other potential sources of chronic pelvic pain (CPP), many of them nongynecologic should be ruled out. Exclude psychiatric, musculoskeletal, gastrointestinal, and urinary tract sources.

○ **In counseling a patient regarding hysterectomy, what points should be discussed?**

The patient should be told:

- what organs are to be removed
- what route is to be used
- how long she will need to recuperate
- what risks she must accept
- what benefits she can expect
- how long the operation will take
- whether she will need to take hormones afterward
- what effects hysterectomy will have on sexuality

○ **What risks should be discussed with a 38-year-old woman undergoing abdominal hysterectomy for 16-week size fibroid tumors?**

- Anesthesia complications.
- Hemorrhage (with need for transfusion).
- Infection (wound, vaginal cuff, urinary tract).
- Pulmonary embolus.
- Injury to the bladder, ureters, or bowel.
- Pneumonia and atelectasis.

○ **What risks should be discussed with a 58-year-old woman undergoing vaginal hysterectomy for uterine prolapse?**

- Anesthesia complications.
- Hemorrhage.
- Infection in the vaginal cuff or urinary tract.
- Pulmonary embolus.
- Injury to the ureters, bladder, or rectum.
- Fistulae.
- Pneumonia and atelectasis.
- Potential need for laparotomy in case of unexpected findings.

○ **What preoperative testing should be done in patients scheduled for hysterectomy?**

- A thorough history and physical will reveal special needs as well as help in the evaluation of potential risks.
- Each patient should have normal cervical cytology or complete evaluation of abnormal cytology to exclude invasive malignancy.
- A complete blood count will give the opportunity to correct anemia and identify thrombocytopenia.
- A urine examination for blood and leukocytes is done.
- An EKG is generally done in healthy women older than age 35.

- A chest film is ordered for smokers and those with suspected pulmonary disease.
- Under special circumstances, IVP, CT scan, mammogram, pulmonary function tests, colonoscopy, cystoscopy, or consultation from other medical specialists may be needed.

○ **When should IVP be done preoperatively?**

When the pelvic disease is extensive or located where the ureters may be compromised, such as with large adnexal masses or very large leiomyomata, or when extensive dissection is anticipated. Also, IVP should be done in women with Mullerian anomalies, since urinary collecting system anomalies are common in this group. If a previous pelvic operation may have injured the urinary tract, a preoperative IVP will help identify this.

○ **When should a "bowel prep" be done before hysterectomy?**

All hysterectomy patients should be instructed to eat light meals the day before surgery, and to remain NPO for 8 hours prior to surgery. Enemas may be given at home. A full mechanical bowel prep with electrolyte solution and antibiotics is reserved for those in whom bowel involvement is suspected—patients with bowel complaints, extensive endometriosis, or suspected ovarian cancer.

○ **What is the most frequent complication of hysterectomy?**

Infection. The most common organisms are those found in normal vaginal flora.

○ **Does pretreatment for bacterial vaginosis before hysterectomy reduce the rate of postoperative cuff cellulitis?**

No. Even though BV is associated with an increased risk of postoperative cuff cellulitis, pretreatment for BV does not appear to reduce this risk.

○ **What incisions are appropriate for abdominal hysterectomy?**

A midline lower abdominal incision should be used in cases of suspected malignancy to facilitate access to the upper abdomen. For benign indications, a transverse Pfannenstiel incision is the most commonly used. A Maylard or Cherney incision may be used, if exposure is difficult with the Pfannenstiel.

○ **When performing an abdominal hysterectomy, what should be done before making an incision?**

After induction of anesthesia, the bladder is emptied and a pelvic examination is performed. The abdominal skin and vagina are then prepped and draped. Failure to perform an examination under anesthesia can result in the wrong incision being chosen, or an inappropriate operation being done.

○ **Which patients undergoing hysterectomy should receive perioperative antibiotic prophylaxis?**

All patients undergoing hysterectomy should receive antibiotic prophylaxis. The target in administering antibiotic prophylaxis is to have the antibiotic present in tissue prior to incision and then throughout the procedure. The antibiotic chosen should have a spectrum broad enough to cover the typical organisms found during the procedure—gram positive for skin, and gram negative for abdominopelvic organisms.

○ **From a historical perspective, why are most abdominal hysterectomies total rather than subtotal, and how has this changed?**

Before 1950, cervical carcinoma was the most common female genital cancer in the US. Although this is still true worldwide, the incidence of cervix cancer in the US has fallen dramatically. Cervical stump cancer is difficult to treat and carries a poor prognosis. Therefore, before widespread Pap smear screening, it was felt that the cervix should almost always be removed. Recently, there has been renewed interest in subtotal hysterectomy because it is technically easier, and is associated with fewer surgical risks. Some have advocated cervical preservation to improve sexual (orgasmic) function, but the literature is divided as to whether any significant benefit exists in this area.

○ **What is the role of laparoscopic-assisted vaginal hysterectomy (LAVH)?**

LAVH is associated with faster postoperative recovery and less pain than abdominal hysterectomy. However, LAVH offers no advantages over simple vaginal hysterectomy (VH) when VH can be done. LAVH has its chief utility in detecting and possibly correcting pelvic adhesive disease that would otherwise make vaginal hysterectomy more technically difficult and potentially dangerous. A further use of laparoscopic assistance is the ligation of the infundibulopelvic ligaments when they are technically difficult to reach via the vaginal approach.

○ **When using a self-retaining retractor in a transverse incision, one must be aware of what potential nerve injury?**

The lateral femoral cutaneous nerve.

○ **What should be done immediately after the peritoneal cavity is entered?**

Pelvic washings should be obtained, if needed, and a thorough exploration of the abdomen and pelvis should be carried out.

○ **Which ligament is divided first in performing abdominal hysterectomy?**

The round ligament. In cases where severe anatomic distortion or adhesions are found, the round ligament will almost always be identifiable, and can be followed to the uterus.

○ **If the adnexa are to be left in, where should the next clamps be placed?**

On the tube and utero-ovarian ligament, as close to the uterus as possible. A window can be made in the peritoneum inferior to the fallopian tube; a clamp is then placed across the tube and the utero-ovarian ligament, just next to the uterus. This preserves the blood vessels located in the broad ligament as much as possible.

○ **What must be identified and located prior to clamping the infundibulopelvic ligament?**

The ureter. The most common site of ureteral injury is at the pelvic brim near the infundibulopelvic ligament, and the most common procedure during which it is injured is abdominal hysterectomy.

○ **When is the ureter most likely to be injured?**

During attempts to obtain hemostasis.

○ **Why are the anterior and posterior broad ligament peritoneum incised prior to clamping the uterine vessels?**

This procedure, often referred to as "skeletonizing" the uterine vessels, aids in avoiding injury to the ureters and bladder, and provides a smaller pedicle that is less likely to slip out of a clamp.

○ **What is the purpose of incising the anterior leaf of the broad ligament?**

To facilitate dissection of the bladder from the lower uterine segment. In order to perform a total abdominal hysterectomy, the bladder must be completely mobilized.

○ **Where are the ureters located when the uterine vessels are being clamped?**

The ureter passes underneath the uterine artery ("water under the bridge") very close to the level of the internal cervical os. If the bladder has been mobilized, and the uterine vessels skeletonized, the ureter will be approximately 1.5 to 2 cm inferior and lateral to the uterine vessel clamps.

○ **Why are the uterine arteries usually doubly clamped abdominally, while they are only singly clamped during a vaginal hysterectomy?**

Double clamps are useful abdominally because there is a danger of tissue slipping out of a single clamp and the uterine artery retracting. Attempts at re-clamping a retracted vessel may result in injury to the ureter. When operating vaginally, there is not enough room between the ureter and the uterine artery to safely apply two clamps. Curved Heaney clamps are designed to be used as single vascular clamps.

○ **What structures must be avoided when clamping the uterosacral ligaments?**

The pelvic portion of the ureter and the anterior rectal wall.

○ **What mistake in performing a total abdominal hysterectomy is most likely to result in a vesicovaginal fistula?**

Inadequate lateral and inferior mobilization of the bladder can result in unrecognized bladder injury and formation of a vesicovaginal fistula.

○ **What is an intrafascial total abdominal hysterectomy, and what are the advantages of this technique?**

An intrafascial hysterectomy is one in which the cervix is removed by placing the cardinal ligament clamps inside the pubovesicocervical fascia. This is done by making a V-shaped incision in the pubovesicocervical fascia anterior to the cervix just below the internal os. The fascia can then be reflected laterally. This is a safer technique, since it avoids most bladder and ureteral injuries. It is appropriate only with benign disease.

○ **What is the purpose of suspending the vaginal cuff after removing the uterus?**

To avoid vaginal vault prolapse and enterocele formation later on.

○ **How is the vaginal cuff suspended after total abdominal hysterectomy?**

The posterior vaginal cuff is sutured to the uterosacral ligaments. In a patient with a deep cul-de-sac, a posterior cul-de-sac obliteration may also be performed using the Moschcowitz or Halban technique.

○ **At what point in abdominal hysterectomy do the most urinary tract injuries take place?**

During removal of the cervix.

○ **Besides careful surgical technique, what can be done to reduce the risk of undiagnosed urinary tract injuries at the time of hysterectomy?**

Intraoperative cystourethroscopy is a low-risk, simple procedure that can identify undiagnosed injury to the urinary tract. Routine use of cystourethroscopy at the time of pelvic surgery is controversial, but should be considered for procedures in which the risk of urinary tract injury is 1% to 2% or greater.

○ **When performing a subtotal hysterectomy, at what point is the uterus amputated from the cervix?**

After ligation of the uterine vessels, the uterus is amputated just below the internal os.

○ **How is the cervical stump closed?**

A V-shaped or conical-shaped portion of the cervical stroma is removed to facilitate closure. The remaining endocervix may be cored out or cauterized. Then the cervical stump is closed and suspended using the round ligaments. The cervix may be cauterized transvaginally at the end of the case.

○ **Some surgeons inject a dilute solution of Pitressin into the vaginal mucosa just before beginning a vaginal hysterectomy. In whom must this be avoided?**

In hypertensives and patients with cardiac arrhythmias.

○ **What maneuvers during vaginal hysterectomy facilitate entry into the posterior cul-de-sac without injury to the rectum?**

Upward (anterior) and outward (caudad) traction applied to the cervix along with retraction of the posterior vagina places the cul-de-sac peritoneum on tension, making entry into the correct space easier.

○ **What should be done if the rectum is inadvertently entered during attempted entry into the cul-de-sac?**

The rectum should be repaired in layers at that time.

○ **What should be done if fluid is encountered when opening the posterior cul-de-sac?**

Approximately 75 to 100 mL of peritoneal fluid is a normal finding. However, if a much larger collection of fluid is encountered, the operator should carefully explore the exposed pelvis for findings that might necessitate an abdominal approach.

○ **What maneuvers can be used to help identify the anterior cul-de-sac?**

Moving the cervix up and down will help identify the point of attachment between the vagina and cervix. Strong downward traction on the cervix helps identify the relatively avascular plane between bladder and cervix. A foley bulb can help to identify the location of the bladder. Methylene blue can also be placed in the bladder. Often, a finger can be passed over the uterus from the posterior cul-de-sac to help identify the proper space. However, as long as the bladder is dissected off of the cervix, entry into the anterior cul-de-sac can be delayed.

○ **What should be done if the bladder is inadvertently entered while trying to enter the anterior cul-de-sac?**

The bladder should be closed at that point.

○ **How can ureteral injuries best be avoided while performing vaginal hysterectomy?**

By maintaining downward (outward) traction on the cervix, by carefully dissecting the bladder off the cervix, and by placing clamps as close to the cervix and uterus as possible.

○ **What maneuvers can be used vaginally to facilitate removal of a large uterine fundus?**

The size of the uterus can be reduced by coring, wedging, morcellating, or bisecting the fundus after the uterine arteries have been ligated. Care must be taken to avoid injury to a loop of bowel that may be adherent to the uterus.

○ **What is the most common reason for inadequate vaginal vault support after vaginal hysterectomy?**

Failure to recognize and repair an enterocele. An enterocele should always be checked for by placing a finger into the posterior cul-de-sac.

○ **What is the advantage of closing the peritoneum after vaginal hysterectomy?**

Peritoneal closure extraperitonealizes the pedicle stumps. Thus, postoperative bleeding is more likely to present vaginally and be recognized earlier than if it occurs intraperitoneally. Also, peritoneal closure can incorporate ligation of an enterocele sac.

○ **How should the vaginal vault be supported after vaginal hysterectomy?**

The uterosacral ligaments are used to support the vaginal vault. Often a modified McCall's culdoplasty is performed. With uterine prolapse, the uterosacral ligaments may be attenuated, and need to be shortened in order to provide adequate support.

○ **Do the ovaries continue to function normally after hysterectomy?**

Yes. In almost all women undergoing hysterectomy prior to the natural menopause, the ovaries continue to produce normal levels of hormones in a cyclic fashion until the natural age of menopause.

○ **In women 40 to 64 years of age undergoing hysterectomy, how many undergo elective oophorectomy?**

50% to 66%.

○ **What does the term "incidental" oophorectomy indicate?**

Incidental oophorectomy refers to removal of the ovaries at the time of surgery performed for another indication, occurring by chance or without consequence. This is in contrast to prophylactic oophorectomy, when removal of the ovaries is performed for future benefit.

○ **In women undergoing prophylactic oophorectomy at the time of vaginal hysterectomy, in what percentage of patients can the ovaries be removed successfully?**

65% to 97%. Laparoscopic assistance can be used to facilitate the removal of the majority of the remainder.

○ **How often does ovarian cancer occur in hysterectomy patients with retained ovaries?**

Approximately 0.1% of these women develop ovarian cancer. This represents a relative risk of approximately 0.6 as compared to women who have not had a hysterectomy. Stated another way, of those women who develop ovarian cancer, between 4% and 14% have had an antecedent hysterectomy during which the ovaries were not removed.

○ **Why would hysterectomy reduce the risk of ovarian cancer?**

Several possibilities exist. These include the opportunity to examine the ovaries at the time of hysterectomy and remove the ones that are abnormal. Protection of the ovaries from environmental carcinogens, a possible reduction or alteration in ovarian blood flow, or more frequent prior use of oral contraceptives could also be mechanisms.

○ **After hysterectomy with ovarian conservation, how many patients will require a subsequent operation for ovarian or tubal pathology?**

Approximately 1% to 2%.

○ **If granulation tissue forms at the vaginal cuff, how should this be treated?**

This granulation tissue can be easily treated in the office by touching it with silver nitrate.

○ **How should prolapse of a fallopian tube be recognized and treated?**

This rare complication is usually recognized when suspected granulation tissue fails to go away with silver nitrate treatment or when the "granulation tissue" seems to have a canal. This tissue can be excised vaginally, and the cuff then closed. Most often, this is done in the operating room.

○ **In the US, what is the most common cause of genitourinary tract fistula?**

While most fistulae worldwide are the result of obstetric trauma, the most common cause in the US is pelvic surgery. Most follow an abdominal hysterectomy for benign disease.

CHAPTER 32 Menopause

Keren Hancock, DO

EPIDEMIOLOGY

○ **What is the definition of menopause?**

12 months of amenorrhea after the final menstrual period.

○ **What is the definition of perimenopause?**

The period of time immediately before and after menopause, ending prior to completion of 12 months after the last menstrual period.

○ **What is the definition of climacteric?**

The transition from the reproductive stages of life to the postmenopausal years, a period marked by waning ovarian function.

○ **What is the mean age for menopause?**

51.4 years.

○ **What percentage of their lifetime will most women spend in postmenopausal life?**

30%. Given a life expectancy of 75 years and a median age of 51 for menopause.

○ **What causes earlier menopause?**

Smoking, some women who had hysterectomies, malnourishment, living in high altitudes, mosaic Turner's, and genetic predisposition.

○ **How much earlier does menopause occur in smokers?**

Approximately 2 years.

○ **What percentage of women will undergo premature menopause (before age 40)?**

1%.

○   **What percentage of women will undergo late menopause (after age 55)?**

5%.

○   **What percentage of women will undergo early menopause (between ages 40 and 45)?**

5%.

○   **What is the weight of the postmenopausal ovary?**

5 g.

○   **What histological changes occur in the ovary with menopause?**

Lack of follicles and a prominent stroma.

○   **What are the common changes associated with estrogen depletion?**

Menstrual cycle changes, cardiovascular disease, osteoporosis, genitourinary atrophy, vasomotor psychological and sexual symptoms.

HORMONE PRODUCTION

○   **What happens to the menstrual cycle with age?**

Initially, the follicular phase and cycle decrease and then increase prior to menopause, and luteal phase defects may occur.

○   **What happens to gonadotropin levels in the <u>premenopausal</u> years?**

FSH increases (as a result of decreased inhibin production from granulosa cells) and LH remains the same.

○   **Why can not FSH levels be suppressed in menopause?**

Inhibin production from granulosa cells is lost. Inhibin normally suppresses FSH levels prior to menopause.

○   **What FSH values are indicative of menopause?**

Levels greater than 35 IU/L, but may vary based on laboratory.

○   **What are the expected changes in gonadotropin levels after menopause?**

FSH increases 10- to 20-fold and LH increases 3-fold, reaching a maximum 1 to 3 years after menopause.

○   **Which hormones decline as a result of menopause?**

Estrogen, androstenedione, and progesterone.

○   **Which hormones decline as a result of age?**

Dehydroepiandrosterone (DHEA), dehydroepiandrosterone sulfate (DHEA-S), and testosterone.

○ **What is the level of dehydroepiandrosterone sulfate (DHEA-S) in a 70 year old compared to peak levels in a 25 year old?**

10% to 20% of peak.

○ **Where is most of the postmenopausal androstenedione produced?**

The adrenal gland.

○ **What is the production rate of estradiol (E_2) in postmenopausal women?**

6 μg/d, decreased from 80 to 500 μg/d in reproductive age women.

○ **What is the production rate of estrone (E_1) in postmenopausal women?**

40 μg/d, decreased from 80 to 300 μg/d in reproductive age women.

○ **What is the circulating estradiol (E_2) level in women after menopause?**

10 to 20 pg/mL (40 to 70 pmol/L).

○ **What is the primary source of estrogen in postmenopausal women?**

Peripheral conversion of adrenal and ovarian androgens by extraglandular aromatase.

○ **What is the predominant estrogen of the postmenopausal woman?**

Estrone (E_1).

○ **What is the biological potency of estrone?**

It is only one third as potent as estradiol.

○ **What happens to progesterone production in menopause?**

Progesterone is no longer produced.

○ **What hormone is secreted more by the postmenopausal ovary than the premenopausal ovary?**

Testosterone. Prior to menopause, the ovary contributes 25% of circulating testosterone; and in menopause, the ovary contributes 40% of circulating testosterone.

○ **Why is the postmenopausal ovarian contribution of testosterone increased?**

Elevated gonadotropins stimulate the stromal tissue to secrete testosterone.

○ **Although the ovary produces increased testosterone in menopause, why is the total amount of testosterone not increased?**

Androstenedione is reduced, adrenal testosterone is reduced.

○   **Does serum testosterone change over the menopausal transition?**

No.

○   **What is the cause of mild hirsutism in menopause?**

Increased free androgen to estrogen ratio as a result of decreased SHBG and estrogen.

○   **What increases aromatization of androgens to estrogens?**

Age and weight. Aromatase activity increases twofold in the perimenopausal period and adipose tissue is a rich source of aromatase.

○   **In which tissues has aromatase been identified?**

Liver, fat, muscle, and certain hypothalamic nuclei.

CARDIOVASCULAR DISEASE

○   **What is the leading cause of death for women?**

Heart disease, followed by malignancies, cerebrovascular disease, and motor vehicle accidents.

○   **How many deaths are attributed to cardiovascular disease in women older than age 50?**

Greater than 50%.

○   **How high does the risk of coronary heart disease increase after menopause?**

It doubles.

○   **What are the risk factors for cardiovascular disease?**

Hypertension, smoking, diabetes, hypercholesterolemia, obesity, and family history.

○   **How many years are women later than men in the onset of coronary heart disease?**

10 years.

○   **How many years are women later than men in the incidence of myocardial infarction and sudden death?**

20 years.

○   **What cholesterol fraction is associated with atherosclerosis in women?**

HDL is more closely associated than LDL.

○   **How important are triglycerides in predicting coronary risk?**

Triglycerides are uniquely predictive in older women, especially at levels above 400 mg/dL.

○   **What contributes to cardioprotection in women?**

Higher high-density lipoproteins (HDL), 10 mg/dL higher than in men, an effect of estrogen.

○ **What are the changes in cholesterol fractions at the age of menopause?**

HDL decreases, LDL increases, and the average cholesterol increases to levels higher than in men.

○ **What is estrogen's effect upon lipids and lipoproteins?**

It increases HDL and decreases total cholesterol and LDL.

○ **What lipoprotein independent mechanisms of estrogen may protect against cardiovascular disease?**

Vasodilatation, decreased platelet aggregation, decreased smooth muscle cell proliferation of arterial vessels, direct inotropic actions on the heart, antioxidant activity, favorable impact on clotting mechanisms, inhibition of intimal thickening, inhibition of macrophage foam cell formation, improved glucose metabolism, and decreased insulin levels.

○ **How does estrogen decrease LDL levels?**

It increases hepatic LDL catabolism and increases LDL receptors.

○ **How does estrogen increase HDL levels?**

It inhibits hepatic lipase activity.

○ **How does estrogen replacement therapy exert an antioxidant cardioprotective effect?**

It inhibits LDL oxidation and resultant endothelial vasospasm.

○ **What other antioxidants may decrease the risk of coronary artery disease?**

Vitamin E and beta-carotene (the prohormone of vitamin A).

○ **Are estrogen and progesterone receptors present in the vascular tree?**

Yes, in the endothelium and smooth muscles of arterial vessels.

○ **How does estrogen exert a cardioprotective effect through the vasculature?**

Vasodilatation and decreased peripheral resistance.

○ **How does estrogen exert cardioprotection via endothelium-dependent mechanisms?**

Augmentation of nitric oxide and prostacyclin leading to vasodilation and decreased platelet aggregation.

○ **What direct effects does estrogen have on the heart?**

Increases left ventricular diastolic filling and stroke volume, delaying age-related decreases in compliance.

○ **What effect does acute administration of estradiol have on myocardial ischemia in women with coronary artery disease?**

Signs of ischemia on electrocardiograms are delayed and exercise tolerance is increased.

○ **What effect does estrogen have on body fat distribution?**

It prevents the tendency to increase central body fat with aging.

○ **What is the relationship between truncal adiposity and coronary heart disease?**

An increased waist to hip circumference ratio is associated with an increased risk of coronary heart disease. Truncal adiposity is associated with an androgenic state, hypertension, insulin resistance, hyperinsulinemia, and an atherogenic lipid profile, all risk factors for coronary heart disease.

○ **What lipid profiles are correlated with women who have a central body fat distribution?**

Positive correlation with increases in total cholesterol, triglycerides, and LDL, and negative correlation with HDL.

○ **What effect does <u>oral</u> estrogen have on diabetes?**

The Nurses Health Study documented a 20% decreased risk of non-insulin-dependent diabetes in current users of estrogen.

○ **Does postmenopausal estrogen replacement therapy adversely affect hypertension?**

No.

○ **What did the PEPI trial demonstrate regarding HRT and cardiovascular disease risk factors?**

Estrogen as well as estrogen progestin combinations had a favorable impact on cardiovascular risk factors, an increase in HDL, a decrease in LDL, as well as prevention of the age-related increase in fibrinogen.

○ **In the PEPI trial, which progesterone combined with conjugated equine estrogen had the most favorable effect on HDL?**

Cyclic micronized progesterone resulted in a significantly greater increase in HDL than either sequential or cyclic medroxyprogesterone acetate.

○ **What did the Women's Health Initiative (WHI) show regarding cardiovascular risk of hormone replacement therapy (HRT)?**

An increase in coronary events with Prempro and no significant difference with Premarin.

CHAPTER 33 Osteoporosis

Keren Itancock, DO

○ **What is osteoporosis?**

A progressive, systemic skeletal disease characterized by low bone density and micro-architectural deterioration of bone tissue, leading to an increase in bone fragility and susceptibility to fracture. (World Health Organization)

○ **In what type of bone is resorption more prevalent?**

Trabecular bone.

○ **What type of bone is predominantly present in the spinal column?**

Trabecular bone.

○ **What is the role of osteoclasts?**

They absorb and remove osseous tissue, forming lacuna.

○ **What is the role of osteoblasts?**

They deposit the osseous matrix called osteoid. (B is for build).

○ **When is maximal skeletal mass obtained?**

The third (20s) and fourth (30s) decade.

○ **At what age does bone resorption exceed formation?**

40, by approximately 0.5%.

○ **After menopause, what is the percentage of bone loss per year?**

2.5% to 5% for the first 4 years, then 1% to 1.5% annually.

○ **What is the most important factor associated with bone loss?**

Age.

○   **What medications are associated with bone loss?**

Corticosteroids, thyroid hormone, anticonvulsants, and heparin.

○   **What is the differential diagnosis of osteoporosis?**

Menopause, thyrotoxicosis, glucocorticoid excess, hyperparathyroidism, multiple myeloma, leukemia or lymphoma, alcoholism, long-term heparin therapy, immobilization, and metastatic cancer.

○   **What preventive measures can be taken for osteoporosis early in life?**

Improved calcium intake, diet, exercise, avoidance of alcohol and smoking, and maintenance of normal menstrual cycles.

○   **What is the most common site of fractures in menopause?**

Vertebral fractures, they account for 50% of all fractures.

○   **What is the expected loss in height as a result of vertebral fractures in untreated postmenopausal women?**

2.5 inches (6.4 cm).

○   **What percentage of patients will die within 1 year after hip fracture?**

20%, caused by complications of prolonged immobilization.

○   **How does estrogen therapy help maintain bone mass?**

A direct effect on osteoblasts, improved intestinal absorption of calcium, and decreased renal excretion of calcium.

○   **What is the total calcium requirement to minimize bone loss in postmenopausal women <u>not</u> taking estrogen replacement?**

1,500 mg.

○   **What is the total calcium requirement to minimize bone loss in women on estrogen replacement therapy?**

1,200 mg.

○   **In addition to calcium, in women older than age of 70, what other supplementation should be included for osteoporosis fracture prevention?**

Vitamin D 800 IU, especially if in Northern latitudes.

○   **Does skim milk have less calcium than whole milk?**

No. Since calcium is water soluble, skim milk has more calcium than whole milk.

○   **What disease process can be unmasked with high calcium supplementation?**

Asymptomatic hyperparathyroidism.

○ **What other agents are known to reduce bone resorption?**

Calcitonin, fluoride, androgens, bisphosphonates (etidronate disodium, risedronate, alendronate), and SERMs (selective estrogen receptor modulators such as raloxifene).

○ **Why is not calcitonin more widely used for osteoporosis?**

It is expensive and must be administered parenterally or nasally, and it is effective only against vertebral fracture reduction.

○ **How often are vertebral compression fractures asymptomatic?**

60% to 66% of the time.

○ **How many osteoporotic fractures occur each year in the US?**

Approximately 1.3 million.

○ **How many of these are vertebral fractures?**

Approximately 50%. Hip fractures account for another 25%.

○ **What is the chance a 50-year-old Caucasian woman will suffer a hip fracture at some time in her life?**

16% to 18% (versus 5% for men).

○ **What percentage of bone is resting at any one time?**

88%.

○ **What percentage of bone is remodeling (forming or resorbing) at any one time?**

12%.

○ **What percentage of bone mass is formed in a young woman between the ages of 13 and 16?**

Almost 50%.

○ **When does bone loss accelerate?**

After menopause, and the rapid loss continues for approximately 5 years. Accelerated bone loss has also been observed in women 2 to 3 years prior to the cessation of menstruation; the rate of bone loss was correlated to an elevation of FSH and bone turnover markers.

○ **What percentage of bone mass is lost during this time?**

20%.

○ **Are osteoporotic fractures more common than heart attack, stroke, and breast cancer combined?**

Yes.

○ **What percentage increase in mortality is seen after hip fracture?**

24%.

○ **What percentage of hip fracture survivors are incapacitated for an extended time?**

50%.

○ **In women who have a vertebral fracture, what percentage will have another fracture within a year?**

19%. After one vertebral fracture, there is a 5-fold increased risk for a second vertebral fracture and almost a 2-fold increased risk for a hip fracture.

○ **Does a hip fracture increase the risk of a second hip fracture?**

Yes.

○ **Which is more common, a fall causing a hip fracture or a fracture causing a fall?**

A fall causing a fracture is much more common.

○ **What are risk factors for osteoporosis?**

Family history, early menopause (younger than 45), race: Caucasian or Asian, low body weight, smoking, excessive alcohol use, lack of exercise, low calcium intake, low vitamin D intake, poor health, impaired vision, natural menopause, surgical menopause, glucocorticoids.

○ **What are the secondary causes of osteoporosis?**

Low vitamin D intake, low calcium intake, irritable bowel syndrome, diabetes

Malabsorption syndromes, hyperparathyroidism, hyperthyroidism, malnutrition, liver disease, glucocorticoids, heparin, rheumatoid arthritis, osteoarthritis.

○ **Can the diagnosis of osteoporosis be made using a symptom complex?**

No. Symptoms present only when fractures occur. Treatment must be instituted before this happens.

○ **What is the most accurate technique available for measuring bone density?**

Dual energy absorptiometry (DXA) measuring the hip and spine.

○ **What hip areas are routinely assessed for BMD using a DXA scan?**

The femoral neck, trochanter, Ward's triangle, and intertrochanter.

○ **Who should have tests for bone mineral density (DXA scan)?**

All women 65 years or older without risk factors.

All postmenopausal women younger than 65 with risk factors.

All postmenopausal women younger than 65 with a history of fracture.

All postmenopausal women considering therapy for osteoporosis.

All women on estrogen/progestogen therapy for a prolonged period. (National Osteoporosis Foundation Guidelines.)

○ **What areas are most reproducible on DXA?**

A-P spine, femoral neck.

○ **What is the ideal screening interval for DXA?**

Every 2 years.

○ **How is osteoporosis diagnosed?**

By DXA scan, measuring bone mineral density (BMD) of the lumbar spine and hip (a central DXA), and it is reported using T-scores.

○ **Can a peripheral DXA (heel, finger, wrist) be used to diagnose osteoporosis?**

No. These are used to screen for osteoporosis. The diagnosis is made by central DXA.

○ **Can a peripheral DXA be used to predict fracture risk?**

Yes. (NORA Trial.)

○ **What is the T score?**

A measurement of BMD, which indicates the number of standard deviations above or below the average peak bone mass in a young woman.

○ **What does the T score indicate?**

A T score of -1.0 is one standard deviation below peak bone mass, and represents approximately a 10% loss in bone mass at the site measured.

○ **What is the Z score?**

This number indicates the number of standard deviations from average bone mass compared to a population of the same age. If there is a significant variance, one should look for secondary causes of osteoporosis.

○ **Does the T score correlate with fracture risk?**

Yes. For each T score below normal, the risk of fracture doubles at that site. (A T score of -1.0 doubles the fracture risk compared to a T score of 0.0).

○ **How does age relate to fracture risk and T score?**

As age increases, fracture risk increases at the same T score.

○ **Does the T score fully explain the fracture risk at one particular site?**

No. There are other characteristics that impact bone strength that are difficult to measure.

○ **What impacts bone strength?**

Bone quality, bone turnover, and microarchitecture.

○ **Can you see a normal T score at one site and osteoporosis at another site in the same patient?**

Yes.

○ **What T score is considered normal?**

Above –1.0. (WHO)

○ **What T scores suggest low bone mass, or osteopenia?**

Between –1.0 and –2.5.

○ **What T score represents osteoporosis?**

Lower than –2.5.

○ **What is severe osteoporosis?**

A T score of –2.5 or below with a previous fracture.

○ **When should treatment be started for osteoporosis?**

When the T score at the A-P spine or hip is –2.0 or lower without risk factors, or –1.5 or lower with risk factors. (NOF Guidelines.)

○ **What are biochemical markers of bone formation?**

Bone-specific alkaline phosphatase and osteocalcin.

○ **What are the biochemical markers for bone resorption?**

Pyridinoline, N-telopeptides, and C-telopeptides.

○ **Are biochemical markers usually used in individual patients to help diagnose osteoporosis?**

No. They are used more in research in large groups of patients to evaluate how effective a drug is regarding its effect on bone.

○ **What therapies are currently available to treat osteoporosis?**

Alendronate, risedronate, and ibandronate, which are bisphosphonates.
Raloxifene, a selective estrogen receptor modulator (SERM).
Calcitonin nasal spray.

○ **What therapy is presently used only to prevent osteoporosis?**

Estrogen-progestin therapy.

○ **In the Women's Health Initiative Trial, what effect did estrogen plus progestin have on fracture risk?**

There was a reduction in fractures of the spine and hip in patients who took estrogen plus progestin compared to placebo.

○ **How do the present treatments work?**

They are antiresorptive agents, affecting the osteoclasts so that less bone is resorbed, allowing the osteoblasts to build bone mass.

○ **Are other agents available?**

Yes. Teriparatide, a form of PTH. This functions as an anabolic agent.

○ **Is it necessary to supplement an osteoporosis therapy drug with calcium and vitamin D to obtain maximal fracture protection?**

Yes.

○ **How important is it for a patient at risk for osteoporosis to exercise, specifically walking and upper body strengthening?**

Extremely important. This reduces the risk of falling and thus lowering the risk of fracture.

○ **Is long-term steroid use a risk factor for osteoporosis?**

Yes.

○ **How soon after starting steroids does one see significant bone loss?**

3 months.

○ **What percentage of patients taking prednisone 7.5 mg or greater develop an osteoporotic fracture?**

50%.

○ **Can lower doses of steroids also increase risk of fracture?**

Yes.

○ **Does age or gender impact fracture risk if a person is on steroids?**

No.

○ **How do steroids affect bone?**

They cause a toxic effect on osteoblasts that shortens their lifespan. Calcium absorption is blocked through the intestine. Calcium is also lost by the kidney, decreasing serum calcium. This causes PTH to be secreted, thereby increasing bone resorption.

○ **How soon after treatment is started should a repeat DXA be done?**

1 to 2 years. The sensitivity of DXA is such that it would take this long to see a meaningful change. One exception is a patient on steroids. In this situation, the DXA can be done as early as 6 months.

○ **What change would you expect to see after 1 to 2 years of treatment?**

The DXA should show stabilization or improvement of BMD.

○   **What if there is a significant loss (greater than 4% to 5%) at 2 years?**

Check the Z score. If it is lower than expected, evaluate for secondary causes of osteoporosis.

○   **What logical steps can be suggested to a patient to prevent falls?**

Safeguard the home by removing electrical wires from the floor.

Remove throw rugs.

Improve lighting.

Evaluate the patient's vision.

○   **How does urinary incontinence increase the risk of hip fracture?**

Any leakage of urine causes the floor to become more slippery resulting in a fall.

○   **T/F Smoking one pack per day throughout adulthood may reduce bone density by as much as 10% by menopause?**

True.

○   **What percentage of patients with hip fractures have histological evidence of osteomalacia, the classic manifestation of vitamin D deficiency?**

30%.

○   **What is the largest source of dietary vitamin D?**

Milk.

GENITOURINARY CHANGES

○   **What genitourinary tissues are estrogen sensitive?**

The vagina, vulva, urethra, and trigone of the bladder.

○   **What vaginal symptoms are related to atrophy?**

Dryness, dyspareunia, and recurrent atrophic vaginitis.

○   **What causes dyspareunia in aging women?**

Decreased vaginal lubrication and elasticity.

○   **Is vaginal estrogen therapy more effective than moisturizers and lubricants?**

Yes.

○   **How much greater is the potency of vaginal conjugated estrogens than that of oral conjugate estrogens?**

Four times greater.

○ **What effect do "night sweats" (hot flushes at night) have?**

Interruption of sleep patterns and thus a decline in sleep quality and length.

○ **What is the most common vulvar symptom of menopause relieved with estrogen replacement?**

Burning and pruritus secondary to atrophy.

○ **Pruritus is also the presenting complaint of vulvar dystrophies. What percentage of vulvar dystrophies are squamous cell carcinomas?**

5% on initial examination, another 5% may develop squamous cell carcinomas within 3 to 5 years after hypertrophic vulvar dystrophy is diagnosed.

○ **What is the most common cause of postmenopausal bleeding?**

Vaginal atrophy.

○ **Why does vaginitis increase during the postmenopausal years?**

Because of estrogen deficiency, the vaginal pH increases from 3.5–4.5 to 6.0–8.0, predisposing to colonization of bacterial pathogens.

○ **What cervical changes are associated with menopause?**

Stenosis, atrophy, erosion, and ulcers.

○ **What changes occur in the squamocolumnar junction and transformation zone?**

They migrate up into the endocervical canal.

○ **What urethral conditions can develop as a result of estrogen deficiency?**

Ectropion (urethral caruncle), diverticula, and urethrocele.

○ **What is the most common problem in menopause related to urethral changes?**

Urethral syndrome, consisting of burning, frequency, hesitancy, nocturia, and urgency associated with sterile urine cultures.

○ **How is the urethral syndrome treated?**

Estrogen therapy.

○ **What urinary symptoms are associated with atrophy?**

Dysuria, urgency, and recurrent urinary tract infections.

○ **Does bacteriuria increase in menopause?**

Yes. The incidence of bacteriuria increases from 4% in reproductive age women to 7%–10% in postmenopausal women.

○   **Is urinary stress incontinence related to estrogen deficiency?**

Yes, urethral shortening and decreased urethral closing pressures associated with atrophy may contribute to urinary incontinence.

○   **Can urge incontinence be treated with estrogen therapy?**

Yes.

○   **Can estrogen therapy improve urinary stress incontinence?**

There are conflicting data, but the best available evidence suggests estrogen therapy is not effective.

○   **What is the best initial therapy for urinary stress incontinence?**

Kegel exercises.

○   **What other treatments exist for urinary stress incontinence?**

Duloxetine (SNRI), collagen injections, surgery.

VASOMOTOR AND PSYCHOLOGICAL SYMPTOMS

○   **What is a hot flush?**

Sudden onset of warmth and reddening of the skin beginning in the head spreading to the neck and chest, sometimes concluded by profuse perspiration, lasting a few seconds to several minutes. It is often accompanied by palpations and feelings of anxiety.

○   **What is the physiology of the hot flush?**

It originates in the hypothalamus and represents thermoregulatory instability in response to estrogen fluctuation.

○   **Do hot flushes subside with time?**

Yes, the incidence of flushes are 80% at 1 year and 20% at 5 years.

○   **What physiologic changes are associated with hot flushes?**

An LH surge, an increase in body surface temperature and skin conductance followed by a decline in core body temperature.

○   **What is the frequency of hot flushes?**

Usually several times a day. Can range from 1–2 daily to 1 per hour.

○   **Are hot flushes more common at night?**

Yes.

○   **How does estrogen exert its effects on improving "quality of life" in postmenopausal women?**

Alleviation of hot flushes and improved quality of sleep leading to improved mood, memory, and quality of life.

○ **What alternatives to estrogen are partially effective in treating hot flushes?**

Clonidine, medroxyprogesterone acetate, methyldopa, SSRIs, gabapentin, black cohosh.

○ **What alternatives to estrogen are <u>ineffective</u> in treating hot flushes?**

Bellergal, propranolol, vitamin E, and soy extracts.

○ **What alternatives to estrogen are currently recommended for the treatment of hot flushes?**

Transdermal clonidine 100 μg weekly, Effexor 37.5 to –75 mg qd, black cohosh.

○ **Are there any safety data on black cohosh?**

Yes, for use up to 6 months.

DUB AND ENDOMETRIAL CANCER

○ **What is the first diagnostic test recommended for postmenopausal bleeding if the uterus is normal?**

Endometrial biopsy.

○ **In the perimenopausal period, after exclusion of gynecological causes of dysfunctional uterine bleeding, what endocrine gland should be evaluated?**

The thyroid gland.

○ **What endometrial thickness on ultrasound requires biopsy and is associated with an extremely low risk of endometrial cancer?**

4 mm.

○ **How do you treat simple hyperplasia in <u>peri</u>menopause?**

Monthly oral progestin therapy, repeat biopsy in 6 months, if hyperplasia persists, D&C.

○ **How effective is monthly progestin therapy in treating simple hyperplasia?**

95% to 98% of the time.

○ **What is the incidence of endometrial hyperplasia after 1 year of unopposed estrogen (conjugated estrogen 0.625 mg or its equivalent)?**

20% incidence of hyperplasia, predominantly simple hyperplasia.

○ **When DUB in perimenopause is diagnosed, what are the treatment options?**

Observation, oral contraceptives, progestational agents.

○ **What is the incidence of <u>adenomatous</u> or <u>atypical</u> hyperplasia in unopposed estrogen users?**

10% per year.

○   **What percentage of complex endometrial hyperplasia eventually progresses to frank cancer?**

10%.

○   **What percentage of atypical endometrial hyperplasia will progress to cancer within 1 year?**

20% to 25%.

○   **What is the time required for endometrial hyperplasia to progress to cancer?**

5 years.

○   **What is the risk of endometrial cancer in postmenopausal women not on hormone replacement therapy?**

4 per 1000 (0.4%).

○   **What is the risk of endometrial cancer in postmenopausal women with abnormal uterine bleeding?**

20%.

○   **How much higher is the risk of endometrial cancer in patients on unopposed estrogen compared to the general population?**

2 to 10 times higher, depending on dose and duration of exposure.

○   **How long does the risk of endometrial cancer persist after discontinuation of estrogen?**

10 years.

○   **What characteristics of endometrial adenocarcinoma are present in patients on estrogen therapy?**

Most lesions are low grade and early stage, and associated with better survival.

○   **What is the 5-year survival rate in women whose uterine cancer was diagnosed while they were taking estrogen replacement therapy?**

95%.

○   **How does progesterone counter effect estrogen on endometrial growth?**

It decreases estrogen receptors, induces enzymatic conversion of estradiol to an excreted conjugate, estrone sulfate, and suppresses estrogen induced oncogene transcription.

BREAST AND OVARIAN CANCER

○   **What is the leading type of cancer in women?**

Breast cancer (32%).

○   **What is the leading cause of cancer deaths in women?**

Lung cancer. Breast cancer is second.

○ **Is there an increased risk of breast cancer associated with estrogen replacement therapy?**

There may be a slightly increased risk of breast cancer especially with long duration of use (5 or more years in users of continuous combined therapy).

○ **Do estrogen users have improved breast cancer survival?**

Yes, this is probably as a result of earlier diagnosis but this is controversial after the results of the WHI.

○ **Does estrogen use affect breast cancer tumor differentiation?**

Yes, women on estrogen develop better differentiated tumors.

○ **What is the diagnosis of an adnexal mass in menopause?**

Cancer, until proven otherwise.

○ **What type of adnexal mass may be managed conservatively, with serial ultrasounds?**

Clear fluid filled cysts without septations, less than 5 cm.

○ **What is the risk of breast and ovarian cancer in BRCA carriers?**

50% to 80% and 40% to 60%, respectively.

○ **What is the third leading cause of cancer deaths in women?**

Colon cancer.

○ **What is the recommended screening for colon cancer?**

Colonoscopy in women older than 50, every 10 years. Alternatives are yearly hemoccults with sigmoidoscopy or barium enema every 5 years.

○ **Who should be offered genetic screening for BRCA mutation?**

Women with a history of a first-degree relative with premenopausal breast cancer, or a family history of several women with breast and/or ovarian cancer, or women with premenopausal breast or ovarian cancer.

○ **What can be recommended for BRCA protection for mutation-positive women?**

Prophylactic oophorectomy in the late 40s or the long-term use of OCP.

○ **Is oophorectomy 100% protective in these women?**

No, approximately 2% to 3% of women get primary peritoneal cancer.

HORMONE REPLACEMENT THERAPY

○ **What is the oral micronized estradiol dose equivalent to conjugated estrogens 0.625 mg?**

1 mg.

○ **What is the transcutaneous 17 β-estradiol dose equivalent to conjugated estrogens 0.625 mg?**

0.05 mg.

○ **What is the estrone sulfate dose equivalent to conjugated estrogens 0.625 mg?**

0.625 mg.

○ **What is the esterified estrogen dose equivalent to conjugated estrogens 0.625 mg?**

0.625 mg.

○ **What type of estrogen is present in Premarin?**

Conjugated estrogens (estrone, equilin, and 17 α-dihydroequilin).

○ **What type of estrogen is present in the transdermal patch and Estrace?**

Estradiol.

○ **What type of estrogen is present in Ogen?**

Estropipate.

○ **What type of estrogen is present in Estratab?**

Esterified estrogens.

○ **What is the daily dose of norethindrone equivalent to 2.5 mg medroxyprogesterone acetate?**

0.35 mg.

○ **Can intravaginal estrogen be absorbed and have systemic effects?**

Yes, atrophic mucosa absorbs estrogen readily.

○ **What herbs contain estrogen-like compounds?**

Ginseng, black cohosh, and red clover.

○ **What is the sequential method of hormone replacement administration?**

Estrogen on days 1 to 25 or days 1 to 30 and medroxyprogesterone acetate 5 mg or norethindrone 0.5 mg for 13 days of estrogen administration per month.

○ **What is the recommended dose of micronized progesterone for sequential therapy?**

200 mg for 14 days every month.

○ **What is the continuous combined method of hormone replacement therapy?**

Daily estrogen and daily progestins, either medroxyprogesterone 2.5 mg, norethindrone 0.35 mg, or 100 to 200 mg micronized progesterone.

○ **What concentration differences of estrogen exist in the portal system versus the periphery after oral estrogen administration?**

The estrogen concentration is four to five times higher in the portal system.

○ **Does the first pass effect occur for transdermal estrogen administration?**

No.

○ **What are some of the adverse symptoms associated with the dose of progesterone in sequential hormone replacement therapy?**

Withdrawal bleeding, breast tenderness, bloating, fluid retention, and depression.

○ **What percentage of women on sequential hormone replacement will have progestin withdrawal bleeding?**

80% to 90%.

○ **What percentage of women will experience breakthrough bleeding on continuous hormone replacement therapy?**

40% to 60% in the first six months, 20% after one year.

○ **What is the origin of breakthrough bleeding in continuous hormone replacement therapy?**

Progestational dominance resulting in an atrophic endometrium.

○ **What evaluation should be performed for breakthrough bleeding in patients on continuous therapy?**

Observation for the first six months, then consider endometrial biopsy, or hysteroscopy and D&C to rule out fibroids and polyps.

○ **What are some conservative treatment alternatives to overcome breakthrough bleeding on continuous HRT?**

Observation, sequential therapy, or a progestin IUD. A progestin IUD will suppress the endometrium.

○ **Is the addition of progestin required in women on estrogen replacement who undergo endometrial ablation?**

Yes.

○ **What are some causes of chronic estrogen exposure predisposing patients to a higher risk of endometrial changes?**

Obesity, DUB, anovulation and infertility, hirsutism, high alcohol intake, hepatic disease, diabetes, and hypothyroidism.

○ **When should endometrial biopsies be performed prior to initiating HRT?**

Patients at high risk of endometrial changes associated with chronic estrogen exposure and a history of previous unopposed estrogen therapy, or patients with abnormal bleeding.

○ **When is an endometrial biopsy recommended when breakthrough bleeding occurs on HRT?**
Women who have used unopposed estrogen in the past, an endometrial thickness greater than 5 mm or after one year of amenorrhea on HRT.

○ **How should women who take unopposed estrogen be followed?**
Endometrial sampling or vaginal probe ultrasound yearly.

○ **Why is the estrogen progesterone combination sometimes recommended in hysterectomized women with endometriosis?**
Adenocarcinoma has occurred in patients with endometriosis on unopposed estrogen.

○ **What are some of the potential benefits of androgen replacement?**
Improved well being and sexual behavior.

○ **What negative effects does testosterone replacement therapy have?**
Hirsutism and adverse effects on lipids.

○ **Patients with what stage of endometrial cancer can safely take estrogen replacement therapy?**
Stage 1 grade 1, low-grade adenocarcinoma.

○ **What conditions are not contraindications for HRT?**
Controlled hypertension, diabetes, and varicose veins.

○ **Does estrogen replacement therapy promote fibroid tumor growth?**
No.

○ **What gynecological malignancies are not contraindications to HRT?**
Ovarian, cervical, and vulvar.

○ **What effect does estrogen therapy have on colorectal cancer?**
It significantly decreases the risk of colorectal cancer.

○ **Does estrogen therapy improve visual acuity?**
Yes, possibly because of the beneficial effect on lacrimal fluid and protection against lens opacities.

○ **What effect does estrogen therapy have on oral complaints common in menopause?**
It relieves oral discomfort, burning, bad taste, and dryness. It also decreases gingival inflammation, bleeding, and tooth loss.

○ **What effect does estrogen therapy have on skin?**

It prevents the age-related declines in skin collagen and thickness.

○ **What effect does estrogen therapy have on muscle strength?**

It prevents the age-related decline in handgrip strength.

○ **What are contraindications to estrogen therapy?**

Estrogen-sensitive cancers, chronically impaired liver function, undiagnosed genital bleeding, acute vascular thrombosis, neurophthalmologic vascular disease, and known or suspected pregnancy.

○ **What disorders may be aggravated by estrogen?**

Seizure disorders, familial hyperlipidemias (high triglycerides), and migraine headaches.

○ **What effect does estrogen alone or in combination with progestin have on clotting factors in menopause?**

It prevents menopause related increases in clotting factors (fibrinogen, factor VII, and plasminogen activator inhibitor) and does not alter antithrombin.

○ **When is a history of venous thromboembolism <u>not</u> a contraindication to estrogen therapy?**

A thromboembolic event related to trauma.

○ **Is there an increased risk of gallbladder disease with estrogen therapy?**

Estrogen therapy may increase the risk of gallbladder disease by 1.5- to 2.0-fold.

○ **How is estrogen believed to induce cholelithiasis?**

Estrogen alters bile salts leading to stone formation.

○ **What effect does <u>oral</u> estrogen replacement have on triglyceride levels?**

It increases triglyceride levels.

○ **What route of estrogen administration does not affect triglycerides?**

Transdermal.

○ **What complications can be precipitated by estrogen administration in women with elevated triglycerides?**

Pancreatitis and severe hypertriglyceridemia.

○ **How should estrogen be administered to women with triglyceride levels between 250 and 750 mg/dL?**

A nonoral route of estrogen with careful surveillance of triglyceride levels.

○   **How quickly do triglyceride levels increase after estrogen replacement administration?**

Triglycerides increase quickly and can be measured between 2 and 4 weeks.

○   **What triglyceride levels are an absolute contraindication to estrogen therapy?**

Greater than 750 mg/dL.

○   **What effect does estrogen have on Alzheimer disease?**

According to the NHS, Alzheimer disease is less frequent among HRT users and cognitive function in affected individuals is improved. However in WHI study, dementia was found to be more frequent in HRT and ET users older than 65 years, although the difference was not statistically significant.

CHAPTER 34 Preoperative Evaluation and Preparation for Gynecologic Surgery

Denise Hartman, MD

○ **Which prescribed medications commonly interfere with anesthesia or surgery?**
Monoamine oxidase inhibitors, nicotinic acid, insulin, corticosteroids, and anticoagulants.

○ **How often do allergic reactions to radiologic contrast media occur during intravenous pyelogram?**
Overall 5% to 8%, with life-threatening reactions occurring in 0.1%.

○ **To what criminal violation would a physician be vulnerable for performing surgery without patient consent?**
Assault and battery.

○ **What is the single most significant reversible risk factor for pulmonary complications?**
Tobacco smoke, which quadruples the risk for pulmonary complications.

○ **What is considered a normal forced expiration?**
FEV in one second should be >75% of the predicted normal volume.

○ **What are the three most common chronic obstructive pulmonary diseases?**
Chronic bronchitis, emphysema, and asthma.

○ **What is the predictive value of history in diagnosing coronary artery disease?**
90%.

○ **What is the sensitivity of stress test for coronary artery disease?**
75% to 80%.

○ **After a myocardial infarction, how long should gynecologic surgery be deferred?**
Usually at least 6 months to decrease reinfarction and mortality.

○ **What is the single most significant predictor of cardiac complications in the surgical patient?**

The presence of congestive heart failure.

○ **When are cardiac rhythm disturbances such as premature ventricular contractions associated with increased surgical risk?**

When accompanied by decreased left ventricular function.

○ **What is the most common perioperative time period for myocardial infarction?**

Postoperative day 3 to 4.

○ **What are indications for digitalization preoperatively?**

Clinical congestive heart failure, poor left ventricular function, or atrial arrhythmias.

○ **What is the most common valvular abnormality of the heart?**

Mitral valve prolapse.

○ **Which arrhythmias are associated with mitral valve prolapse?**

Ventricular ectopic beats, atrial tachyarrhythmias, bradyarrhythmias, and rarely sudden death.

○ **How should patients with bioprosthetic valves be managed preoperatively?**

Coumadin should be stopped 2 days prior to surgery so that the prothrombin time decreases to 15 seconds; the Coumadin should be restarted as soon as it is deemed safe.

○ **What is the recommended endocarditis prophylaxis for gynecological surgery?**

Ampicillin 2 g IV or IM and gentamicin 1.5 mg/kg (80 mg maximum) IV approximately 1 hour prior to surgery and repeated 8 hours later.

○ **Which patients scheduled for hysterectomy are at risk for abnormal intravenous pyelograms?**

Patients with pelvic inflammatory disease, endometriosis, pelvic relaxation, lateral projections of uterine myomas, fixed adnexal masses, and prior abdominal surgery.

○ **What is the anesthesiology classification of surgical risk?**

The Dripps-American Society of Anesthesiologists' Classification of surgical risk ranging from Class 1 (normal healthy patient) to Class 5 (moribund patient not expected to survive 24 hours with or without operation).

○ **Which group of hysterectomy patients is most helped with prophylactic antibiotics?**

The premenopausal patient undergoing vaginal hysterectomy to decrease vaginal cuff cellulitis.

○ **What is obstructive lung disease?**

Reduction and prolongation of air flow during expiration.

○ **What is restrictive lung disease?**

Reduction in volume of air-containing tissue, affecting the volume of air that can be inspired.

○ **What is a confirmation that anatomical shunting is the cause of hypoxemia?**

By the inability to raise the PaO_2 above 55 mm Hg after breathing 100% oxygen for 30 minutes.

○ **What does high PCO_2 represent?**

Usually hypoventilation.

○ **What does low PaO_2 represent?**

Ventilation-perfusion mismatch, diffusion defect, or anatomical shunting.

○ **What food allergy may suggest an iodine allergy?**

Allergy to shellfish.

○ **If allergy to iodine is suspected, and yet an intravenous pyelogram is necessary, what can be done?**

Corticosteriod preparation help to prevent life-threatening anaphylaxis.

○ **What pertinent family history may play a role in the preoperative evaluation of a patient?**

A family history of bleeding disorders or malignant hyperthermia, which can be inherited as an autosomal dominant disorder, can be important.

○ **What laboratory evaluation should be performed on a routine preoperative work-up?**

A complete blood count with hemoglobin level and platelet count is essential. Chemistries and/or coagulation studies are rarely helpful unless the patient has significant medical history.

○ **What components should go into the preoperative discussion with the patient?**

The nature and extent of the disease; the likely results if untreated; the extent of the proposed operation and potential modifications, anticipated benefits, risks, and alternative management options; and expected success rate of the surgery.

○ **What is the purpose of the preoperative counseling of the patient?**

Provide informed consent, allows the patient to have questions answered, to work through emotions, and build trust.

○ **What effect does preoperative nutritional preparation have?**

Optimizing nutritional, fluid, and electrolyte status leads to more rapid recovery, better wound healing, and less postoperative infection.

○ **What components are necessary to calculate the caloric needs of a surgical patient?**

Height, weight, sex, age, activity level, type of surgery, and extent of disease.

○   **In consideration of nutritional status, what variables are related to increased surgical morbidity and mortality?**

Generally, hypoalbuminemia (≤2.5 mg/dL) and unintended weight loss (≥10%).

○   **What are the advantages and disadvantages of enteral nutritional supplementation?**

Advantages: easy and inexpensive. Disadvantages: high osmolarity can lead to vomiting or diarrhea, or electrolyte disturbances, and cannot be used with bowel obstruction.

○   **What is the most common side effect of peripheral parenteral nutrition?**

Phlebitis because of the high osmolarity solution.

○   **What is the most common complication associated with total parenteral nutrition?**

Catheter infection, which can be reduced with meticulous care of the catheter.

○   **What is the amount and distribution of total water in an average woman?**

Total water constitutes 50% to 55% of body weight with 40% to 66% in the intracellular compartment, and 20% to 33% in the extracellular compartment (1/4 is in the plasma and 3/4 in the interstitium).

○   **What are the primary electrolytes contributing to the osmolarity in the extracellular fluid compartment?**

Sodium and chloride.

○   **How can one calculate the serum osmolarity?**

$2 \times Na + [Glucose (mg/dL)/18] + BUN (mg/dL)/2.8$.

○   **What conditions are associated with hyponatremia and extracellular fluid excess?**

Cardiac failure, liver failure, and renal dysfunction.

○   **What preoperative conditions predispose to hypokalemia?**

Significant gastrointestinal fluid losses, prolonged diuretic use, and prolonged parenteral potassium-free fluids.

○   **What risk factors place the hysterectomy patient at risk for postoperative infection?**

Low socioeconomic status, surgical duration greater than 2 hours, malignancy, obesity, malnutrition, immunosuppression, and increased number of procedures performed.

○   **What is the optimal timing of prophylactic antibiotic administration?**

30 minutes prior to the actual incision time.

○   **What are the advantages of lower bowel preoperative preparation?**

Greater exposure in the abdomen and pelvis, and if the rectosigmoid is entered, the decrease in formed stool decreases the bacterium inoculum. Preoperative enemas also hasten the return of normal bowel function postoperatively and decrease the incidence of fecal impaction immediately postoperatively.

○ **What is the timing and dosage of heparin for deep venous thrombosis (DVT) prophylaxis?**

5000 units subcutaneously given 2 hours prior to surgery and continued every 8 to 12 hours postoperatively.

○ **Does prophylactic low-dose heparin affect the APTT or increase bleeding complications?**

Up to 10% to 15% of normal patients develop a prolonged APTT after 5000 u is given subcutaneously. Also, increase in bleeding complications and hematoma formation may occur.

○ **How do pneumatic compression stockings compare with heparin in the prevention of DVT?**

They are similar to heparin. The stockings must be placed intraoperatively, and particularly in patients with malignancy, should be maintained for 5 days.

○ **What is the most common cause of death in diabetes patients?**

Cardiovascular disease, which accounts for more than half of deaths in diabetics.

○ **What are risk factors for postoperative mortality in diabetics?**

Serum creatinine >2.0 mg/dL, vascular disease, and onset of diabetes prior to age 40.

○ **What would be optimal preoperative insulin management for a diabetic patient in poor control?**

Admission one to two days prior to surgery for glucose control, likely by insulin drip. There is a threefold increase in morbidity and a doubling in mortality if an operation is performed in a diabetic patient with poor control.

○ **What is the most common etiology for hyperthyroidism?**

Graves' disease.

○ **What should be the preoperative care for a newly diagnosed hyperthyroid patient?**

One regimen is PTU (propylthiouracil) 100 to 200 mg every 6 hours as well as propranolol 10 to 80 mg every 6 to 8 hours initiated at least 2 weeks prior to surgery and continued postoperatively.

○ **What anesthetic concerns arise in the hyperthyroid patient?**

Tracheal compression or deviation caused by the enlarged thyroid, tachycardia exacerbated by medications, and thyroid storm.

○ **How should the patient recently diagnosed with hypothyroidism be handled preoperatively?**

Slow replacement with levothyroxine is imperative to avoid cardiovascular collapse.

○ **What prior steroid use constitutes potential concern for adrenal insufficiency caused by surgery?**

As little as three days of steroid use, equivalent to prednisone 25 mg/d in the last year.

○ **How can one test for preoperative pituitary-adrenal axis insufficiency?**

ACTH 250 μg can be administered and the maximum cortisol response measured.

○ **How would one handle a patient with Addison disease or chronic steroid use?**

Hydrocortisone 100 mg IM on call to the OR, then 50 mg IV/IM in the recovery room, then give every six hours for three doses, then taper to a maintenance dose over the next three days.

○ **What is the relationship between chronic hypertension and perioperative morbidity/mortality?**

No increased adverse results unless accompanied by cardiac disease.

○ **What is the greatest risk factor for the development of postoperative pulmonary complications?**

Chronic obstructive pulmonary disease (COPD).

○ **What factor predisposes patients with COPD to postoperative pneumonia and atelectasis?**

The impaired ability for effective cough and clearance of secretions.

○ **What preoperative arterial blood gas findings are associated with postoperative pulmonary complications?**

PaO_2 values less than 70 mm Hg, and $PaCO_2$ values greater than 45 mm Hg.

○ **What preoperative measures for COPD patients help to minimize postoperative pulmonary complications?**

Chest physiotherapy, bronchodilators, and antibiotics for patients with positive sputum cultures.

○ **What duration of smoking cessation is necessary to significantly lower the incidence of pulmonary complications?**

2 months.

○ **How should patients with liver disease and elevated prothrombin time be prepared in the preoperative stage?**

The etiology of liver insufficiency should be investigated. Vitamin K 10 mg intramuscularly for three days should correct the prothrombin time. Electrolytes, LFTs, BUN, serum creatinine, platelet count, and PTT should be checked.

○ **How should a patient be evaluated when the platelet count is discovered to be less than 100,000/mm³?**

An etiology should be sought, and a bleeding time should be obtained.

○ **What is the most common inherited condition leading to platelet dysfunction?**

Von Willebrand disease.

○ **What is the role for preoperative screening for coagulation defects?**

Only seriously ill patients and those with history of bleeding should be tested.

○ **What screening test should be used when suspecting diabetes mellitus or glucose intolerance?**

A 2 hour 75 g glucose tolerance test.

○ **In what age group is the highest incidence of major surgeries being performed?**

Between 60 and 69 years of age.

○ **What type of musculoskeletal evaluation should be performed in the preoperative phase?**

Back, hip, or lower extremity pathology should be assessed since patients often need to be in the dorsolithotomy position.

○ **What measures can be taken to avoid neurological injury to operative patients?**

Proper positioning and padding.

○ **What duration of gonadotropin releasing hormone agonist use has been associated with the maximum decrease of uterine leiomyomata size?**

3 months.

○ **What is the role of endometrial sampling before hysterectomy?**

Endometrial sampling is not routinely done but when there is suggestion of endometrial abnormality.

○ **What are the two most common causes of thrombocytopenia?**

Laboratory error and collagen vascular diseases.

○ **What medications have been shown to cause platelet dysfunction?**

Aspirin, amitriptyline, nonsteroidal anti-inflammatory agents, and high doses of penicillin and carbenicillin.

○ **When patients are noted to have increased bleeding times because of medications, what should be done in the preoperative period?**

The medications should be discontinued for 7 to 10 days before undergoing surgery.

○ **What is the most common method of diagnosing a platelet dysfunction?**

By history and physical examination (easy bruisability, sustained bleeding from cuts, bleeding with brushing teeth, petechiae on examination).

○ **How do platelet counts correlate with surgical hemorrhage?**

A platelet count greater than $100,000/mm^3$ is adequate for surgical hemostasis.

○ **What preoperative granulocyte count is associated with surgical morbidity?**

Less than $1,000/mm^3$.

○ **What FEV_1 value is correlated with postoperative pulmonary complications?**

An FEV_1 value of <1 liter.

○ **When should preoperative chest radiographs be performed?**

Age older than 60, a history of smoking, pulmonary disease, surgery for malignancy to exclude pulmonary metastases, and patients who present with cardiac or pulmonary signs or symptoms.

○ **What fraction of the United States population is affected by asthma?**

Approximately 5%.

○ **Why has morbidity and mortality because of asthma increased in the recent years?**

This is probably because of under-diagnosis and under-treatment.

○ **What should be the preoperative work-up of an asthmatic patient?**

Pulmonary examination, chest x-ray, pulmonary function testing should be performed with and without bronchodilators (arterial blood gases in select cases).

○ **What role do corticosteroids have in the management of asthma?**

In curtailing the significant inflammatory component of asthma, which is not treated by beta-agonists.

○ **What are the most common etiologic factors leading to end-stage renal disease?**

Glomerulonephritis, hereditary factors (e.g., polycystic kidney disease), renovascular disease like diabetes, and hypertensive disease.

○ **What type of anemia is the most common in patients with renal insufficiency?**

Normocytic normochromic.

○ **What measures may be employed for patients with renal insufficiency and anemia?**

Recombinant erythropoietin can help correct the anemia if surgery can be delayed for several weeks.

○ **What preoperative measures can reduce coagulation problems in patients with chronic renal insufficiency?**

Cryoprecipitate, desmopressin, and conjugated estrogen have been given to shorten the bleeding time.

○ **When should dialysis-dependent patients be dialyzed before surgery?**

Within 24 hours of surgery.

○ **What classification has been used to predict liver disease and risk assessment for surgery?**

The Child's classification taking into account serum bilirubin, albumin, ascites, encephalopathy, and nutritional status.

○ **In patients with ascites and hydrothorax, when should preoperative thoracentesis and paracentesis be considered?**

When massive ascites and hydrothorax cause marked pulmonary or abdominal symptoms.

○ **How does viral hepatitis affect timing of surgery?**

Perioperative morbidity approaches 12%, and mortality 9.5%. Thus, surgery should be deferred until convalescence, if possible.

○ **What therapy do patients with Mobitz type I (Wenckebach) second-degree heart block need prior to surgery?**

No preoperative therapy needed.

○ **In patients with pacemakers, what preoperative preparation is advised?**

Demand pacemakers should be converted to fixed-rate mode by passing a magnet over the pacemaker.

○ **What is the classic history of a patient with severe aortic stenosis?**

Exercise dyspnea, angina, and syncope.

○ **What physical examination findings are suggestive of cardiovascular disease?**

Hypertension, JVD, laterally displaced point of maximal impulse, irregular pulse, third heart sound, pulmonary rates, heart murmurs, peripheral edema, or vascular bruits.

○ **What is the typical murmur of aortic stenosis?**

Systolic murmur at the right sternal border that radiates into the carotid arteries.

Postoperative Care of the Gynecologic Patient

CHAPTER 35

Denise Hartman, MD

○ **How does postoperative stress affect sodium and water balance?**

Surgical stress can induce high levels of antidiuretic hormone (ADH) and aldosterone leading to water and sodium retention.

○ **How much fluid is usually sequestered in patients with a postoperative ileus?**

One to three liters.

○ **When in the postoperative period does third spacing of fluid begin to resolve?**

Usually after 3 to 4 days, when the ADH and aldosterone levels normalize.

○ **What is the most common fluid and electrolyte disorder in the postoperative period?**

Fluid overload because of excess isotonic intravenous fluids.

○ **How much fluid should be replaced for insensible losses in patients with fever and hyperventilation?**

Up to 2 liters of free water can be lost a day as a result of perspiration and hyperventilation. These losses are difficult to monitor, so trend in body weight can be useful.

○ **What is the most common acid-base abnormality encountered in the postoperative period?**

Alkalosis caused by nasogastric suction, hyperventilation, and hyperaldosteronism.

○ **What is considered marked alkalosis, and what dangers does this entity pose?**

A pH greater than 7.55 can induce seizures and cardiac arrhythmias, especially with hypokalemia.

○ **How does metabolic acidosis affect the cardiovascular system?**

Decreased myocardial contractility, venodilation with hypotension, and responsiveness to defibrillation.

○ **What are the indications for bicarbonate administration in postoperative metabolic acidosis?**

A pH less than 7.2, or severe cardiac complications because of acidosis.

○ **What methods of postoperative pain control are the most effective?**

Intraspinal anesthetics and/or narcotics administered in the epidural or intrathecal space; continuous subcutaneous infiltration of anesthetic solution via implanted catheter.

○ **What are the advantages of epidural rather than intrathecal analgesia?**

Epidural analgesia can provide extended pain relief (greater than 24 hours) whereas intrathecal analgesia is limited to one dose because of the risk of CNS infection, the development of headaches, and respiratory depression.

○ **What is the most serious complication associated with epidural postoperative analgesia?**

Respiratory depression occurring in less than 1% of patients.

○ **What is the mechanism of postoperative halothane-induced hepatitis?**

A halothane metabolite via an autoimmune process induces hepatitis. Risk factors include familial history and obesity.

○ **When does halothane-induced hepatitis typically occur?**

Usually, one to two weeks after the exposure to halothane.

○ **What is the definition of febrile morbidity in a postoperative patient?**

Temperature greater than or equal to 100.4°F (38°C) on two separate occasions at least 4 hours apart excluding the first 24 hours.

○ **When should blood cultures be obtained on the postoperative febrile patient?**

Blood cultures are of little value in immunocompetent patients unless the temperature is >102°F.

○ **How should the postoperative patient with costovertebral tenderness and fever be evaluated?**

The urine should be examined for evidence of infection. If infection is not evident, then an intravenous pyelogram should be considered to assess for ureteral damage or obstruction.

○ **Should prophylactic antibiotics be routinely used when patients have indwelling Foley catheters?**

Not unless the patient is immunocompromised.

○ **What is the most common postoperative site of infection?**

Intravenous catheter-related infections have a reported incidence of 25% to 35%. Urinary tract infections are much less frequent with the greater use of prophylactic antibiotics.

○ **When should a chest film be performed for the febrile postoperative patient?**

In the presence of pulmonary findings or risk factors for pulmonary complications.

○ **How often should intravenous catheters be changed?**

Every 72 hours, after which time the risk of catheter-related phlebitis increases greatly.

○ **What is the relationship between preoperative shaving and wound infection?**

Preoperative shaving increases the rate of wound infection.

○ **Does vaginal cuff cellulitis need intravenous antibiotics?**

It is present to some extent in most patients who have undergone hysterectomy, and is usually self-limited. However, when fever, leukocytosis, and pelvic pain are present, antibiotics are indicated.

○ **What are the most common bacteria isolated from pelvic abscesses in the postoperative patient?**

E. coli, *Klebsiella*, and *Bacteroides* species.

○ **What tissues are involved in necrotizing fasciitis?**

The dermis and subcutaneous tissue with necrosis of the superficial fascia, without muscle involvement.

○ **What are predisposing factors to the development of necrotizing fasciitis?**

Diabetes mellitus, trauma, alcoholism, immunocompromised state, hypertension, peripheral vascular disease, intravenous drug use, and obesity.

○ **What is the primary treatment for necrotizing fasciitis?**

Extensive surgical debridement down to the fascia.

○ **What are the characteristics of a drug-induced postoperative fever?**

The patient appears well, without tachycardia, occasionally with eosinophilia.

○ **What is the biggest risk factor for the development of a postoperative urinary tract infection?**

The presence of an indwelling urinary catheter.

○ **What fraction of postoperative febrile morbidity result from an infectious etiology?**

20%.

○ **What is the most common cause of postoperative fever in the first 48 hours?**

Atelectasis.

○ **What is the most common complaint associated with retained sponge or laparotomy pad?**

A tender infected pelvic mass.

○ **What is the etiology of pseudomembranous colitis?**

Broad-spectrum antibiotics such as clindamycin select *C. difficile* to predominate in the bowel. *C. difficile* releases an exotoxin.

○ **How is pseudomembranous colitis treated?**

Oral vancomycin <u>or</u> metronidazole.

○ **How long following laparotomy can a pneumoperitoneum normally be found?**

Up to 7 to 10 days following surgery.

○ **What is the most common cause of small bowel obstruction following surgery?**

Adhesions to the operative site.

○ **What are the barrier agents proven in controlled studies to safely reduce the incidence and severity of postoperative adhesions?**

Hyaluronic acid with carboxymethylcellulose (HAL-F, Seprafilm) and oxidized regenerated cellulose (Interceed).

○ **What findings indicate the need for immediate surgery for small bowel obstruction?**

Worsening symptoms, leukocytosis, acidosis, and fever may indicate bowel ischemia.

○ **What is the most common cause of postoperative colonic obstruction in gynecological patients?**

Pelvic malignancy, most likely caused by advanced ovarian cancer.

○ **What is the most common gynecological process associated with both bowel ileus and obstruction?**

Severe pelvic inflammatory disease.

○ **Which parts of the gastrointestinal tract recover first after intraperitoneal surgery?**

The small intestine recovers after several hours, the stomach after 24 to 48 hours, and the large intestine after 48 to 72 hours.

○ **When are the symptoms of postoperative small bowel obstruction most likely to present?**

5 to 7 days postoperatively.

○ **What is the most common etiology for rectovaginal fistulas following gynecological surgery?**

Surgical trauma associated with extensive adhesions in the posterior cul-de-sac or scar tissue in the rectovaginal septum.

○ **Where do most pulmonary emboli arise?**

The deep venous system of the legs.

○ **When do the majority of deep venous thromboses develop relative to surgery?**

Within the first 24 hours of surgery.

○ **How should a deep venous thrombosis be managed in a postoperative patient?**

Intravenous heparin for 7 to 10 days, then oral Coumadin for at least three months.

○ **What is the most definitive method of diagnosing pulmonary embolism?**
Pulmonary angiography.

○ **What is the most common sign associated with pulmonary embolism?**
Tachypnea, presents more than 90% of the time.

○ **What percentage of acute iliofemoral thrombosis will lead to pulmonary embolus?**
40% of these patients will develop pulmonary embolism.

○ **Once a deep venous thrombosis has been diagnosed, what activity should the patient perform?**
The patient should have leg elevation and strict bed rest to prevent embolization of the clot.

○ **What is the initial procedure of choice for diagnosing deep venous thrombosis?**
Duplex ultrasonography.

○ **What is Virchow's triad?**
Stasis, coagulability, and endothelial wall damage.

○ **How do intermittent compression devices help in preventing deep venous thrombosis?**
Decreasing venous stasis and also decreasing coagulability (increasing fibrinolysis).

○ **How can postoperative pneumonia be differentiated from atelectasis?**
Pneumonia usually presents with a purulent productive cough, high fever, and coarse rales over the infected area.

○ **How is adult respiratory distress syndrome (ARDS) distinguished from congestive heart failure or pulmonary edema?**
A Swan-Ganz catheter is helpful showing a low pulmonary capillary wedge pressure.

○ **Which blood product is the most volume efficient method of increasing fibrinogen?**
Cryoprecipitate has a volume of 40 mL vs fresh frozen plasma (200 mL).

○ **What is the most sensitive indicator of decreased volume status caused by intraperitoneal hemorrhage?**
Decreased urine output, which precedes tachycardia and hypotension.

○ **What is the primary goal in the management of a patient in hypovolemic shock?**
Adequate oxygenation and ventilation, followed by fluid replacement.

○ **How much blood must be lost for a young woman to demonstrate signs of shock?**
At least 20% of blood volume.

○ **What are risk factors associated with femoral neuropathy following gynecological surgery?**

Thin patient, self-retained retractor with deep blades, and a transverse skin incision.

○ **What is the best way to close a fascial dehiscence?**

A mass closure with through-and-through monofilament nylon or a Smead-Jones closure.

○ **What is the most common sign of wound disruption?**

Spontaneous serosanguineous fluid from the abdominal incision.

○ **When diffuse erythema surrounds a wound infection within the first 24 hours postoperatively, what is the most likely etiology?**

Beta-hemolytic streptococci, needing prompt intravenous antibiotics.

○ **How should granulation tissue at the vaginal vault apex following hysterectomy be treated?**

Chemical cautery, cryocautery, or electrocautery.

○ **In operative cases, where the risk of wound infection is high, what measure can be used to decrease the risk?**

Delayed primary closure of the wound decreases wound infections from 23% to 2%.

○ **Where do rectovaginal fistulas usually occur following gynecological surgery?**

After hysterectomy, the fistula occurs in the upper third of the vagina; after a posterior repair, the fistula is usually in the lower third of the vagina.

○ **When do the majority of rectovaginal fistulas present in the postoperative period?**

7 to 14 days postoperatively.

○ **How is a prolapsed fallopian tube diagnosed?**

Watery discharge, postcoital spotting, coital pain, or lower abdominal pain within the first few months following hysterectomy.

○ **In what situations are suprapubic catheters useful?**

When prolonged drainage of the bladder is anticipated such as after a radical hysterectomy.

○ **What is the treatment for ARDS?**

Treatment of the underlying etiology, ventilatory support and PEEP, and careful fluid management.

○ **What is the treatment for cardiogenic pulmonary edema?**

Assessment of volume status and cardiac ischemia, oxygen, diuretics, afterload reduction.

○ **What are the postoperative pulmonary changes that predispose patients to atelectasis?**

Decrease in vital capacity and functional residual capacity, discomfort from sighing and deep breathing, and impairment of the mucociliary clearing mechanism.

○ **What is the most common postoperative complication in patients with mitral stenosis?**

Pulmonary edema because of excess fluid administration.

○ **Why is sinus tachycardia to be avoided in postoperative patients with aortic stenosis?**

Decrease in ventricular filling in diastole exacerbates inadequate cardiac output.

○ **What is the most important aspect in diagnosing myocardial infarction in the postoperative patient?**

A high degree of suspicion, since only 50% of postsurgical patients have chest pain.

○ **What is the most sensitive indicator of postoperative myocardial infarction?**

The creatinine phosphokinase MB isoenzyme level.

○ **In patients with coronary artery disease, what constitutes significant hypotension, and puts the patient at risk for myocardial infarction?**

33% to 50% decrease in systolic blood pressure for at least 10 minutes.

○ **What should be the management of patients who have been on beta-blockers during the intraoperative and postoperative period?**

Continuing these agents, since removal can lead to severe rebound with hypertension and angina.

○ **What precautions should be taken for patients with pacemakers?**

Electrocautery devices can trigger demand type pacemakers. Therefore, the electrode should be placed as far from the pacemaker as possible. Also, a magnet should be used to convert the pacemaker from the demand to a fixed pacing mode.

○ **How does intermittent positive pressure breathing (IPPB) therapy compare with incentive spirometry in the prevention of atelectasis in high-risk patients?**

Incentive spirometry is as effective, cheaper, and has less complications.

○ **What glucose value is targeted in the postoperative diabetic patient?**

Less than 180 to 240 mg/dL to prevent glucosuria, dehydration, and leukocyte inhibition.

○ **What are the indications for mechanical ventilation in a postoperative patient?**

Acute respiratory acidosis, ARDS, and progressive symptomatic hypoxemia unresponsive to oxygen supplementation.

○ **What is the difference between assist-control (AC) and intermittent mechanical ventilation (IMV)?**

With assist control (AC), the ventilator will provide assistance to any inspiration initiated by the patient; if necessary, provide additional breaths so that the total number of breaths per minute meets the designated set rate. Intermittent mechanical ventilation provides only a set number of assisted ventilations and does not provide assistance to breaths initiated by the patient. IMV is useful in patients who hyperventilate or those being weaned from the ventilatory support.

○ **What is the most common renal problem in a postoperative patient?**

Oliguria, defined as less than 25 mL/h urine output.

○ **How might postoperative prerenal oliguria be differentiated from acute renal failure?**

Prerenal azotemia tends to have a low fractional excretion of sodium, usually less than 1%. This is calculated by: (Urine sodium × Plasma creatinine) × 100/(Plasma sodium × Urine creatinine).

○ **What are the indications for dialysis in a postoperative patient who develops acute renal failure?**

Volume overload, hyperkalemia unresponsive to potassium binders, alteration in mental status, and a pericardial friction rub.

○ **How should hypertensive patients who have been taking diuretic medications be managed in the postoperative phase?**

Diuretics can cause volume and electrolyte disturbances, and usually are not needed in the first two postoperative days.

○ **What gynecological surgeries predispose to postoperative inability to void?**

Operations involving the urethra or bladder.

○ **What surgery is associated with the majority of vesicovaginal fistulas?**

Total abdominal hysterectomies for benign indications.

○ **How does a low albumin level reflect on nutritional status?**

A low albumin level reflects a depletion of visceral proteins of at least 3 weeks' duration.

○ **What protein level gives a more immediate picture of nutritional status?**

The transferrin level, which has a half-life of 8 to 9 days, provides a more recent protein assessment.

○ **What are the indications for total parenteral nutrition?**

No oral intake for 7 to 10 days, especially if nutritionally compromised.

○ **When is peripheral alimentation useful?**

Patients who are in a noncatabolic state and who require nutritional support for less than 7 days.

○ **What is the most common etiology of postoperative hemorrhage arising from the vaginal vault following hysterectomy?**

Improperly ligated vaginal artery at the lateral vaginal angle.

○ **When does hemorrhage from cervical conization typically occur?**

Usually in the first 24 hours or 7 to 14 days later when the cervical sutures lose their tensile strength.

○ **How much crystalloid should be administered per milliliter of blood loss in the initial treatment of hemorrhagic shock?**

3 mL of crystalloid per l mL of blood loss.

○ **What is the most common cause of shock in the perioperative period?**

Inadequate hemostasis related to hemorrhage.

○ **After intravascular fluid equilibration, what change in hematocrit usually corresponds to a blood loss of 500 mL?**

Usually a reduction of the hematocrit of 3% to 5%.

○ **What is the mechanism whereby hypogastric artery ligation helps in pelvic hemorrhage?**

Decrease in the pulse pressure, allowing a stable clot to form over the injured pelvic vessels.

○ **What flow of blood is required to visualize a bleeding vessel for angiographic embolization?**

At least 1 mL/min.

○ **Which artery is most likely to be injured in performing a transverse muscle cutting incision (Maylard incision)?**

The inferior epigastric artery.

○ **In performing a hypogastric artery ligation, what structure is most likely to be injured?**

The hypogastric vein.

○ **Gynecologic procedures that carry a significant risk of postoperative infection include:**

Vaginal hysterectomy, abdominal hysterectomy, surgical treatment of pelvic abscess, pregnancy termination, or radical surgery of gynecologic cancers.

○ **Factors that place patients at risk for posthysterectomy infection include:**

Low socioeconomic class, duration of surgery greater than two hours, presence of malignancy, and increased number of surgical procedures performed.

○ **The antibiotic class most well suited for prophylaxis in gynecologic surgery:**

1st and 2nd generation cephalosporins.

○ **A urinary tract infection is defined as:**

Growth of $>10^5$ organisms/mL of urine.

○ **Most UTIs are caused by the growth of which bacteria?**

E. coli, Klebsiella, Proteus, Enterobacter, and *Staphylococcus.*

○   **Symptoms of a wound infection most commonly occur after what postoperative day?**

Fourth.

○   **Standard therapy for intra-abdominal abscess:**

Surgical evacuation and drainage combined with administration of ampicillin, gentamycin, and clindamycin.

○   **When is a second dose of prophylactic antibiotics indicated?**

If the operation lasts more than 3 hours or the EBL is greater than 1500 cc.

○   **What prophylactic antibiotics should be used, if the patient is allergic to penicillins or cephalosporins?**

Clindamycin, doxycycline, or metronidazole.

○   **The organisms most likely to cause postabortive endometritis include:**

Neisseria gonorrhoeae, *Chlamydia trachomatis*, and *Streptococcus agalactiae*.

○   **What antibiotics should be used to avoid postabortive endometritis?**

Doxycycline, ofloxacin, and ceftriaxone.

○   **What type of fascial closure technique has been shown to result in the lowest incidence of wound dehiscence and hernia formation?**

A loosely approximated mass closure by using a slowly absorbable monofilament suture with a suture:wound length ratio of at least 4:1 (achieved by placing suture 1.5 cm from fascial edge with 1 cm between each placement).

○   **What are the four stages of would healing?**

Inflammation.
Epithelialization (migration).
Fibroplasia.
Maturation.

○   **What is the duration of each of these stages?**

Inflammation: completed within three days in absence of infection.
Epithelialization: completed within 48 hours of surgery.
Fibroplasia: collagen production begins on second postoperative day, maximum rate at 5 days postoperatively, and continues for at least 6 weeks. Angiogenesis occurs during this stage.
Maturation: 80% or original tissue strength is restored by 6 weeks postoperative, appearance of normal skin at 180 days, remodeling continues for years.

CHAPTER 36 Urinary Tract Injuries

Vincent Lucente, MD

○ **What is the overall incidence of urologic injury during gynecologic procedures, and what urologic organ is most commonly injured?**

The exact incidence of accidental lower urinary tract injury during obstetric and gynecologic procedures is hard to assess because most cases are unreported. Most authors report an overall incidence of 0.2% to 2.5%. Bladder injuries outnumber ureteral injuries, with a ratio of 5.3:1. A recent review that included 47 studies and more than 120,000 patients estimated the incidence of bladder and ureteral injury to be 2.6/1,000 and 1.6/1,000, respectively.

○ **What is the incidence and major cause of urethral injury?**

Urethral injury is rare. Formerly, obstructed labor or instrumented deliveries were the major causes of urethral injury resulting in fistula in the US and are still in developing countries. In the US, most urethral injuries resulting in fistula result from complications after excision of a diverticulum, including failed repair, hematoma, or infection. Urethral injury may occur during anterior colporrhaphy or traumatic catheterization, especially if a rigid catheter is used.

○ **What is the leading cause of bladder injury resulting in vesicovaginal fistula?**

Hysterectomy.

○ **True or False: An abdominal hysterectomy has a lower risk of ureteral injury than a vaginal hysterectomy?**

False. Seventy-five percent of ureteral injuries occur during abdominal hysterectomy, and 25% during vaginal hysterectomy. The rate of ureteral injury during abdominal hysterectomy is 0.5% to 1%, and during vaginal hysterectomy is 0.1%.

○ **What is the leading cause of ureteral injury?**

Abdominal hysterectomy for benign causes.

○ **What are the signs that a bladder injury may have occurred?**

The first indication that a bladder injury has occurred during surgery is the appearance of fluid in the wound. Appearance of fluid in the vagina 3 to 12 days postoperatively is a late sign of vesicovaginal fistula.

329

○ **At what times during an abdominal hysterectomy is the bladder at greatest risk?**

(1) Incising the parietal peritoneum—failure to drain the bladder before entering the peritoneal cavity increases this risk.

(2) Entering the vesicouterine fold—if the fold is entered too low, the dome of the bladder may be injured.

(3) Separating the bladder from the uterine fundus, cervix, or upper vagina—adhesions from previous surgery, endometriosis, irradiation, or pelvic inflammatory disease can cause the bladder to be densely adherent to the lower uterus and upper vagina. Sharp dissection with Metzenbaum scissors pointed away from the bladder will decrease this risk.

(4) Entering the anterior vagina and suturing the vaginal vault. Grasping the edges of the vaginal cuff in preparation for repair will prevent bladder injury here. In addition, suturing the vaginal cuff in an anterior to posterior direction will decrease the risk of bladder injury.

○ **Where is the most common location of a bladder injury during entry into the peritoneal cavity?**

Bladder dome.

○ **What is the most common location of a bladder injury during vaginal hysterectomy?**

Supratrigonal portion of the bladder base.

○ **How is the correct plane between the bladder and cervix recognized during vaginal hysterectomy?**

Firm downward traction on the cervix with gentle countertraction of the bladder with a right-angled retractor should reveal the correct plane, which is *white and relatively avascular.*

○ **Once a bladder injury is suspected, how is it diagnosed?**

Use a Foley catheter to instill 400 to 600 cc of sterile milk or sterile water and methylene blue into the bladder and watch for this colored fluid in the surgical field.

○ **How should a bladder injury be repaired?**

Careful assessment of the extent of injury with intraoperative cystoscopy should be performed. Intravenous indigo carmine should be administered to assure ureteral patency and absence of damage to the ureters. In addition, ureteral catheter placement makes ligation of the ureters during repair less likely. A continuous multilayer closure with 3-0 delayed absorbable suture on a small tapered needle with inversion of the mucosa on the first layer should be performed. The suture line should be tested by distending the bladder with sterile milk (especially during vaginal repairs) and additional sutures placed to until the repair is watertight.

○ **What should the postoperative management of a cystotomy repair include?**

Bladder decompression for 7 to 10 days. Consider prophylactic antibiotic suppression. Performing a voiding cystourethrogram to assure that the bladder is completely healed prior to removing the indwelling catheter is recommended by some authors; however, care should be taken as to not over distend the bladder during the study. Ureteral catheterization is not necessary for injuries at the dome that do not involve the ureters.

○ **What injury to the urinary tract is the most difficult to recognize?**

Injury to ureter.

○ **What injury to the urinary tract produces the most serious complications?**

Injury to ureter.

○ **Where is the most common site of ureteral injury?**

Approximately 80% to 90% of all ureteral injuries occur in the distal portion of the ureter from the uterine artery to the ureterovesical junction.

○ **At what sites is the ureter at greatest risk?**

At the infundibulopelvic ligament near the pelvic brim, in the base of the broad ligament where the ureter passes beneath the uterine vessels, along the sidewall above the uterosacral ligaments, and as the ureter passes through the cardinal ligament and turns anteriorly and medially to enter the bladder.

○ **What types of ureteral injury can occur?**

(1) Crushing injury from misapplication of surgical clamps; (2) ligation with suture, partial or complete transection; (3) angulation with partial or complete obstruction; (4) ischemia from stripping of the adventitia and decreased blood supply to that part of the ureter; (5) resection of a segment of ureter intentionally or unintentionally.

○ **What pelvic conditions may predispose to ureteric injury?**

Lateral displacement of the cervix by tumors or large fibroids, masses adhering to the peritoneum overlying the ureter, intraligamentary tumors, retroperitoneal tumors, abscesses in the broad ligament, cervical cancer.

○ **What technique should be used to mobilize masses that may involve the ureter?**

Open the retroperitoneal space lateral to the mass, identify the ureter, and dissect the mass away from the ureter under direct visualization.

○ **Where does ureteral injury most often occur during abdominal surgery?**

Where the ureter crosses beneath the uterine artery lateral to the cervix. This happens most often when trying to gain hemostasis.

○ **True or False: Using ureteral stents prevents intraoperative injury to the ureters.**

False.

○ **What techniques protect against ureteral injury at the time of vaginal hysterectomy?**

Ureteral injury occurs rarely in vaginal hysterectomy, despite the fact that downward traction on the uterus pulls the ureter downward. Clamping the uterine vessels at a right angle to the vessel and as close to the uterus as possible will decrease the risk of ureteric injury.

○ **What percentage of ureteral injuries are recognized at the time of surgery?**

20% to 30%.

○ **What should be done when ureteral injury is suspected?**

Administer 5 mL of indigo carmine IV, followed by cystoscopy to verify bilateral excretion of the dye from each ureteral orifice.

○   **What should be done when a ureteral injury is diagnosed?**

Consult a urologist or a urogynecologist. Attempts to place stents will be made to identify the area of injury if it is not already apparent. Further management will depend on the degree and location of the trauma.

○   **What is the most common cause of ureterovaginal fistula?**

Unrecognized clamp injury or suture ligation of the ureter.

○   **What should be done, if the ureter is included in a clamped or ligated vessel?**

The clamp should be removed and the ureter inspected. If the damage is minor, the area of injury should be drained extraperitoneally. A suture should simply be removed. If after removal of a clamp or suture the ureter appears pale, ureteral catheterization for 7 to 10 days should be performed to allow revascularization.

○   **How should a partially transected ureter be managed?**

Repair with several interrupted sutures of 4-0 delayed absorbable sutures over a ureteral stent with retroperitoneal drainage.

○   **How should a total transected ureter be managed?**

Management of a total transection depends on location. If the transection occurs within 5 cm of the vesicoureteral junction, ureteroneocystostomy (direct re-implantation of the ureter into the bladder wall) should be performed. If the transection is higher and the ureter will not reach the bladder without tension, a psoas hitch is performed. The bladder is mobilized and secured to the psoas muscle and a tension-free ureteroneocystostomy is performed. If the ureter is transected above the pelvic brim, a ureteroureterostomy is performed. Both ends of the ureter are spatulated for 5 mm and approximated without tension over a silastic catheter with interrupted 4-0 delayed absorbable suture. The stent should be left in place for 2 to 3 weeks. The repair should be drained extraperitoneally.

○   **What is a patient at risk for after ureteroneocystostomy, and how can this be prevented?**

Vesicoureteral reflux. This can be prevented by tunneling the ureter in the submucosa of the bladder (Politano and Leadbetter technique).

○   **What postoperative symptoms are associated with ureteral injury?**

Flank pain or tenderness, fever, sepsis, ileus, abdominal distension, unexplained hematuria, urine leakage through the vagina or skin, urinoma, oliguria or anuria, elevated serum creatinine.

○   **What should be done if ureteral injury is suspected postoperatively?**

IVP.

○   **What should be done if IVP shows obstruction or hydronephrosis?**

Attempts to pass a ureteral catheter past the point of obstruction should be made. If successful, the catheter should be left in place for 14 to 21 days. Follow-up IVP should be performed after catheter removal.

○   **What should be done if a catheter cannot be passed past the ureteral obstruction?**

Immediate ureteral repair or percutaneous nephrostomy. If percutaneous nephrostomy is performed, the injury may resolve spontaneously, thus definitive surgery should be deferred for 8 weeks. However, when unintentional ureteral ligation is performed in a healthy patient and is discovered within 10 to 14 days of surgery, immediate repair consisting of ureteroneocystostomy can be performed.

○ **How long can an obstructed, uninfected kidney survive?**

7 to 158 days.

○ **What is the leading cause of litigation in gynecology?**

Failure to recognize a urinary tract injury. Patients do quite well with intraoperative urinary tract injury repair, but suffer tremendously when these repairs go undiagnosed.

CHAPTER 37 Genital Prolapse

Oren Azulay, MD

○ **Urethroceles appear to be more common in women with what type of bony pelvis?**
Gynecoid.

○ **Pus expressed through the urethral meatus on palpation of the urethra may indicate the presence of what defects?**
Infected urethral diverticulum or infected Skene's glands.

○ **What defect in vaginal support is frequently found in conjunction with a cystocele?**
Rectocele and/or urethrocele.

○ **What defect of pelvic support result from a weakened cul-de-sac of Douglas?**
Enterocele.

○ **What structures are most important in prevention of posthysterectomy enterocele formation?**
Uterosacral-cardinal ligament complex, pubocervical fascia, and rectovaginal fascia.

○ **The contents of an enterocele may include omentum but always include what structure?**
Small intestine.

○ **How is prolapse of the pelvic organs to the introitus classified?**
Second degree or grade 3.

○ **Although ulcers of the vagina associated with complete prolapse are rarely malignant, they should be biopsied. What is the most common cause?**
Stasis.

○ **Name three types of nonoperative management of cystoceles?**
Pessaries, Kegel's exercises, and estrogen.

○ **Name two conditions that may mimic a cystocele.**

Urethral diverticula and inflamed Skene's glands.

○ **What forms the intermediate layer of the pelvic floor between the endopelvic fascia and the urogenital diaphragm?**

Levator ani.

○ **What structure is located on the pelvic sidewall approximately halfway between the pubic bones and the sacrum?**

Ischial spine.

○ **What two band of fibrous tissue are located on the pelvic wall between the spines and pubic bones?**

Arcus tendineus fasciae pelvis and arcus tendineus muscularis levator ani.

○ **What muscle overlies the sacrospinous ligament?**

Coccygeus muscle.

○ **Trunks of what nerve cross the surface of the piriformis muscle?**

Sciatic nerve.

○ **The cardinal ligaments arise from what region?**

Greater sciatic foramen.

○ **The uterosacral ligaments originate from what region?**

Second, third, and fourth sacral vertebrae.

○ **What muscles support the pelvic viscera?**

Pubococcygeus and iliococcygeus.

○ **Vesical neck support is provided by what structure and it's attachment to the fascial arch (arcus tendineus musculi levatori ani)?**

Pubovesical Fascia.

○ **What are the most frequent symptoms of uterine prolapse?**

Fullness of the vagina, sensation of something "falling out" or a protrusion at the introitus.

○ **Marked degrees of uterine prolapse may compress the ureters resulting in what abnormality of the ureters?**

Hydroureter.

○ **Name three management strategies for uterine prolapse.**

Expectant, surgical, and pessaries.

○ **Name three medical conditions that may make uterine prolapse worse with time.**

Chronic cough, obesity, and chronic constipation.

○ **Name two urological findings that are contraindications to expectant management of uterine prolapse.**

Hydroureter, hyronephrosis.

○ **The standard Le Fort procedure is contraindicated in the postmenopausal patient with a desire to preserve what function?**

Coital function.

○ **The sacrospinous ligament fixation is a procedure used as treatment for or prophylaxis against what condition?**

Vaginal prolapse.

○ **Failure to recognize and repair what defect results in prolapse of the vaginal vault after hysterectomy?**

Failure to suspend vaginal cuff with cardinal and uterosacral ligaments complex.

○ **The need to "splint" the vagina to defecate is indicative of what defect?**

Rectocele.

○ **Most women with a rectocele have a concomitant defect of what structure?**

Perineal body.

○ **Disorders of what sacral nerves may be responsible for uterine prolapse?**

S1 to S4.

○ **Inflatable, Smith - Hodge, and donut are types of what device?**

Pessaries.

○ **What is the name of the operation combing anterior and posterior colporrhaphy with amputation of the cervix and use of the cardinal ligaments to support the anterior vaginal wall and bladder?**

Manchester–Fothergill.

○ **The Miya hook is an instrument commonly used in what procedure?**

Sacrospinous ligament fixation.

○ **Femoral hernias are more common in which gender?**

Females.

○ **Inguinal hernias are more common in which gender?**

Males.

○ **What technique of examination is useful in distinguishing between enterocele, vaginal prolapse, and rectocele?**

Rectovaginal examination with the patient standing.

○ **Operative injury to what nerve results in the patient experiencing footdrop?**

Common peroneal.

○ **Injury to the sciatic nerve presents what clinical picture?**

Weakness during knee flexion.

○ **A patient who experiences pain in the medial groin, inner thigh, or labia after bladder suspension may have entrapment of what nerve?**

ilioinguinal.

○ **Saphenous nerve injury is manifested by what symptoms?**

Pain, burning, or aching in the calf.

○ **What nerve injury results in weakness of the thigh on adduction?**

Obturator.

○ **Quadriceps weakness and gait impairment may be indicative of injury to what nerve?**

Femoral.

○ **Rectal prolapse is more common in multiparous or nulliparous women?**

Nulliparous.

○ **What is the name of the defect that is present when the pubocervical fascia separates from its attachment to the fascia covering the obturator internus and levator ani muscles?**

Paravaginal defect.

○ **A hernia through the Canal of Nuck may be confused with what cystic lesions?**

Gartner duct cyst or Bartholin cyst.

○ **What complication of ovarian malignancy can cause a cystocele?**

Ascites.

○ **Name a group of women more likely than Asian women to develop prolapse?**

Caucasian.

○ **The anterior separation in the levator ani is known by what term?**

Levator hiatus.

○   **McCall sutures have what purpose?**

Posterior cul-de-sac obliteration to prevent enterocele formation.

○   **If the uterosacral-cardinal ligament complex is too attenuated to use for vaginal suspension, what other structures can be used?**

Sacrospinous ligament or iliococcygeus fascia and longitudinal ligament of sacrum.

○   **During repair of the perineal body constriction of the posterior fourchette may result in what patient complaint?**

Dyspareunia.

○   **What should be the basic principle in the management of pelvic organ prolapse?**

Individualization.

○   **Since pelvic organ prolapse is thought to be in many instances a result of vaginal delivery, it is best to defer surgical treatment until when?**

Until childbearing is complete.

○   **Name three problems apart from infection and hemorrhage that may be the result of ventral suspension of the vagina.**

Urethral or ureteral kinking and enterocele development.

○   **Name two approaches to paravaginal repair.**

Abdominal (open or laparoscopy) and vaginal.

○   **When compared to each other, is an abdominal or vaginal paravaginal repair more easily accomplished and durable?**

Abdominal.

○   **What vaginal complication results from excessive trimming of vaginal mucosa in an anterior colporrhaphy?**

Vaginal shortening or stenosis.

○   **Anterior colporrhaphy is indicated for correction of a cystocele caused by what type of vaginal wall defect?**

Anterior midline.

○   **The Moschowitz or Halban techniques, although different are used to accomplish what?**

Cul-de-sac obliteration to prevent enterocele.

○   **To what structure is the distal posterior wall of the vaginal fused?**

Perineal body.

○   **Name two defects resulting from anterior vaginal prolapse.**

Cystocele and cystourethrocele.

○   **Patient with symptoms of pelvic organ prolapse should be evaluated in what positions?**

Sitting, standing, and lithotomy.

○   **Name three urologic complications of anterior colporrhaphy.**

Incontinence, ureteral injury, cystotomy, vesicovaginal fistula, and urethral injury.

○   **Wide sheets of anterior and posterior vaginal epithelium are removed and the denuded walls are then approximated in what procedure?**

Le Fort.

○   **What is the common name of the arcus tendineus fascia pelvis?**

White line.

○   **What are the three goals in the management, whether operative or non-operative, of genital prolapse?**

Relief of symptoms, restoration of anatomy, and preservation or restoration of normal function.

○   **What is the most common defect in cystocele?**

Paravaginal defect.

○   **Describe supporting system of vagina**

Apex of the vagina is suspended with uterosacral-cardinal ligament complex, majority of midvagina is attached with white line of fascia pelvic up to the level of ischial spine, and base of the vagina is fused with perineal body and pubic bone.

○   **Name the muscle groups of the pelvis.**

Iliopsoas, obturator internus, piriformis, ischiococcygeal, iliococcygeal, puborectalis, coccygeus, and urogenital diaphragm.

○   **What is the specific defect seen in prolapse of the vaginal vault after hysterectomy?**

Failure of vaginal cuff suspension with uterosacral-cardinal ligament complex.

○   **What is the specific defect seen in enterocele?**

Disruption of cervical ring between pubocervical fascia and rectovaginal fascia.

○   **What other condition beside prolapse of pelvic organ should be evaluated before corrective surgery?**

Urinary incontinence.

○   **What suture material is used for surgical correction of pelvic organ prolapse?**

Permanent suture.

○   **What are possible risk factors for prolapse?**

Genetic predisposition, parity more with vaginal birth, advancing age, elevated intra-abdominal pressure, obesity, prior pelvic surgery, and connective tissue disorders.

○   **Are symptoms of urgency, incontinence, or frequency related to degree of prolapse?**

No. Most incontinence improves with worsening prolapse.

○   **What is the best position for examination?**

Supine position with heels in stirrups with full Valsalva. Standing position with straining can be attempted as well. In women with pessaries, remove pessary first. Following a standard examination, always perform a single blade examination, which allows site-specific evaluation.

For enterocele detection, the best position is a standing position with one leg elevated while performing a rectovaginal examination.

○   **What systems are used to evaluate prolapse?**

Baden-Walker System and pelvic organ prolapse quantification (POPQ).

○   **What are the grades of the Baden-Walker System?**

Grade 0: Normal position for all anatomical markers.

Grade 1: Descent halfway to the hymen.

Grade2: Descent to the level of the hymen.

Grade3: Descent halfway past the hymen.

Grade 4: Maximum possible descent at all markers.

○   **What are the grades of the POPQ system?**

All measurements are in reference to the hymen level. Measurements above the hymen are recorded as negative numbers, while measurements beyond the hymen are designated at positive values.

Measurements are of the following:

Point Aa: Midline anterior wall, 3 cm proximal to urethral meatus.

Point Ba: Most proximal part of anterior vaginal wall, anterior fornix.

Point Ap: Midline of posterior vaginal wall.

Point Bp: Furthest and the most dependent in the posterior vaginal wall.

Point C: Anterior cervix, most dependent in anterior wall.

Point D: Deepest point in the posterior fornix (uterosacral ligament level).

TVL: Total vaginal length is the distance from hymen the point D (without prolapse).

Genital hiatus (GH): Distance from midurethra to posterior hymen.

Perineal body (PB): Distance from posterior hymen to midanus.

○   **Does estrogen have a role in treatment or prevention of prolapse?**

No.

○ **What are the considerations in selecting synthetic meshes?**

Pore size and subsequent rates of infection, vaginal vs abdominal approach and degree of mesh erosion, and presence of chemical coating and subsequent failure rates.

○ **What is the most common site of prolapse?**

Anterior vaginal wall prolapse (40% of evaluated prolapse).

○ **Is there a relationship between prolapse and incontinence?**

Not direct relationships, but it is found that up to 40% of patients with prolapse will develop incontinence. Upon evaluation in office, always reduce prolapse and evaluate for different types of incontinence (beneficial for patient to consider two procedures at the same time).

○ **What are some of the factors physicians should discuss with patients when deciding surgical vs medical therapy?**

Desire to have intercourse
Durability
Recovery time
Types of complication rate.
Surgical candidacy
Foreign body risks

○ **In a patient with apical defect, is there a benefit of vaginal sacrospinous suspension vs abdominal sacrocolpopexy?**

There are no clear studies. Recently, various small randomized trials have been done, showing similar patient satisfaction at a distant follow-up care; though, objective findings of anatomical prolapse outcome are more superior with the abdominal approach. Each patient must be evaluated individually and have a full disclosed discussion of all possible treatment regiment and true long term success rates.

○ **What is the success rate of sacrospinous ligament suspension?**

63% to 97%.

○ **What is the Michigan modification?**

Modifying the sacrospinous ligament suspension, in the sense that all four vaginal walls are attached to the ligament reducing anterior wall prolapse after procedure.

○ **What are the complications of sacrospinous ligament suspension?**

Pudendal hemorrhage, bowel/bladder injury, and possible entrapment of the sciatic nerve causing severe pain in the posterior leg/gluteal area. (Upon diagnosis, remove stitches immediately.)

○ **What are the possible treatments in hemorrhage from middle sacral artery/venous plexus during sacral colpopexy?**

Sterile thumbtacks, ligation (if vessel is visualized), bone wax, various thrombogenic materials (Gelfoam, FLOSEAL, Surgicel, thrombin, and arista), and finally abdominal packing with VAC closure and re-exploration in 48 hours.

○   **What is the CARE trial?**

Colpopexy and urinary reduction efforts study. This study randomized women to have colpopexy with and without incontinence surgery. Study showed that the group with the incontinence procedure had clinically significant lower rates of SUI postoperatively, thus, proposing to perform Burch prophylactically.

○   **Is fecal incontinence a symptom of posterior wall prolapse?**

No.

○   **Which pessary is specifically designed to correct rectoceles?**

Gehrung pessary.

○   **What are the possible complications of pessary use?**

Urinary retention, vaginal irritation, new onset urinary incontinence, vaginal ulceration, recurrent UTIs, and abnormal discharge (foreign body reaction).

CHAPTER 38 Urinary Incontinence and Urodynamics

Vincent Lucente, MD

○ **What is urinary incontinence?**

The International Continence Society defines urinary incontinence as the "demonstrable involuntary loss of urine that is socially or hygienically unacceptable to the patient or detrimental to her physical well-being."

○ **What is the prevalence of urinary incontinence?**

One of the risk factors for developing urinary incontinence is age, thus as the population ages, the prevalence of incontinence will increase. The prevalence of incontinence also depends on the population under study. Studies have reported overall rates ranging from 8% to 41%, and in the nursing home population, the prevalence is as high as 70%.

○ **What risk factors predispose someone to the development of urinary incontinence?**

Sex: Urinary incontinence is two to three times more common in women than in men.

Age: The prevalence of urinary incontinence increases with age, with a 30% greater prevalence for each 5-year increase in age.

Childbirth: The risk of developing stress incontinence increases with parity. Urge incontinence is not related to parity.

Menopause, smoking and obesity are also risk factors for the development of urinary incontinence.

○ **There are four main types of established urinary incontinence in women. What are they?**

Genuine stress incontinence

Detrusor overactivity (formerly know as detrusor instability)

Mixed incontinence

Overflow incontinence

○ **What is genuine stress incontinence (GSUI)?**

The involuntary loss of urine secondary to increase in intra-abdominal pressure (coughing or bearing down) without a bladder contraction. The International Continence Society defines GSUI as the involuntary loss of urine, occurring when in the absence of a detrusor (bladder) contraction, the intravesical pressure exceeds intraurethral pressure.

○   **What is detrusor overactivity incontinence?**

Detrusor overactivity is also known as overactive bladder or urge incontinence. It is the involuntary loss of urine following a strong urge to void. Detrusor overactivity can be associated with a bladder contraction without associated incontinence.

○   **What is mixed urinary incontinence?**

Urinary urge incontinence (UUI) and GSUI occurring together in the same patient.

○   **What is overflow incontinence?**

The involuntary loss of urine secondary to bladder over distension. The hydrostatic pressure within the bladder rises above the urethral pressure and a "decompression" of pressure occurs often leaving a high-volume residual, as there is no detrusor contraction.

○   **What are some causes of overflow incontinence?**

Bladder atony (postepidural, diabetic neuropathy).
Outflow obstruction (vaginal or uterine mass, prolapse, gravid uterus with extreme retroversion).
Decreased bladder compliance (interstitial cystitis, postradiation fibrosis).

○   **What type of incontinence is associated with urinary retention?**

Overflow incontinence.

○   **What are three rare causes of urinary incontinence?**

Ectopic ureter
Fistulas
Urethral diverticulum

○   **What should always be ruled out when a patient presents with complaints of incontinence?**

Reversible causes of incontinence.

○   **What are the reversible causes of incontinence?**

Remember the mnemonic "DIAPPERS":
Delirium
Infection
Atrophy
Pharmacologic (e.g., diuretics, alpha-blockers, calcium channel blockers, etc.)
Psychological (depression)
Excessive fluid intake
Restricted mobility (functional incontinence)
Stool impaction

○   **What should be included in the basic evaluation of a patient with incontinence?**

A detailed history including precipitating factors, size of incontinence, leakage episodes (small leaks with exertion suggest stress incontinence, leakage of large amounts preceded by urgency suggests overactive bladder), requirement for protective garments, etc., physical examination including neurologic exam, urinalysis with culture, if indicated, assessment of urethral mobility, and simple cystometry. For those patients with any voiding symptoms a post-void residual should also be obtained. If the patient describes symptoms of mixed incontinence or fails initial therapy, she should be referred to a specialist for complex cystometry.

○ **How is urethral mobility assessed?**

The "Q-tip test" is an office-based assessment of urethral mobility (which is a risk factor for stress incontinence). A cotton swab is placed in the urethra to the level of the vesical neck and the measurement of the axis change with strain is performed with a goniometer. Hypermobility is defined as a change in angle with Valsalva of greater than 30 degrees.

○ **What is simple cystometry?**

Simple cystometry is the evaluation of bladder filling. It examines the pressure-volume relationship during filling. It is a "single channel" measurement, in that only bladder pressure is being measured. It can be done without urodynamic equipment using a "hand held" system. A 50 mL syringe without its piston or bulb is attached to the catheter and held above the bladder. The bladder is then gradually filled by gravity in 50 mL increments and the patient's first sensation of filling (normal values vary, usually the patient senses this, when asked), first sensation of urgency (normal range 150–250), and maximum bladder capacity (normal 300–500) are noted. Any rise in the column of water in the syringe resulting from inappropriate bladder contractions (the patient inadvertently bearing down may also cause this). The standing stress test may then be performed after the patient's catheter is removed.

○ **What is the Standing Stress test and how is it performed?**

The cough stress test involves, filling a patient's bladder to at least 300 mL or symptomatic fullness and having the patient cough while standing, while the urethral meatus is visualized. If urine leakage is observed, the test is positive. This test is an indicator of stress incontinence.

○ **What is intrinsic sphincter deficiency (ISD)?**

The "intrinsic" factors that contribute to urethral closure are deficient. They include the striated external urethral sphincter, the longitudinal smooth muscle and the vascular-elastic component. The condition very often results in urine leakage with very minimal activity.

○ **How is intrinsic sphincter deficiency diagnosed?**

By complex multichannel cystometry (urodynamic testing). GSUI in the absence of urethral hypermobility (failure of extrinsic support) is most often considered by definition because of ISD. Maximum urethral closure pressure less than 20 cm H_2O and/or Valsalva leak-point pressures less than 60 cm H_2O. A positive empty stress test (stress test done after patient has emptied her bladder) is also a sign of ISD.

○ **What population is at risk for ISD?**

Women of advanced age, a history of previous radiation, previous failed incontinence procedure, or spinal cord injury.

○ **Why is the distinction between GSUI and ISD important?**

There is a higher failure rate (33%–54%) with conventional urethral suspension procedures in patients with ISD. These patients should be treated with suburethral slings or bulking agents.

○   **What is urodynamic testing (UDT)?**

Urodynamics means observation of the changing function of the lower urinary tract over time. Most often, the focus of these tests is on the changes in pressure in the bladder and urethra as the bladder is filled with fluid and as the patient performs Valsalva maneuvers.

○   **When is urodynamic testing indicated?**

When surgical treatment is planned, whenever objective findings do not correlate with the patient's symptoms, and in clinical trials.

○   **What is complex cystometry?**

Complex cystometry usually refers to subtracted or multichannel cystometry. That is, the pressure in the bladder (intravesical pressure) is additive; it is the sum of the pressure in the abdomen and the pressure generated by the bladder itself (detrusor pressure). With complex cystometry, you are able to subtract the effects of increases (or decreases) in abdominal pressure from the vesical pressure, to get a true detrusor pressure. This allows the clinician to determine the exact cause of an elevated vesical pressure, which may result from a bladder/detrusor contraction, or a simple cough, position change, or other Valsalva maneuver by the patient.

Small pressure transducers are placed in the bladder and urethra, and one is placed in the vagina or rectum (to estimate abdominal pressure). The bladder is filled and the pressure diagram is analyzed for bladder contractions (increases in detrusor pressure not vesical pressure). The same sensations noted with simple cystometry are noted (first sensation, first urge, maximum capacity). The patient is then asked to bear down, and assessments of stress incontinence and intrinsic sphincter deficiency are performed. If the patient demonstrates incontinence with bearing down, the pressure at which the leakage occurred is called the Valsalva leak point pressure. Valsalva leak point pressures less than 60 cm H_2O indicate ISD.

Because there are pressure transducers in the bladder and urethra, urethral closure pressures can be calculated. This is the difference between the vesical pressure and the urethral pressure at the area of maximum urethral closure pressure (MUCP). UCP less than 20 cm H_2O indicate ISD.

○   **What are the classic findings on UDT with stress incontinence?**

On Valsalva, there is an increase in abdominal and vesical pressures, the detrusor pressure remains the same (no increase) and there is urinary leakage. Urethral pressure may increase slightly, but it is less than the vesical pressure, thus the urethral closure pressure is negative, allowing urinary leakage.

○   **What are the classic findings on UDT with detrusor overactivity?**

On filling the bladder with fluid, there is an increase in vesical pressure and abdominal pressure has little or no increase in pressure. The true detrusor pressure (vesical pressure–abdominal pressure), therefore, is positive (represented by an increased pressure curve on the tracing). This increase in pressure is usually associated with a sense of urgency. If there is associated incontinence, then the diagnosis of detrusor overactivity incontinence or urge incontinence is made. The urethral pressure should stay the same or may increase, if the patient attempts to suppress the urge to void.

CHAPTER 39

Pediatric and Adolescent Gynecology

Hipolito Custodio III, MD

○ **List five indications for vaginoscopy in a female child.**

(1) Recurrent vulvovaginitis

(2) Persistent bleeding

(3) Suspicion of foreign body

(4) Suspicion of neoplasm

(5) Congenital anomalies

○ **What strategies could be employed if a bimanual examination could not be performed in a child or adolescent?**

(1) A rectal–abdominal examination in the dorsal lithotomy position.

(2) Inserting a cotton-tip swab in the vagina to evaluate for agenesis or a transverse septum.

(3) Ultrasonography.

○ **List five ways in which the vagina of a child is different from the vagina of an adult.**

(1) Thinner epithelium

(2) Neutral pH

(3) Lack of glycogen

(4) Lack of lactobacilli

(5) Insufficient level of antibodies to help resist infection

○ **What is the initial endocrinologic change associated with the onset of puberty?**

The occurrence of episodic pulses of LH, occurring during sleep.

○ **What is the last endocrinologic event of puberty?**

The activation of the positive gonadotropin response to increasing levels of estradiol, which results in the midcycle gonadotropic response.

○ **What is the relation between the age of menarche and the onset of ovulatory cycles?**

Adolescents with an early menarche at less than 12 years of age achieve ovulatory cycles sooner, with 50% of cycles being ovulatory within a year of menarche. Women with later onset of menarche could take 8 to 12 years before their cycles become fully ovulatory.

○ **When is the normal length of the menstrual cycle established?**

The normal cycle length is usually established by the sixth year after menarche.

○ **What is the differential diagnosis of irregular menses in an adolescent?**

(1) Pregnancy.

(2) Endocrine: Diabetes, PCOS, Cushing syndrome, thyroid disease, premature ovarian failure, late onset congenital adrenal hyperplasia.

(3) Tumors of the ovaries, adrenals, or a pituitary prolactinoma

(4) Acquired disorders: Stress-related hypothalamic dysfunction, exercise-induced amenorrhea, eating disorder.

○ **When is it appropriate to initiate cervical screening in adolescents?**

Cervical screening is recommended at least 3 years after the first sexual intercourse, or no later than age 21. Screening at less than 3 years after first intercourse may result in the over diagnosis of cervical lesions, which often spontaneously regress. Moreover, there is little risk in adolescents, of missing an important cervical lesion within 3 to 5 years of HPV exposure.

○ **What alternative recommendations can be made in the management of abnormal cervical cytology or histology in adolescents?**

ASCUS with positive high-risk HPV, as well as LSIL, may be managed by repeating cytology twice at 6- and 12 months, or repeating HPV testing in 12 months. Also a finding of CIN 2 may be followed up in four- or six-months' time with either cytology or colposcopy.

○ **Is parental consent needed for colposcopy in an adolescent minor?**

Colposcopy is considered as an evaluation for a sexually-transmitted infection; therefore, parental consent is not required.

○ **How effective is LEEP in the treatment of CIN 2/3 in adolescents?**

Treatment of CIN 2/3 with LEEP is associated with a 55% recurrence rate in women aged 14 to 21 in a colposcopy clinic in Alabama. In this study, the reported rate of CIN 2/3 was 35% among patients with an ASCUS Pap, 36% among LSIL patients, and 50% in HSIL. Of the 192 patients, who underwent LEEP for biopsy-proven CIN2/3, none were diagnosed with cervical carcinoma. The procedure is thus overly aggressive therapy, given the transient nature of HPV infections in adolescents.

○ **Describe the temporal pattern of serum antibody titers in adolescents and young women after immunization with the human papillomavirus-16 vaccine.**

A study done among women aged 16 to 23 showed a peak in serum antibody geometric mean titers at 7 months after vaccination, which declined through month 18 and then remained stable between months 30 and 48. There were no cases of CIN 2-3 observed among vaccine recipients up to 3.5 years after administration.

○ **What are the guidelines for human papillomavirus vaccination?**

(1) Vaccination should be routinely offered between the ages of 9 and 26.

(2) Women with a previously abnormal Pap can still benefit from vaccination.

(3) Completion of a vaccination series can be done during pregnancy, but vaccination initiation is not recommended.

(4) Vaccination may be initiated in lactating women.

(5) Vaccination is not contraindicated in immunocompromised women.

○ **What is the most common gynecologic complaint among adolescents?**

Dysmenorrhea is the most common complaint among adolescent girls. It is also the leading cause of repeated short-term absences from school in this age group.

○ **What is the most common cause of dysmenorrhea in adolescents?**

Most cases of dysmenorrhea in adolescents have no underlying pelvic pathology, and are thought to be the result of the uterine release of prostaglandins during menstruation. The remaining 10% have an underlying pathology, which is most commonly endometriosis. Other causes are obstructing Mullerian anomalies and pelvic inflammatory disease.

○ **What is the usual presentation of endometriosis in adolescents?**

Pelvic pain is the primary reason adolescents with endometriosis seek medical attention. This presents as an acquired, progressive dysmenorrhea, usually with both cyclic and acyclic components.

○ **Describe the appearance of endometriotic lesions on laparoscopy, in an adolescent.**

Endometriotic lesions in adolescents are usually red, clear, or white, in contrast to the powder-burn lesions commonly seen in adults.

○ **What are the treatment guidelines for endometriosis in adolescents?**

(1) NSAIDS and continuous combination hormone therapy is considered first line treatment.

(2) GnRH agonists with add-back are reserved for failure of hormonal treatment because of concern over its potential to retard bone growth.

(3) Surgery should be used to preserve fertility.

(4) A multidisciplinary pain management service should be provided, including support groups.

○ **What is the role of empiric treatment with GnRH agonists for endometriosis in adolescents?**

A trial of a GnRH agonist is reasonable in adolescents 18 years or older who do not have an ovarian mass or tumor. In younger adolescents, a diagnostic or therapeutic laparoscopy is the preferred first step in treatment, if pain persists despite medical therapy.

○ **What factors influence the treatment of congenital syphilis?**

(1) Identification of syphilis in the mother.

(2) Adequacy of maternal treatment.

(3) Presence of clinical, laboratory, and radiographic evidence of syphilis in the infant.

(4) Comparison of maternal and infant nontreponemal serologic titers.

○ **What are the components of a complete evaluation of infants, born to mothers with syphilis?**

    (1) Quantitative nontreponemal test (RPR/VDRL) in the infant's serum.

    (2) Physical examination for nonimmune hydrops, jaundice, hepatosplenomegaly, rhinitis, rash, or pseudoparalysis.

    (3) Pathologic examination of the cord and placenta, with specific fluorescent antitreponemal antibody staining.

    (4) Dark-field examination or direct fluorescent antibody staining of suspicious lesions or body fluids.

    (5) Cerebrospinal fluid examination for VDRL, cell count, and protein.

○ **How high should an infant's RPR/VDRL titers be in order to be diagnostic for congenital syphilis?**

Greater than fourfold of the corresponding maternal titers.

○ **What is the expected time rate of decrease of RPR/VDRL titers in infants of syphilitic mothers who did not have a congenital infection?**

Nontreponemal titers should be decreased by age 3 months, and negative by age 6 months.

○ **What is the threshold for the diagnosis of congenital syphilis using a treponemal antibody test?**

A reactive TP-PA or FTA-ABS by age 18 months is diagnostic for congenital syphilis. Maternal transplacental antibodies are no longer present in the infant's serum beyond age 15 months.

○ **What is the usual presentation of neonatal chlamydia infection?**

Neonatal *Chlamydia trachomatis* infection results from perinatal exposure to the mother's infected cervix. The initial infection involves the mucous membranes of the eye, oropharynx, urogenital tract and rectum. It most commonly presents as conjunctivitis at age 5 to 9 days, but could also present as a subacute afebrile pneumonia at age 1 to 3 months.

○ **What is the treatment for chlamydia infection in infants and children?**

Oral erythromycin is the drug of choice for infants. Either oral azithromycin or oral doxycycline is appropriate agent for children older than 8 years of age.

○ **What is the role of ocular silver nitrate and ocular antibiotic ointments in neonatal prophylaxis?**

Neonatal ocular silver nitrate or antibiotic ointments are not effective in preventing neonatal transmission of *Chlamydia trachomatis*. However, they do prevent gonococcal opthalmic infection.

○ **What is the treatment of choice for gonorrhea in infants and children?**

Ceftriaxone IV/IM is the agent of choice for infants; however, exudates must be cultured and tested for antibiotic susceptibilities. Spectinomycin is also suitable for children. Fluoroquinolones are not recommended because of concern over potential damage to cartilage.

○ **Which infections are diagnostic of sexual abuse in infants and children?**

Gonorrhea, chlamydia, HIV and syphilis are considered diagnostic for sexual abuse. The presence of trichomonas, condyloma or herpes is considered highly suspicious for abuse. Conversely, bacterial vaginosis is considered inconclusive.

○ **What situations indicate the need for STD testing in children?**

   (1) Signs and symptoms consistent with STD, such as vaginal discharge or pain, genital itching or odor, urinary symptoms, genital ulcers or lesions, even if there were no suspicion for abuse.

   (2) A suspected assailant is known to have an STD or high-risk behavior.

   (3) Evidence of genital, oral, or anal penetration.

   (4) The patient or a parent requests testing.

○ **What is the recommendation for the presumptive treatment of sexually abused or assaulted children?**

   Presumptive treatment for STD is not recommended for several reasons. The incidence of STD is low after abuse. Prepubertal girls also have a lower risk for ascending infection compared to adolescents and adults. Lastly, regular follow-up of children can usually be ensured.

○ **What are the present trends in hepatitis B infection in adolescents and children?**

   The incidence of hepatitis B infection has fallen from 260,000 cases per year during the 1980s to 78,000 cases in 2001. The greatest decrease in incidence is noted in adolescents and children—a result of hepatitis B vaccination.

○ **What percentage of sexually active adolescents report consistent condom use?**

   45%.

○ **What is the effect of over-the-counter availability of emergency contraception through the pharmacy on the frequency of its use among adolescents?**

   A study of 2117 patients, from San Francisco, aged 15 to 24 showed that pharmacy access did not improve the overall frequency or promptness of emergency contraceptive use, when compared to clinic access. However, condom users were twice as likely to use emergency contraception if they could obtain it over-the-counter, possibly because a high proportion of women in this subgroup did not have an established relationship with a clinic physician.

○ **What is the effect of access to emergency contraception on the sexual behavior of adolescents?**

   Adolescents as a group are more likely to rely on condoms rather than hormonal methods for contraception, and are more likely to engage in unprotected intercourse than adults. Adolescents with access to emergency contraception were more likely to use it more frequently; however, their behavior in terms of the rates of unprotected intercourse, condom use, STD acquisition, and pregnancy was similar to those adolescents who did not have access to emergency contraception.

○ **What are the components of proper STD counseling for adolescents?**

   (1) Discussing what constitutes responsible and consensual sexual behavior.

   (2) Saying that abstinence is the only completely effective way of preventing pregnancy and STD.

   (3) Reinforcing correct and consistent condom use.

○ **What are the risk factors in adolescents that make them more susceptible to STD infection?**

   (1) Cervical ectropion, presenting a large area of exposed columnar epithelium

   (2) Immature local immunity.

   (3) Lack of foresight to understand the consequences of sexual acts

   (4) Need for peer approval.

(5) Use of alcohol or drugs

(6) Presence of tattoos or body piercings.

○ **40% of all Chlamydia cases present in sexually active adolescents ages 15 to 19 years. What is the incidence of infection in this population?**

1 in 10.

○ **What are the indications for annual screening for HIV and syphilis in adolescents?**

(1) Diagnosis of a sexually transmitted infection.

(2) Multiple partners or a high-risk partner.

(3) Engaging in sex for drugs or money.

(4) Recreational intravenous drug use.

(5) Admission to jail or a detention facility.

(6) Residing in an area of high prevalence for HIV or syphilis.

○ **What are the important components of the initial examination of an adolescent victim of sexual assault?**

(1) Gonorrhea and chlamydia testing from penetration sites

(2) Wet mount or swab culture for trichomonas, candida, or bacterial vaginosis

(3) Serum tests for HIV, hepatitis B, and syphilis

○ **When is it appropriate to repeat serologic testing for HIV in adolescent victims of sexual abuse?**

Repeat evaluation is recommended at 6 weeks, 3 months, and 6 months after the assault if the initial testing is negative, but HIV infection in the assailant cannot be ruled out.

○ **What is the appropriate prophylaxis given to adolescent victims of sexual assault?**

(1) Postexposure vaccination for hepatitis B, without hepatitis B immune globulin.

(2) Empiric antibiotics for gonorrhea, chlamydia, trichomonas, and bacterial vaginosis; ceftriaxone, metronidazole, azithromycin, or doxycycline are all appropriate agents.

(3) Emergency contraception.

○ **Under what circumstances is it indicated to give post exposure prophylaxis for HIV?**

(1) High-risk behavior in the assailant

(2) Multiple assailants

(3) Mucosal lesions on the assailant

(4) Vaginal or anal penetration

(5) Ejaculation on mucous membranes

○ **What is the differential diagnosis of a patient presenting with vaginal agenesis?**

(1) Mullerian agenesis

(2) Congenital absence of vagina with present uterine structures

(3) Androgen insensitivity

(4) 17-hydroxylase deficiency

(5) Low-transverse vaginal septum

(6) Imperforate hymen

○ **Describe the characteristics of a patient with Mullerian agenesis.**

(1) Normal breast development

(2) Normal secondary sexual characteristics and body proportions

(3) Presence of body hair

(4) Presence of hymenal tissue

(5) Normal ovarian hormonal and oocyte function

(6) 46 XX karyotype

○ **What tests are useful in differentiating Mullerian agenesis from androgen insensitivity in a pubertal female?**

(1) Serum testosterone is in the male range in androgen insensitivity

(2) Ultrasound studies show ovarian tissue in Mullerian agenesis

(3) The karyotype is 46 XY in androgen insensitivity

○ **What is the role of MRI in the evaluation of Mullerian agenesis?**

About 2% to 7% of patients with Mullerian agenesis have active endometrium present in the Mullerian structures. MRI is useful in assessing for the presence of functional endometrium, if the ultrasound is equivocal in a patient presenting with chronic or cyclical abdominal or pelvic pain.

○ **What is the role of laparoscopy in vaginal agenesis?**

Laparoscopy is useful in evaluating patients with cyclic abdominal pain. It is useful in identifying the presence of obstructed hemiuteri and in the surgical removal of these structures.

○ **What congenital anomalies are associated with Mullerian agenesis?**

(1) Inguinal hernia

(2) Renal agenesis

(3) Pelvic kidney

(4) Scoliosis

○ **What is the first line approach to the creation of a neovagina?**

The nonsurgical creation of a neovagina using dilators in a recumbent position is the primary approach. Many patients report dilation using the bicycle seat stool to be awkward and uncomfortable. Adherence to the treatment protocol is improved by providing the patient with a "buddy" who has successfully had vaginal dilation.

○ **Describe the steps in the creation of a neovagina using the Abbe-McIndoe operation.**

(1) Dissection of the space between the bladder and the rectum.

(2) Placement into the space of a mold covered with split-thickness skin graft.

(3) Regular postoperative use of vaginal dilators, until regular coitus is assured.

○ **Name the important components of an annual examination for patients after the creation of a neovagina.**

Examination for vaginal strictures or stenosis.

Screening for STD, when appropriate.

Inspection for malignancies for both bowel- and skin neovaginas.

Inspecting bowel neovaginas for colitis or ulceration.

○ **What is the most common cause of breast asymmetry in an adolescent?**

Normal variation in the development of the breasts is the most common cause of asymmetry, with 25% of cases persisting to adulthood. Biopsy should almost always be avoided in prepubertal girls or during early puberty to avoid causing potentially irreversible damage to the breast bud.

○ **What is the usual presentation of mastalgia in an adolescent?**

Cyclic breast pain that is worse premenstrually is characteristic. Symptoms might also include mild breast swelling or palpable nodularity in the upper outer quadrants, consistent with fibrocystic changes.

○ **What are the characteristic findings in benign mammary ductal ectasia in an adolescent?**

(1) Bloody or dark-brown nipple discharge.

(2) Dilation of mammary ducts.

(3) Periductal fibrosis and inflammation.

(4) Breast mass.

○ **How should the clinician counsel an adolescent patient who asks about nipple piercing?**

(1) Describe the associated risks of infection, bleeding, breast pain, hematoma formation, cyst formation, allergic reaction, or keloid formation.

(2) Describe the risk of forming a breast abscess, even up to 5 months after piercing.

(3) Define the risks of transmission of HIV, hepatitis B, and hepatitis C.

(4) Reiterate the need for hepatitis B and tetanus immunization prior to piercing.

○ **Which are the contraindications against nipple piercing in adolescents?**

(1) Alcohol or drug abuse

(2) Anticoagulant therapy

(3) Diabetes

(4) Heart valve disease

(5) History of chronic or acute infections

(6) Immune suppression

(7) Metal allergies

(8) Steroid therapy

○ **At what age, should adolescents be taught to perform regular breast self-examination?**

Starting at age 19. It is generally not recommended to teach younger adolescents to examine their breasts regularly, because those who identify breast masses on self-examination are likely to have multiple physician visits, invasive testing, and unwarranted surgery. However, early breast self-examination should be taught to those with a high risk for breast cancer, such as a personal history of malignancy. Daughters of BRCA-1 and BRCA-2 carriers should start examining their breasts at age 18. Adolescents, who have had chest radiotherapy, should examine themselves starting from 10 years after radiation exposure.

○ **Describe the four types of female genital cutting or circumcision?**

  (1) Type I: excision of the prepuce with or without removal of all or part of the clitoris.

  (2) Type II: removal of the clitoris and part or all of the labia minora.

  (3) Type III: removing part or all of the external genitalia and sewing together the remaining edges to leave a small neointroitus (infibulation).

  (4) All other forms, such as burning, pricking, or scraping.

○ **What are the criteria that would allow an Institutional Review Board to waive the requirement for parental permission in research involving adolescents?**

  (1) When only minimal risk is involved.

  (2) If waiving parental permission does not adversely affect the welfare of the adolescent.

  (3) When research could not practically be done without a waiver.

  (4) When subjects will be provided with pertinent information after participation.

○ **In which areas of adolescent research may parental permission be waived?**

  (1) Sexually transmitted infections

  (2) Birth control use

  (3) High risk sexual behavior

  (4) HIV prevention

  (5) Pregnancy

  (6) Family planning

○ **What is the most frequent gynecologic disease of children?**

  Vulvovaginitis.

○ **Adhesive vulvitis does not require treatment unless what condition occurs?**

  Voiding is compromised.

○ **What conditions are included in the differential diagnosis of persistent or recurrent vulvovaginitis?**

  (1) Foreign body

  (2) Pin worms

  (3) Primary vulvar skin disease

  (4) Ectopic ureter

  (5) Child abuse

○ **Name three common organisms that cause prepubertal vulvitis.**

  (1) Candida

  (2) Pinworms

  (3) Group A β-hemolytic streptococcus

○   **What is the classic symptom of *Enterobius vermicularis* infestation?**

The classic presentation of pinworm infestation is nocturnal itching of the vulvar and perianal areas.

○   **What medication is used to treat pinworms?**

Mebendazole.

○   **What is the most common foreign body found in the vagina of a child?**

Toilet paper.

○   **List the differential diagnosis of persistent vaginal bleeding in a preadolescent female.**

(1) Neoplasia

(2) Precocious puberty

(3) Ureteral prolapse

(4) Trauma

(5) Sexual assault

(6) Vulvovaginitis

(7) Exposure to exogenous estrogen

(8) Shigella infection

(9) Group A and beta-hemolytic streptococcal infection.

(10) Foreign body in vagina.

○   **What percentage of all neoplasms in premenarcheal children are ovarian tumors?**

1%.

○   **75% of ovarian neoplasms in children that necessitate surgery are found to have what pathologic diagnosis?**

Benign teratoma.

○   **Precocious puberty is defined as the appearance of any sign of secondary sexual maturation at age of more than how many standard deviations below the mean?**

2.5 SD.

○   **Which type of precocious puberty involves premature maturation of hypothalamic pituitary ovarian axis and includes normal menses, ovulation and the possibility of pregnancy?**

GnRH dependent precocious puberty.

○   **Which type of precocious puberty involves premature female sexual maturation and uterine bleeding but without associated ovulation?**

GnRH independent precocious puberty.

○   **Breast hyperplasia is a normal physiologic phenomenon in the neonatal period and may persist for how many months?**

Up to 6 months of age.

○ **Anatomically, most central nervous lesions associated with precocious puberty are located in what region of the brain?**

Hypothalamus, in the region of the third ventricle, tuber cinereum, or mammillary bodies.

○ **What blood tests would be appropriate in the evaluation of a female child with precocious puberty?**

Serum level of FSH, LH, prolactin, TSH, estradiol, testosterone, dehydroepiandosterone sulfate (DHEAS), hCG, androstenedione, 17-hydroxyprogesterone, triiodothyronine, and thyroxine.

○ **In childhood, what percentage of ovarian neoplasms necessitating surgery are benign?**

75% to 85%.

○ **What percentage of cases of true precocious puberty are secondary to a life threatening central nervous system disease?**

30%.

○ **What percentage of precocious puberty is caused by idiopathic (constitutional) development?**

70%.

○ **What are the goals of medical therapy in precocious puberty?**

(1) Reduce gonadotropin secretion.

(2) Reduce or counteract peripheral actions of sex steroids.

(3) Decrease the growth rate to normal.

(4) Slow skeletal maturation.

○ **What percentage of all cases of sexual abuse of children involve a family member as the perpetrator?**

80%.

○ **What nonhormonal diagnoses should be differential for heavy bleeding at menarche?**

(1) Blood dyscrasias (von Willebrand disease, prothrombin deficiency).

(2) Platelet dysfunction (leukemia, idiopathic thrombocytopenic purpura, hypersplenism).

○ **If a pediatric patient has an asymptomatic transverse vaginal septum, what condition might occur at the time of puberty?**

Hematocolpos or hematometrium.

○ **If a pediatric patient has an asymptomatic imperforate hymen, what condition might occur at the time of puberty?**

Hematometra and hematosalpinx, causing a menstrual blood bulge behind the imperforate hymen.

○ **You are examining a neonate. Labial fusion is noted. What other portion of the physical examination may most likely assist you in your analysis of this condition?**

Groins and labial folds should be palpated for evidence of gonads.

○ **What is the most common cause of labial fusion?**

Congenital adrenal hyperplasia. The most common form is caused by an inborn error of metabolism involving 21-hydroxylase.

○ **What complaints might a pubertal patient with an imperforate hymen describe?**

Cyclic cramping but no menstrual flow.

○ **Name a rare variant of embryonal rhabdomyosarcoma that most often presents in infancy and adolescence.**

Sarcoma botryoides is a rare tumor of the vagina that most often presents before 8 years of age, although cases have been reported among adolescents. The tumor grossly forms multiple polypoid masses resembling a cluster of grapes. Histologically, they appear as malignant pleomorphic cells in a loose myxomatous stroma and occasional "strap cells," eosinophilic rhabdomyoblasts with characteristic cross striations. To confuse matters further, there is a benign entity called pseudosarcoma botryoides found in infants that resembles sarcoma botryoides. Grossly, these polyps do not have a grape-like appearance and histologic examination demonstrates an absence of strap cells.

○ **List the criteria for the diagnosis of anorexia nervosa in an adolescent female.**

(1) Refusal to maintain normal weight for age and height (less than 85% recommended level).

(2) Morbid fear of becoming fat.

(3) Disturbance of body image.

(4) Absence of menstruation for three consecutive cycles.

○ **List some of the laboratory findings found in anorexia nervosa.**

(1) Prepubertal levels of follicle-stimulating hormone and luteinizing hormone.

(2) Diminished response to gonadotropin-releasing hormone.

(3) Postmenopausal levels of estrogen.

(4) Absence or reversal of normal circadian rhythm of plasma cortisol.

(5) Reduction of metabolic clearance rate of cortisol.

(6) Incomplete suppression of adrenal corticotropin and cortisol by dexamethasone.

○ **List the criteria for the diagnoses of bulimia nervosa.**

(1) Binge eating at least twice weekly for at least 3 months.

(2) Recurrent inappropriate compensatory behavior to prevent weight gain, such as, self-induced vomiting, laxatives or diuretics, strict dieting or fasting, or vigorous exercise averaging at least twice weekly for 3 months.

(3) Over concern with weight and body shape.

○ **List three physical findings that may be present in a patient with bulimia nervosa.**

(1) Erosion of dental enamel

(2) Calluses on dorsal aspects of the hands

(3) Parotid hypertrophy.

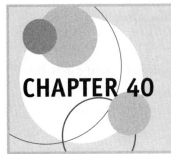

CHAPTER 40 Breast Disorders

Diane M. Opatt, MD and
John S. Kukora, MD

○ **What is Mondor disease?**

Mondor disease is a painful string-like thrombophlebitis within a cutaneous vein of the chest wall or breast. A tender cord is usually palpable and visible in the lateral aspect of the breast. Treatment consists of warm compresses, elevation of the breast in a well-fitting bra, and use of anti-inflammatory medications. Associated thrombophlebitis in other veins is uncommon, and anticoagulant therapy is not indicated. On rare occasion, though, the cause of the phlebitis may be venous occlusion from an adjacent carcinoma. Therefore, any mass near the thrombosed vein should be biopsied. Excision of the thrombosed vein may be required if the process has not resolved spontaneously after 4 to 6 weeks of nonoperative treatment.

○ **What is the most common cause of nipple discharge in the nonlactating breast?**

Fibrocystic changes, which cause serous or watery discharge.

○ **What are other causes of nipple discharge in the nonlactating breast?**

Intraductal papilloma, duct ectasia, galactorrhea, and rarely, carcinoma.

○ **What are the most common types of nipple discharge?**

Milky, multicolored and sticky, purulent, clear or watery, yellow, pink or serosanguinous, and bloody.

○ **What is the most common cause of bloody nipple discharge?**

Intraductal papilloma, a benign process. Since carcinoma can also cause bloody discharge, however, aggressive workup must establish a definitive diagnosis of papilloma and rule out cancer by exclusion.

○ **When do patients typically present with symptoms of an intraductal papilloma?**

When they are perimenopausal.

○ **What is the most important histopathologic feature that distinguishes a benign papilloma from a papillary carcinoma?**

The presence of a myoepithelial layer.

○ **Is there an increased risk of carcinoma in a patient with a single, central, intraductal papilloma?**

Most experts agree that there is no significant increased risk.

○ **Is there an increased risk for development of carcinoma in a patient with multiple intraductal papillomas?**

The risk is similar to that of patients with atypical ductal hyperplasia. Multiple papillomas may be also associated with concurrent atypical ductal hyperplasia, ductal carcinoma in situ (DCIS), or invasive carcinoma.

○ **What condition most commonly causes a greenish nipple discharge?**

Duct ectasia, a common condition in elderly women with concomitant fibrocystic changes in the breast.

○ **What is duct ectasia?**

Periductal mastitis, which is characterized by duct dilatation with associated fibrosis and lymphoplasmacytic inflammation. This condition is typically found in perimenopausal or older women and can mimic carcinoma by causing nipple alterations. Ultrasonography may demonstrate dilated ducts with thickened walls in the central breast.

○ **When is nonpuerperal mastitis most commonly seen?**

After trauma. Other causes include foreign body and malignancy. Since an inflamed breast can mimic inflammatory carcinoma, if symptoms have not resolved promptly with treatment for mastitis, a mammogram must be performed.

○ **What are the contraindications to breast-feeding?**

The following women should not breast-feed: Those who take street drugs or do not control alcohol use; have an infant with galactosemia; are infected with HIV; have active, untreated tuberculosis; are undergoing treatment for breast cancer; are infected with human T-cell lymphotropic virus type I or type II; are undergoing radiation therapy, and take certain medications, such as antiretrovirals or cancer chemotherapy agents.

○ **Does hepatitis B infection preclude breast-feeding?**

No. With appropriate immunoprophylaxis, including hepatitis B immune globulin and vaccine, breast-feeding poses no additional risk for the transmission of the virus.

○ **What are the complications of lactation?**

Mastitis, breast abscess, nipple excoriation, tenderness, and galactocele formation are potential consequences of lactation and breast-feeding.

○ **What condition may result from severe intrapartum or early postpartum hemorrhage?**

Sheehan syndrome (pituitary failure), which is characterized by failure of lactation, amenorrhea, breast atrophy, hypothyroidism, and adrenal cortical insufficiency.

○ **Which vitamin is absent in breast milk?**

All vitamins except vitamin K are found in breast milk.

○ **What is galactorrhea?**

Galactorrhea is the pathologic secretion of milky fluid without associated pregnancy and lactation. Typically, normal milk production should stop within 6 months after the cessation of nursing. Galactorrhea is frequently associated with amenorrhea and may be caused by a host of endocrine disorders or be a consequence of a medication. Galactorrhea should be investigated by measuring serum prolactin levels initially. Hyperprolactinemia is the commonest endocrine cause of galactorrhea and may be the result of a pituitary adenoma or, much less commonly, of ectopic prolactin secretion by a neuroendocrine tumor. Coexisting hyperprolactinemia and hypercalcemia should occasionally undergo additional investigations to exclude the multiple endocrine neoplasia type I syndrome. Hypothyroidism may cause galactorrhea and should be investigated by measurement of serum thyroid stimulating hormone levels. Many hormonal medications and psychotropic medications can directly affect prolactin secretion and inhibition as well as prolactin receptor responsiveness that may occasionally cause galactorrhea. Galactorrhea following the cessation of nursing may be the result of continued nipple stimulation from clothing, exercise, sexual activity, stress, or sleep disorders that may be difficult to identify or mitigate. Bromocriptine administration will frequently diminish hyperprolactinemia from pituitary adenoma or persistent lactation after the cessation of nursing, affecting a cessation of both galactorrhea and amenorrhea.

○ **Breast hypoplasia is generally associated with what conditions?**

Gonadal dysgenesis and Turner syndrome.

○ **How do you counsel a patient regarding future potential for breast-feeding, if plastic surgery is planned?**

Both augmentation and reduction can interfere with duct openings to the nipple and innervation of the breast. This occurs most commonly in breast reduction when the nipple is removed and regrafted. If the subareolar tissue is moved en bloc, then the structure may be preserved and lactation occurs, although perhaps diminished in efficiency. Ideally, such procedures should be deferred until childbearing and breast-feeding are completed. Subpectoral augmentation is less likely to interfere with lactation than intraparenchymal implant placement.

○ **How do you counsel a patient regarding future potential for breast-feeding if reconstructive breast surgery is planned?**

It should be explained to the patient that breast reconstruction after mastectomy returns form, not function. If mastectomy and reconstruction are unilateral, the opposite normal breast can maintain adequate lactation.

○ **A 9-year-old presents with her mother with a complaint of unilateral breast lump and tenderness. What is the proper management?**

Reassurance. This mass represents the breast bud's initial development at thelarche. It frequently is asymmetric in presentation. Surgery and biopsy are contraindicated as any removal of the breast bud or damage to it may result in amastia, or absence of the breast.

○ **What is the preferred radiographic technique to diagnose breast abscess?**

Ultrasound. In some circumstances, percutaneous drainage can also be done at the same time.

○ **What is the workup of a 25-year-old with a palpable breast mass?**

A complete history and physical examination is initially performed. In this age group, the lesion is likely to be a cyst or fibroadenoma. However, risk factors for breast carcinoma are determined such as strong family history. The next step is an ultrasound of the lesion since mammography is not very sensitive in this age group. A cyst aspiration or core needle biopsy is the final step in accurate diagnosis of this lesion.

○ **What is the role of magnetic resonance imaging (MRI) in screening?**

The responsible use of MRI for the evaluation of the breast is focused, primarily on patients with a high probability of breast cancer. This category includes screening in women who are known or likely carriers of a BRCA1 or

BRCA2 mutation. In 2003, the American Cancer Society updated their guidelines for breast cancer screening, stating that women at increased risk for breast cancer might benefit from the earlier initiation of screening, shorter screening intervals, or the addition of screening methods such as MRI. These guidelines recommend annual breast cancer screening by means of MRI for women with approximately 20% or greater lifetime risk of breast cancer, according to risk models that are in large part based on a strong family history of breast or ovarian cancer. Annual MRI screening is also recommended for women who have undergone radiotherapy for Hodgkin lymphoma. The ACS guideline also states that there is insufficient evidence to make a recommendation concerning MRI screening in women with a personal history of breast cancer, carcinoma in situ, atypical hyperplasia, or in women with extremely dense breasts. Breast MRI is becoming more readily available throughout the United States. Centers with the ability to perform an MRI but without the ability to perform an MRI-guided biopsy if a lesion is detected, are under concern. Patients at such facilities who require follow-up evaluation at a center with the capacity to perform the necessary biopsy must undergo a repeat of the entire imaging procedure. The new American Cancer Society guidelines strongly recommend that a center without the capacity to perform MRI-guided breast biopsy should not be performing breast MRI.

○ **What is the role of MRI in diagnosis?**

This is currently a debated issue. If a breast lesion is suspected but not seen on mammography or ultrasound, a breast MRI is a reasonable study to investigate the presence of disease. Many groups feel that a breast MRI is mandatory for every woman diagnosed with breast cancer to rule out the possibility of multicentric disease.

○ **What are the initial imaging studies for a breast mass during pregnancy and lactation?**

Ultrasound is the initial study. An MRI can be performed to further delineate the lesion. Mammography is contraindicated in pregnancy, but may be appropriate for non-pregnant women who are lactating and have a clinically worrisome examination.

○ **What is the cause of axillary swelling and pain during late pregnancy?**

Swelling in the axilla during late pregnancy is often the result of ectopic axillary breast tissue. The condition is initially treated with reassurance and observation. The swelling will usually resolve with the cessation of nursing and lactation. When swelling is persistent and causes discomfort or cosmetic dissatisfaction, ectopic axillary breast tissue can be removed by a subcutaneous resection.

○ **When is core needle biopsy preferred over fine needle aspiration?**

Core needle biopsy (CNB) is preferred for solid lesions. Fine needle aspiration (FNA) is preferred for cyst aspirations. The pathologist cannot differentiate between invasive carcinoma and DCIS from a cytology aspirate obtained by an FNA.

○ **What is the average radiation exposure during a routine mammogram?**

The FDA limits radiation dose for a mammogram to 300 mrad for an average thickness breast per exposure.

○ **Which lymph node groups are most likely to be affected by breast cancer metastases?**

The axillary, supraclavicular, internal mammary, and cervical lymph node basins.

○ **Ductal proliferation is dependent on what hormone?**

Estrogen.

○ **Lobuloalveolar development depends on what hormone?**

Progesterone.

○ **What is the average number of lobes in the mature breast?**

Each breast contains milk glands: 15 to 20 subdivided lobes of glandular tissue surrounded by fatty or fibrous tissue.

○ **A patient with bronchogenic carcinoma may present with what symptom relative to the breast?**

Galactorrhea. Both bronchogenic tumors and renal cell carcinomas may infrequently secrete ectopic prolactin, sufficient to induce lactation.

○ **What are the common causes of a breast abscess?**

Breast abscesses can be divided into the following: lactational, nonlactational, and rare infections. In lactational infections, the patient usually has a cracked nipple or skin abrasion resulting in the ability for the bacteria to enter the breast and infect poorly draining segments. Nonlactational infections generally occur in young women, usually with a history of periductal mastitis. Rare infections, such as tuberculosis, primary actinomycosis, syphilis, mycotic, helminthic, and viral infections can also affect the breast.

○ **How is a lactational breast abscess diagnosed and treated?**

Lactational breast abscess typically presents with pain, fever, and localized redness or warmth of the overlying skin that is often difficult to distinguish from mastitis. Clinical palpation will disclose focal tenderness with induration or a palpable mass. The patient should be started promptly on a broad-spectrum oral antibiotic, recognizing that *Staphylococcus aureus* is the most common infecting organism. The patient should be encouraged to continue nursing from both breasts and to apply warm, wet compresses to the tender area several times daily. Mastitis and many abscesses will resolve with antibiotic therapy alone. The patient should be seen several times weekly, to determine if the process is resolving, persisting, or progressing. An ultrasound examination of the breast should be performed if there is no improvement by 48 to 72 hours after starting antibiotic treatment. Whenever a well-defined abscess remains palpable or is demonstrated by ultrasonography, consideration should be given to prompt surgical incision and drainage or ultrasound-guided percutaneous drainage.

○ **What is the most common location of an abscess in a lactating breast?**

The central and subareolar areas.

○ **What is the most common organism found in breast abscess?**

S. aureus and *Streptococcal species* are the most common organisms isolated in puerperal breast abscesses. Nonpuerperal abscesses typically contain mixed flora (*S. aureus, Streptococcal species*, and anaerobes). At least one study established a correlation between cigarette smoking and subareolar breast abscesses.

○ **What structure supports the breast tissue?**

The skin ultimately supports the breast tissue along with a framework of fibrous, semielastic bands of tissue called Cooper's ligaments (after the physician who first identified them). These ligaments partition the breasts into a honeycomb of interconnecting pockets, each containing mammary glands surrounded by lobules of fatty tissue. These ligaments can cause skin dimpling from scar formation in the breast that results from injury or from cancer-associated fibrosis.

○ **What is the name of the staging system for breast development?**

Tanner Stage 1: (Prepubertal) Papilla elevation only.

Tanner Stage 2: Breast buds palpable and areolae enlarge at age 10.9 years (8.9 to 12.9 years).

Tanner Stage 3: Elevation of breast contour; areolae enlarge at age 11.9 years (9.9 to 13.9 years)

Tanner Stage 4: Areolae form secondary mound on the breast at age: 12.9 years (10.5 to 15.3 years).

Tanner Stage 5: Adult breast contour and areola recesses to general contour of breast (>15.3 years)

○ **What glands are present under the areola?**

Montgomery's. These glands secrete lubricating substances and IgA that protect the nipple and areola during nursing. The openings to these glands are found as papillae on the areola. These are called Morgagni's tubercles.

○ **A 45-year-old woman presents with the complaint of a rapidly growing lesion in her right breast, which is ulcerating through the skin near the areola. She had a normal mammogram 1-year-ago and a negative family history of malignancy. On examination, the mass replaces most of the upper outer quadrant of the breast, is firm, and ulceration is present. There is no adenopathy in spite of the large size. What is your initial impression and presumptive diagnosis?**

The likely diagnosis is the rare cystosarcoma phyllodes tumor [Insert Fig. 40.1]. These masses are uncommon, accounting for 0.3% to 0.5% of breast tumors in females. The average patient age at diagnosis is in the 40s. The mean age of women with benign phyllodes tumors is younger than those with malignant phyllodes tumors. This tumor tends to spread hematogenously rather than through the lymphatics.

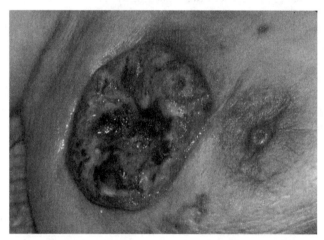

Figure 40.1 *A locally advanced phyllodes tumor with ulceration through the skin.*

○ **What are the main characteristics of phyllodes tumor?**

The gross appearance is that of a circumscribed round to oval nodular mass. Most tumors have a gray-white appearance and often bulge from the surrounding tissue when cut, similar to a fibroadenoma. There is a higher risk in Latino women compared with Caucasian or Asian women. They typically present as palpable masses in the breast. Some patients report continuous or rapid growth of the mass. Shiny, stretched, and attenuated skin with varicose veins can overlie a phyllodes tumor as it pushes against the skin. Skin ulceration can develop from ischemia, secondary to the stretching. Metastasis is uncommon, but when it does occur, spread involves the lung and less frequently, the liver and bones. It does not metastasize to the regional lymph nodes, thus lymph node dissection is unnecessary.

○ **What is the most common benign breast neoplasm?**

Fibroadenoma. Most commonly detected in young women, they are firm, rubbery, and well-marginated on examination. Estrogen stimulates fibroadenoma growth, especially in adolescence or during pregnancy. As transformation into cancer is rare and regression is frequent, current management recommendations are conservative. Enlarging fibroadenomas or those greater than 2 cm should be excised. After menopause, fibroadenomas can atrophy from the lack of estrogen-causing calcifications in a clustered arrangement within a round or elliptical mass on mammogram. This appearance can mimic breast carcinoma and require biopsy.

○ **What is the management of a premenopausal patient who presents with palpable breast mass, not clinically malignant?**

Ultrasound is the initial modality used to establish if the lesion is a cyst. Simple cysts may be observed or aspirated. Complex cysts should be biopsied. Solid masses may be further evaluated by mammogram, especially if the woman is of 30 years or greater. Biopsy should always be performed unless clinical examination and imaging suggest the lesion is a fibroadenoma. Nonbiopsied fibroadenomas should be imaged sequentially at 6 months, 1 year, and 2 years to demonstrate stability.

○ **What is the management of a postmenopausal patient with a palpable breast mass, not clinically malignant?**

In this case, the first test will be a mammogram with possible additional ultrasound or compression and magnification views to clarify the mammographic image. If these studies suggest malignancy, image-guided biopsy should be performed.

○ **What malignant component is rarely found in fibroadenomas?**

Atypical hyperplasia of both ductal and lobular types may be found in a fibroadenoma in less than 1% of the cases. Very rarely, lobular carcinoma in situ (LCIS), DCIS, invasive ductal carcinoma (IDC), or invasive lobular carcinoma (ILC) have been observed in association with a fibroadenoma.

○ **In general, what criteria do you use to evaluate the malignant potential of a cyst aspirate?**

Clear or straw-colored fluid is generally considered benign and is not typically evaluated cytologically, while hemorrhagic fluid has a higher malignant potential and should be sent for cytologic evaluation.

○ **What systemic disease has been associated with the use of silicone breast implants?**

Plaintiffs have successfully litigated claims in tort action that autoimmune phenomena have increased, allegedly because of the leakage of the implant membrane and reaction to the silicone. The FDA, after exhaustive scientific review of the question, has found no evidence that silicone breast implants are harmful and has approved their use for both breast reconstruction and breast augmentation.

○ **Why should the term "fibrocystic breast disease" be avoided on medical records?**

A better term is "fibrocystic change" since these findings are seen histologically in the majority of adult women's breasts as a normal finding. Women should be informed that fibrocystic changes are normal and are not a disease state, so that they are not unduly concerned that they have a health problem. If a woman presents with physical findings suggestive of fibrocystic changes, use the term "nodular thickening" to describe the texture of the breast on examination. Refer to symptoms associated with fibrocystic changes by specific terms such as "mastodynia" or "nipple discharge". Fibrocystic changes seen on mammography are usually diffuse regions of dense breast parenchyma. They can be described as "fibrocystic density" or "fibroglandular density."

○ **What dietary substances are associated with mastalgia?**

Dietary substances chemically classified as methylxanthines are implicated in the causation of mastalgia from several studies that describe improvement of breast discomfort in more than half of affected women when these substances are stringently eliminated from the diet. These substances include caffeine, theobromine, and theophylline that may be present in coffee, tea, soda beverages, and chocolate. They may be found in both prescription and nonprescription medications as well. Cyclic mastalgia has also been linked with high-dietary fat consumption and observed improvement with adherence to a low-fat diet by affected women.

○ **What is the treatment for severe mastodynia?**

In addition to avoidance of dietary methylxanthines and adhering to a low fat diet, patients should be instructed to wear a well-supporting bra and avoid physical activities that exacerbate pain from breast motion. Herbal and prescription medicinal therapies may also be of value. Evening primrose oil at a dose of 3g/d has been associated with improvement in mastalgia. The effect results from increasing essential fatty acid levels by the gamma linolenic acid supplement found in the primrose oil. Adverse effects of its use are low. Androgen therapy may also be useful but is associated with more adverse effects and should be considered a last resort measure. Danazol is the only androgen approved for the treatment of mastalgia and should be administered initially at 100 mg twice daily. The dose may be doubled if no improvement occurs after 2 months. This medication should be discontinued by tapering the dose after 6 months to minimize the risk of adverse events that include oily skin, acne, hirsutism, lowered vocal pitch, hot flashes, abdominal cramps, increased libido, dyspareunia, headaches, nervousness, depression, and venous thromboembolism.

○ **What is mastopexy?**

This refers to the alteration of breast contour by removal of skin only, without actual removal of underlying breast tissue. It is most commonly used for sagging breasts rather than large, pendulous breasts.

○ **How common is breast cancer?**

One in nine women will develop it.

○ **What is the most common congenital abnormality of the breast?**

Polythelia (supernumerary nipples) are the commonest congenital abnormality of the breast. They are identified at birth as 2 to 3 mm pigmented spots that lie on the embryonic milk lines (mammary ridges) that extend from the axilla to the groin on each side of the thoracoabdominal skin. The condition has a slight increased association with renal anomalies, vertebral anomalies, and cardiac rhythm abnormalities.

○ **At what point do the male and female breasts begin to differ histologically?**

Prior to puberty, they are identical; however, after that the female breasts undergo significant development, including lengthening and branching of ducts, proliferation of stroma and fat, and development of lobules.

○ **What is microscopically lacking in the male breast to distinguish it from the female breast?**

Lobules.

○ **What conditions are associated with gynecomastia?**

The most common causes are the following: Puberty, drugs (estrogens, antiandrogens, ketoconazole, metronidazole, cimetidine, omeprazole, ranitidine, methotrexate, alkylating agents, amiodarone, captopril, digoxin, diltiazem, enalapril, nifedipine, spironolactone, verapamil, diazepam, haloperidol, tricyclic antidepressants, reglan, or phenytoin, theophylline), or idiopathic. Other causes include: cirrhosis, malnutrition, primary or secondary hypogonadism, testicular tumors, hyperthyroidism, or renal disease.

○ **What is "witch's milk"?**

It is a folk term for the milk that often comes from the breast of a newborn baby. This temporary phenomenon is a result of the stimulation of the baby's breasts by the mother's hormones that cross the placenta during pregnancy. The ability of the baby's breasts to respond in this fashion is a mark of a baby born at (or near) full-term. The term "witch's milk" is sometimes applied broadly to milk from the nipple at any time other than during nursing.

○ **When is juvenile hypertrophy of the breast most likely to develop?**

This is a rare, bilateral condition, which consists of massive enlargement of the breast and occurs immediately after menarche. Actually, this condition is a hyperplasia although it has been incorrectly termed a hypertrophy.

○ **What are the commonest causes of breast mass in premenopausal women, which are clinically significant?**

Fibroadenoma, fibrocystic changes, cysts, abscess, and carcinoma.

○ **What factors affect fibrocystic changes?**

Although the cause is not completely understood, the changes are believed to be associated with ovarian hormones since the condition usually subsides with menopause and may vary in consistency and symptomatic intensity during the menstrual cycle. Its incidence is estimated to be more than 60% of all women. It is common in women between the ages of 30 and 50 and rare in postmenopausal women. The incidence is lower in women taking birth control pills. Risk factors may include family history and diet (such as excessive dietary fat and caffeine intake), although these are controversial.

○ **Is there an increased risk for subsequent development of cancer in fibrocystic change?**

The risk of development of carcinoma is related to the degree and type of epithelial hyperplasia present. Proliferative or atypical fibrocystic changes increase the risk of breast carcinoma. Assigning a risk for development of breast carcinoma to fibrocystic change must be done with the caveat that this assignment is based on the degree and type of hyperplasia and atypical breast tissue, not the cystic and fibrotic change itself.

○ **What effects does oral contraceptive (OCs) use have as regards the breast?**

Some studies have shown that women who take OCs are less likely to demonstrate fibrocystic changes. A 1996 analysis of worldwide epidemiologic data conducted by the Collaborative Group on Hormonal Factors in Breast Cancer found that women who were current or recent users of birth control pills had a slightly elevated risk of developing breast cancer. The risk was highest for women who started using OCs as teenagers. However, 10 or more years after women stopped using OCs, their risk of developing breast cancer returned to the same level as if they had never used birth control pills, regardless of family history of breast cancer, reproductive history, geographic area of residence, ethnic background, differences in study design, dose and type of hormone, or duration of use.

○ **What histologic pattern of the epithelial component of phyllodes tumor is useful in differentiating it from a fibroadenoma?**

The epithelial component in phyllodes tumor is characteristically "leaf-like" with a branching pattern. The stroma in phyllodes tumor is also more cellular and mitotically active and has more atypical cells, including multinucleated cells.

○ **When are mammary hamartomas most commonly seen?**

These lesions are seen in 2–16:10000 of mammograms and do not usually cause symptoms. The mean age at diagnosis is 45 years.

○ **What are the components of a hamartoma?**

This uncommon, benign breast lesion is also called a fibroadenolipoma and is composed of adipose, glandular, and fibrous tissues. These lesions appear on mammograms as well-circumscribed masses containing both fat and soft-tissue density. A thin radio-opaque line (pseudocapsule) is often seen surrounding a portion of the mass.

○ **What is the name of the benign tumor of the breast, characterized by a proliferation of small, round, tubular structures in a tightly packed, well-circumscribed architecture with a distinct myoepithelial layer?**

Tubular adenoma.

○ **What are some risk factors for development of carcinoma of the breast?**

Risk factors can be divided into two separate groups: Those that one cannot change and those that are associated with lifestyle. Risk factors that cannot be changed include the following: Increasing age, female gender, genetic factors (BRCA1/BRCA2, ataxia-telangiectasia, CHEK-2, Li-Fraumeni syndrome), family history of breast cancer, personal history of breast cancer, Caucasian race, history of abnormal breast biopsy, previous chest irradiation, early menarche, late menopause, and exposure to diethylstilbestrol (DES). Risk factors associated with lifestyle include: Nulliparity, hormone replacement therapy (HRT), alcohol use, obesity and high-fat dietary consumption, and lack of physical activity.

○ **What is the recommended screening for breast cancer?**

The recommendations are different for average-risk and high-risk patients. For average-risk patients, yearly mammograms are recommended starting at age 40 and continuing for as long as a woman is in good health. Clinical breast examination (CBE) should be a part of periodic health examination, about every 3 years for women in their 20s and 30s and every year thereafter for women 40 years and older. Women should know how their breasts normally feel and report any breast change promptly to their physician. Self breast examination (SBE) accomplishes this goal and should be instituted by women starting in their 20s.

Women at increased risk (strong family history, genetic mutation) should start screening at 10 years younger than the age of the youngest affected first-degree relative when they were diagnosed with breast cancer. These women may be screened with mammography, ultrasound, or MRI as appropriate. They should perform SBE monthly and have CBE every 6 months. Depending on the degree of risk, these patients may be enrolled in prevention clinics where they can be closely followed and considered for chemoprevention, or prophylactic surgery.

○ **What mammographic features are most worrisome for the possibility of breast malignancy?**

Any density that is new or increasing in size, in comparison to prior mammographic studies, should be regarded as suspicious and evaluated with ultrasonography and obligates biopsy unless it is shown to be a simple cyst. Clusters of calcifications, especially very fine or linear calcifications, are seen with both invasive ductal carcinoma and ductal carcinoma in situ. Such calcifications are also seen on occasion with atypical ductal hyperplasia and with other benign breast conditions, as well. A stellate or spiculated density is the most ominous mammographic characteristic of invasive carcinoma especially if there are associated clustered calcifications. The rare and benign radial scar lesion of the breast may give an identical stellate appearance as carcinoma, so there is no completely specific sign of malignancy on mammography.

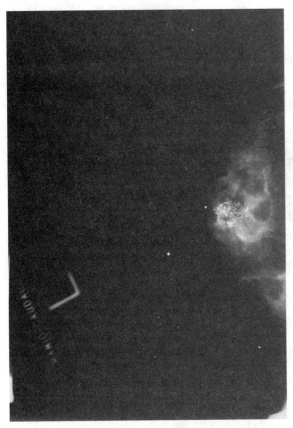

Figure 40.2 *Craniocaudal (CC) view mammogram showing subareolar calcifications. Note the linear, irregular nature of the calcifications, typical of ductal carcinoma in situ (DCIS).*

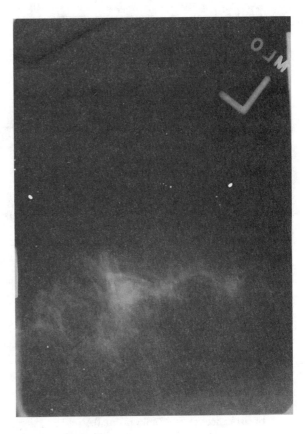

Figure 40.3 *Medial-lateral oblique (MLO) mammogram. Note the asymmetric mass with an irregular, spiculated appearance. This lesion is worrisome for breast carcinoma.*

○ **What unusual diagnostic difficulties are associated with infiltrating lobular carcinoma?**

Infiltrating lobular carcinoma has two insidious characteristics that may contribute to a delay in diagnosis. These tumors tend to arise from a small focus of tumor that permeates extensively throughout the breast without an associated concentrically enlarging central mass. This makes recognition of the central mass difficult or impossible on mammogram even when the overall extension exceeds several centimeters. Additionally, the physical growth characteristics of the tumor do not always produce a suspicious lump recognized by patient or physician. These tumors tend to cause subtle visible foreshortening, asymmetry, or retraction of the breast associated with slight palpable thickening of the parenchyma. Despite normal mammographic appearance in such breasts, biopsy should be performed.

○ **Does papillary carcinoma have a generally good or bad prognosis?**

Good, it is an indolent tumor found in older women, which is largely intraductal.

○ **Based on a pathological classification, how are benign breast disorders divided?**

Non-proliferative lesions

Proliferative lesions without atypia

Atypical proliferative lesions

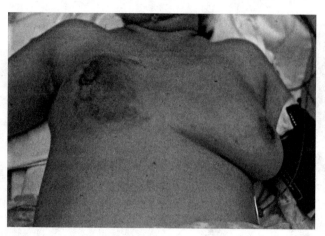

Figure 40.4 *A 54-year-old woman with locally advanced infiltrating lobular right breast carcinoma, exhibiting inflammatory and peau d'orange skin changes. Note the foreshortening and retraction of the right breast.*

○ **What is the risk for subsequent development of invasive carcinoma in patients with non-proliferative and proliferative breast disorders?**

Non-proliferative lesions of the breast: These lesions carry no increased risk for development of carcinoma as long as the patient does not have a strong family history of breast cancer. Included in this category are fibroadenomas, duct ectasia, cysts, apocrine metaplasia, and mild ductal epithelial hyperplasia.

Proliferative breast disorders without atypia: These include intraductal papillomas, sclerosing adenosis, and moderate and florid hyperplasia, among others. There is a slightly increased risk for the development of invasive breast cancer (1.5–2 times normal).

Atypical proliferative lesions: These include both ductal and lobular lesions. These are lesions with some, but not all of the features of carcinoma in situ. The two main types include atypical lobular hyperplasia and atypical ductal hyperplasia (increases the risk by about four times normal).

○ **What is the relative risk of development of invasive carcinoma of the breast in a patient with atypical ductal hyperplasia (ADH)?**

Four to five times.

○ **What is the relative risk of development of invasive carcinoma of the breast in a patient with hyperplasia (mild)?**

1.5 to 2 times.

○ **What is the relative risk of development of invasive carcinoma of the breast in a patient with atypical lobular hyperplasia (ALH)?**

Four to five times. Interestingly, the tumors that develop in these patients are most commonly ductal carcinomas, thus indicative of ALH as a marker for cancer risk rather than a precursor lesion.

○ **What is the risk of developing breast cancer for a person with LCIS?**

These patients have a rate of development of invasive carcinoma of about 1% to 2% per year, with a lifetime risk of 30% to 40%. The risk is bilateral, and the majority of the invasive tumors that develop are actually ductal and not lobular.

○ **Is there a myoepithelial layer in sclerosing adenosis?**

Yes, at least focally.

○ **Is there an increased relative risk of development of invasive breast carcinoma in patients with sclerosing adenosis?**

Yes, a mild one (1.5 to 2 times).

○ **Are there myoepithelial cells present in microglandular adenosis?**

They are typically absent, although they have been described and are seen with the aid of immunostains focally.

○ **What two genes account for the vast majority of inherited breast cancers?**

BRCA1 and BRCA2.

○ **What percentage of breast cancer is genetic?**

5% to 10%.

○ **Where are BRCA1 and BRCA2 located?**

BRCA1 is found on chromosome 17q21, and BRCA2 is found on chromosome 13q12.

○ **Is there a risk of development of other types of malignancies in patients with mutations involving BRCA1 and BRCA2?**

Yes. BRCA1 mutations are associated with a pronounced increased risk of development of ovarian cancer (up to 60% by age 70) and it has risks associated with development of prostate and colon cancer. BRCA2 is associated with the development of male breast cancer, ovarian cancer, and cancer of the bladder, prostate, and pancreas.

○ **What is the risk of development of breast cancer in a patient who has two first-degree relatives with breast cancer?**

Four to six times.

○ **Do the majority of women with a family history of breast cancer have the BRCA1 and BRCA2 genes?**

No, less than 10% do.

○ **How significant is the risk of development of breast cancer in a patient with Cowden disease?**

This is a mutation found on the long arm of chromosome 10, and these patients have up to 50% risk of development of breast carcinoma by the time they reach age 50.

○ **What initial receptors in carcinoma cells should be determined at the time of initial biopsy?**

Estrogen, progesterone, and human epidermal growth factor receptor 2 (HER-2/neu).

○ **How common is the presence of estrogen receptors in carcinoma cells?**

Approximately half of the cases contain estrogen receptors.

○ **Why is it important to determine the presence or absence of estrogen and progesterone receptors in the cytoplasm of tumor cells?**

They are of proven value in determining adjuvant therapy and therapy for patients with advanced disease. If positive, hormonal therapy can be used in the treatment of breast cancer. These hormonal agents can block either the synthesis of hormones or the hormone receptor sites. These agents include tamoxifen (antiestrogen), anastrozole (aromatase inhibitor) among others.

○ **How does the status of HER-2/neu affect the prognosis in breast cancer?**

It is associated with decreased survival when overexpressed in tumor cells, which occurs in 20% of the cancers.

○ **What is HER-2/neu and where is it located?**

It is a proto-oncogene found on chromosome 17q21–22, and it has structural similarity to the epidermal growth factor receptor. Overexpression appears to be associated with a poor prognosis.

○ **What drug can be used as a single agent or can be added to first line chemotherapy in HER-2/neu receptor positive to improve outcome?**

Herceptin (trastuzumab), which is a recombinant, humanized monoclonal antibody directed against the HER-2/neu product. The most significant toxicity of Herceptin is cardiotoxicity.

○ **What is the relative risk of developing invasive breast carcinoma in a patient with atypical ductal hyperplasia and a strong family history of breast cancer?**

Greater than 10 times.

○ **What is the risk of developing breast cancer in association with caffeine consumption and cigarette smoking?**

There is no substantial data to prove a causative effect of either substance.

○ **What structure within the breast gives rise to all carcinomas?**

The terminal duct lobular unit.

○ **What is the most common type of in situ carcinoma and invasive carcinoma?**

Ductal carcinoma accounts for 80% of the in situ lesions and 80% of the invasive lesions.

○ **What are the various treatment options for a patient with breast carcinoma?**

The patient can choose breast conservation therapy (BCT), which consists of lumpectomy plus radiation or mastectomy. To qualify for BCT, the tumor should be less than 5 cm without any associated inflammatory carcinoma, skin nodules, or ulceration, and with a favorable ratio of breast size to tumor size such that the patient would have a good cosmetic result. To address the axilla, the patient may have a sentinel lymph node biopsy, if there is no palpable lymphadenopathy followed by axillary node dissection, if the sentinel node is positive. If there is axillary lymphadenopathy, an axillary lymph node dissection should be performed. Radiation is indicated after mastectomy for tumors greater than 5 cm, chest wall invasion, and/or 4 or more positive lymph nodes. Chemotherapy is used in patients with tumors greater than 1 cm, positive lymph nodes, young age, and aggressive tumor factors. Herceptin is used if the tumor is positive for the HER-2/neu receptor. Antiestrogens are used if the tumor is ER/PR+. In premenopausal women, tamoxifen is used. In postmenopausal women, either tamoxifen or aromatase inhibitors are used.

○ **How is a sentinel lymph node biopsy performed?**

The surgeon may inject a radioactive colloid, blue dye, or both. Different surgeons advocate for various injection sites: peritumoral, subareolar, and intradermal, all of which seem to be equally effective. The tracer travels through lymphatics in the breast to the ipsilateral axillary sentinel node. The sentinel node is any radioactive node, blue node, or a blue lymphatic leading to a nonblue node. The axilla is also palpated for suspicious lymph nodes, which are removed, if identified.

○ **How are sentinel nodes analyzed?**

The sentinel nodes can be sent for frozen section, touch prep, or permanent evaluation. If a positive lymph node is identified while in the operating room, an axillary dissection is performed. Since there are typically less lymph nodes removed with a sentinel node biopsy than with axillary dissection, the pathology lab can more meticulously analyze the tissue. The lymph nodes are serially sectioned and examined.

○ **What nerve injuries can occur after a mastectomy?**

The long thoracic nerve innervates the serratus anterior muscle and injury results in winged scapula. The thoracodorsal nerve can be injured causing paresis of the latissimus dorsi muscle. Injury to the intercostal brachial nerve causes numbness, tingling, or pain on the upper, medial aspect of the ipsilateral arm.

○ **What are the histologic features of Bloom–Richardson, which is used to grade invasive carcinoma of the breast?**

Percentage of tubule formation by the tumor, degree of nuclear pleomorphism, and mitotic rate. Each of these three features are given a score of 1 to 3 (3 is the highest grade) and those three numbers are added to give a total score. A total score of 3 to 5 is grade I, 6 to 7 is grade II, and 8 to 9 is grade III.

○ **What is the best single indicator of breast cancer prognosis?**

The extent of nodal involvement.

○ **What is the characteristic histologic invasion pattern of infiltrating lobular carcinoma?**

These tumors classically invade in a single file fashion and exhibit a "targetoid" or concentric ring formation around normal ducts.

○ **What tumor is characterized by occurrence in younger women, disproportionate occurrence in patients with the BRCA1 gene, circumscription, and sheets of tumor cells with a marked lymphoplasmacytic infiltrate surrounding and extending into the tumor?**

Medullary carcinoma.

○ **What is the prognosis of medullary carcinoma?**

It has an excellent prognosis, better than intraductal carcinoma, with 10-year survivals of up to 90%.

○ **What is the prognosis for tubular carcinoma?**

It is the best of all invasive carcinomas, with a 5-year survival rate approaching 100%.

○ **What is the prognosis for mucinous (colloid) carcinoma of the breast?**

It, too, is excellent. It is more common in older females and has a 10-year survival of up to 90% for the typical mucinous carcinoma.

○　**How common are axillary lymph node metastases in tubular carcinoma?**

Uncommon, occurring in less than 10% of cases.

○　**What is the incidence of bilaterality and multifocality in tubular carcinoma?**

The mean age for those with tubular carcinoma is the sixth decade with a range of 23 to 89 years. In a recent review in a pathology journal, 4% were bilateral and 19% were multifocal.

○　**What is the maximal tumor measurement for a stage I breast carcinoma?**

2 cm or less.

○　**What is the maximal tumor measurement for a stage II breast carcinoma?**

5 cm or less.

○　**How does the presence or absence of hormone receptors in a tumor affect prognosis?**

Tumors with high number of hormone receptors have a slightly better prognosis than those without. Most breast cancers express estrogen receptors, particularly in postmenopausal women.

○　**How does mammary Paget's disease differ from extramammary Paget's?**

While it is uncommon to have underlying adenocarcinoma in extramammary Paget's, Paget's disease of the nipple is characterized by the presence of intraepidermal malignant cells from an underlying invasive ductal carcinoma or comedo DCIS. The clinical presentation is erythema, thickening, crusting, and/or itching of the nipple-areolar complex.

○　**Is there an association with the BRCA1 and BRCA2 genes in male breast cancer?**

There is an association with BRCA2 in some familial breast cancers in males but not BRCA1.

○　**What is the characteristic histologic feature of mucinous (colloid) carcinoma?**

It is characterized by pools of mucin, within which, groups of tumor cells "float".

○　**What does the term "metaplastic carcinoma" describe in breast cancer?**

These are tumors with "sarcomatoid" features or a mixture of malignant epithelial and mesenchymal elements.

○　**What is the most common pure sarcoma to occur in the breast?**

Angiosarcoma.

○　**What is the mean age of development of angiosarcoma of the breast?**

Approximately 40 years.

○　**What factors are associated with the development of angiosarcoma?**

Lymphatic obstruction and radiation.

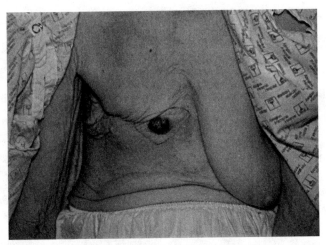

Figure 40.5 *An 85-year-old patient with a 15-year prior right-sided mastectomy and chest wall radiotherapy for locally advanced carcinoma, now exhibits a raised, nodular, purplish mass that is angiosarcoma.*

○ **In general terms, what is the prognosis of angiosarcoma of the breast?**

This neoplasm carries a very poor prognosis, with a 5-year survival rate of 8% to 50%. Up to 90% of the patients with primary breast angiosarcoma die within 2 years of diagnosis. However, more recently, survival (lower tumor grade, smaller lesion size, prompt mastectomy) has improved. Recurrence usually is local, although hematogenous dissemination may occur. Dissemination usually involves the lungs, skin, contralateral breast bone, liver, brain, and ovary, in decreasing frequency. If surgery as primary treatment fails, survival is seriously compromised because adjuvant or palliative treatments are not very effective. The odds for a significant response of metastatic disease to chemotherapy are approximately 35% with rare complete responses. If metastases are amenable to surgical extirpation, surgery should be attempted first for cure and chemotherapy and radiation reserved for either the immediate postoperative period or for the next failure.

○ **Does non-Hodgkin lymphoma occur in the breast?**

Yes, many believe this condition to be a part of the lymphomas related to mucosa-associated lymphoid tissue (MALT).

○ **What is the typical age at presentation for male breast cancer?**

The median age for males diagnosed with breast cancer is 67 years.

○ **In general terms, what is the prognosis of male breast cancer?**

The prognosis is the same for males and females with breast cancer, although men tend to present at later stages than women.

○ **What is the most important aspect of treatment for fibromatosis of the breast?**

As with all fibromatoses, the initial wide excision of the lesion is of paramount importance.

○ **What characteristics differentiate a granular cell tumor?**

Cells with abundant eosinophilic granular cytoplasm, immunoreactivity with S-100 protein, and oval to round cells.

○ **What is the definition of microinvasive carcinoma of the breast?**

This refers to a carcinoma, which is almost exclusively in situ; however, there are one or more separate foci of early invasion by tumor. None of the foci can measure greater than 1 mm in diameter to qualify as microinvasive.

○ **What are some immunohistochemical markers associated with the tumor cells in Paget's disease of the nipple?**

The tumor cells will react with low-molecular weight cytokeratin, epithelial membrane antigen, and HER-2/neu.

○ **What condition can present after trauma to the breast?**

Fat necrosis. It is important because it produces a mass, often accompanied by skin or nipple retraction that is indistinguishable from carcinoma. It produces irregular densities on mammography associated with calcifications in some cases that mimic the appearance of a malignant tumor.

CHAPTER 41   Ethics and Psychiatric Pearls

Hipolito Custodio, MD

○ **What are some principles of medical ethics?**
- *Autonomy:* The promotion of self-determinism or the freedom of the clients to choose their own direction.
- *Beneficence:* Refers to promoting good for others.
- What is in the best interest for the client?
- *Nonmaleficence:* Avoiding doing harm, which includes refraining from actions that risk hurting clients.
- *Justice/fairness:* Refers to providing equal treatment to all the people.
- *Confidentiality:* A person's right to decide how and to whom personal medical information will be communicated.

○ **Is it ethical to release information to insurance companies?**

Yes. This information should be limited to the process of insurance claim.

○ **When can confidentiality be broken?**
- At the patients request
- When child abuse is suspected
- Court mandate
- Duty to warn and protect
- Reportable diseases
- Danger to others

○ **What is an ethical dilemma?**

When two or more ethical principles conflict. An example of this is a patient who wishes to have a treatment that is not indicated. This is a conflict of autonomy and nonmaleficence.

○ **What is a health care proxy?**

This is an individual who acts as a surrogate in making decisions regarding another individual's health care, should the person become unable to do so. This is usually the spouse of the patient.

The health care proxy has, in essence, the same rights to request or refuse treatment that the individual would have, if capable of making and communicating decisions.

○　**What is power of attorney?**

The durable power of attorney allows an individual to make bank transactions, sign Social Security checks, apply for disability, or simply write checks to pay the utility bill while an individual is medically incapacitated (but not to make decisions on health care).

○　**What is a living will?**

A living will specifies that certain medical procedures (CPR, etc.) not be performed in the event that the patient lacks the capacity to decline the procedures.

○　**What is an advance directive?**

This document is a living will or a durable power of attorney for health care.

○　**True or False: A patient who is fully coherent and is a Jehovah's Witness is having a massive lower GI hemorrhage. The patient is an adult and refuses blood products. The physician is legally bound to coerce the patient to receive blood because withholding it may result in the patient's death.**

False. The principle of autonomy dictates that this patient may refuse blood products even if it results in his/her death.

○　**What must be present to decide that a patient has the capacity to make health care decisions?**

The patient must have knowledge of the options and their consequences and an understanding of the costs and benefits of the options relative to a set of stable values.

○　**What condition should always be evaluated before declaring competency?**

Depression.

○　**True or False: A patient who refuses a recommendation by their physician is incapacitated to make health care decisions.**

False.

○　**True or False: It is unethical to withdraw a patient from a ventilator who has end stage COPD and inoperable lung cancer, has sound mind, and requests such a maneuver.**

False.

○　**True or False: A patient with stage I bronchogenic carcinoma has pulmonary edema requiring mechanical ventilation. You explain this to the patient and he agrees with proceeding with intubation and mechanical ventilation. His wife refuses. The physician should not intubate the patient.**

False. The principle of autonomy declares that each individual is the ultimate arbiter of his or her own health care.

○　**In the above patient, what should the physician do next?**

Speak to the wife. It could be that she is unaware that the tumor is potentially curable and that the pulmonary edema can be remedied by medications.

○ **May a physician disclose the content of a medical record to another health care professional in the regular course of treatment?**

Yes.

○ **May a physician disclose the content of a medical record under a court order?**

Yes.

○ **May a physician disclose the content of a child's medical record to school officials who request it?**

No.

○ **In artificial insemination by donor, where the mother is married, who is considered the legal father?**

The mother's husband.

○ **Is there an ethical difference between withholding and withdrawing life-support measures in patients with acute respiratory failure?**

Ethical principles underlying the decision to withhold intubation and mechanical ventilation apply equally when patients or proxies request discontinuance of care for patients who have no hope for an acceptable and meaningful recovery.

○ **Are physicians required to honor properly established advance directives by a patient with severe COPD, to forego intubation and mechanical ventilation?**

Respect for patient autonomy requires a physician to honor such requests or transfer the patient's care to another physician who can honor the patient's directives.

○ **What is the prevalence of alcoholism in the United States?**

10% to 15% is the lifetime prevalence. 10% of men and 3.5% of women have alcoholism.

○ **Does alcoholism has a heritable component?**

Yes, there may be a tendency of father to son inheritance.

○ **What laboratory changes are suggestive of alcoholism?**

AST >2 times the ALT value, vs a 1:1 ratio with other forms of hepatitis.

○ **An alcoholic is brought to the emergency department. He is drowsy but arousable; his AST is 350 and the ALT 150, blood glucose 35 g/dL. The nurses get and IV access and the new ER intern order a glucose solution. The patient starts acting confused and is ataxic. Why?**

In alcoholics, thiamine should be given first, otherwise a Wernicke encephalopathy can be precipitated.

○ **Describe the symptoms of Wernicke's encephalopathy.**

Confusion, nystagmus, and ataxia.

○   **Describe the symptoms of alcohol withdrawal and their temporal relations.**

Hallucinations: Auditory, visual, and tactile occur 24 hours after the patient's last drink.

Autonomic hyperactivity: Tachycardia, hypertension, tremors, anxiety, and agitation occur 6 to 8 hours after the patient's last drink.

Global confusion: Occurs 1 to 3 days after the patient's last drink.

○   **What is the most common mental illness in large cities?**

Substance abuse. Substance abuse is prevalent in rural communities as well, but the addiction percentages are lower. Incidentally, opiate is predominantly a city drug, while marijuana, alcohol, and amphetamines are found in both rural and urban settings.

○   **A patient presents with tearing eyes, a runny nose, tachycardia, piloerection, abdominal pains, nausea, vomiting, diarrhea, insomnia, pupillary dilation and leukocytosis. What is the diagnosis?**

Opiate withdrawal.

○   **Antidote for opiate intoxication is:**

Naloxone.

○   **Treatment for opiate dependence is:**

Methadone.

○   **What are a few substances that might mimic generalized anxiety when ingested?**

Nicotine, caffeine, amphetamine, cocaine, and anticholinergic agents. Alcohol and sedative withdrawal can also mimic this disorder.

○   **Describe the characteristics of normal bereavement and its treatment?**

Uncomplicated grief or bereavement is a normal response. Initially, it can be manifested as a state of shock, followed by suffering and distress, crying, decreased appetite, weight loss, decreased concentration, guilt, hearing the person's voice or feeling the person's presence.

Usually lasts for 6 to 12 months.

○   **Characteristics of pathological grief are:**

Chronic depression, significant impairment, and suicidal ideation.

○   **Why can a patient taking lithium experience polyuria?**

Long-term lithium ingestion can cause nephrogenic diabetes insipidus.

○   **What is dementia?**

Disturbed cognitive function that results in impaired memory, personality, judgment, or language. Dementia has an insidious onset, but it may present as acute, worsened mental state when the patient is facing other physical or environmental stresses.

○ **What is delirium?**

"Clouding of consciousness" that results in disorientation, decreased alertness, and impaired cognitive function. Acute onset, visual hallucinosis, and fluctuating psychomotor activity are all commonly seen. These symptoms are variable and may change within hours.

○ **What are two major causes of dementia?**

Alzheimer disease and multi-infarction.

○ **What conditions may mimic dementia in the elderly?**

Depression (pseudodementia)
Hypothyroidism

○ **Name some treatable causes of dementia.**

Uremia, syphilis, vitamin B12 deficiency, Parkinson syndrome.

○ **Name some over-the-counter and "street" drugs that may produce delirium or acute psychosis.**

Salicylates, antihistamines, anticholinergics, alcohols, phencyclidine, LSD, mescaline, cocaine, and amphetamines.

○ **What are the typical side effects of antipsychotics?**

Autonomic side effects:

- Dry mouth
- Urinary retention
- Orthostatic hypotension
- Sedation

    Extrapyramidal side effects:

- *Dystonic reaction:* The first side effect to appear. Usually hours to days. Characterized by muscle spasm and stiffness. Treatment Benadryl or anticholinergics.
- *Akathisia:* First weeks of treatment. Feelings of restlessness. Treatment with beta-blockers.
- *Parkinsonism:* First months of treatment. Characterized by cogwheel rigidity, shuffling gait and mask like facies. Treatment with antihistamines or anticholinergics.
- *Tardive dyskinesia:* Occurs after years of treatment. Involuntary movements of the tongue, head, limbs, and trunk. Treatment is to discontinue antipsychotic and consider switching.
- *Neuroleptic malignant syndrome:* This is a feared complication. Can occur at any time. Characterized by hyperthermia, rigidity, and increase in creatinine phosphokinase. Treatment includes discontinuation of antipsychotic, aggressive-IV hydration, and dantrolene.

○ **What are the five Kubler-Ross stages of dying?**

(1) Denial

(2) Anger

(3) Bargaining

(4) Depression

(5) Acceptance

    Patients may undergo all or only a few of these stages.

○ **What is an extreme case of factitious disorder?**

Munchausen syndrome. These patients may actually try to cause harm to themselves (e.g., by injecting feces into their veins) and are very accepting or seeking of invasive procedures. Munchausen by proxy is another example. In this disease the patient seeks medical care for another, usually a child.

○ **What is the difference between low-potency and high-potency neuroleptics?**

Low-potency neuroleptics have greater sedative, postural hypotensive, and anticholinergic effects. High-potency neuroleptics have greater extrapyramidal effects.

○ **Why is haloperidol one of the preferred neuroleptics?**

It can be used IM in emergencies plus it has few side effects. It does, however, have a high frequency of extrapyramidal effects.

○ **You are considering chemical restraint. What are your options?**

Benzodiazepines:

(1) Lorazepam (Ativan)

(2) Midazolam (Versed)

(3) Diazepam (Valium)

Sedative hypnotics:

(1) Haloperidol (Haldol)

(2) Droperidol (Inapsine)

Benzodiazepines may be given in combination with the sedative hypnotics to both hasten and potentiate their effect. Titrate, to effect and monitor appropriately.

○ **What may happen when ethanol is combined with an anxiolytic (benzodiazepine)?**

Death resulted from their combined respiratory depressive effects.

○ **What is the life-time prevalence of major depression?**

15%.

○ **What are the diagnostic criteria for major depression?**

Five or more of the following symptoms that have been present for 2 weeks and at least one of the symptoms is depressed mood or loss of interest:

Marked diminished interest or pleasure in all, weight loss or weight gain, insomnia or hypersomnia, psychomotor agitation or retardation, decreased energy, feelings of worthlessness, inability to concentrate, and suicidal ideation.

○ **What should be used to treat a hypertensive crisis caused by the combination of an MAO inhibitor and a sympathomimetic agent?**

An alpha-adrenergic antagonist agent as IV phentolamine or a potent intravenous vasodilator as nitroprusside.

○ **Name some drugs and foods contraindicated in a patient who is taking MAO inhibitors.**

Meperidine (Demerol) and dextromethorphan can cause a sympathomimetic crisis. Other agents to avoid include ephedrine, sympathomimetic amines in cold remedies, amphetamines, cocaine and methylphenidate (Ritalin). Wine and cheese.

○ **List some life threatening causes of acute psychosis.**

WHHHIMP:

Wernicke's encephalopathy

Hypoxia

Hypoglycemia

Hypertensive encephalopathy

Intracerebral hemorrhage

Meningitis/encephalitis

Poisoning

○ **What signs and symptoms suggest an organic source for psychosis?**

Acute onset, disorientation, visual or tactile hallucinations, younger than 10 years or older than 60 years and any evidence suggesting overdose or acute ingestion, such as abnormal vital signs, pupil size and reactivity, or nystagmus.

○ **A 30-year-old female complains of calf pain, a headache, shooting pain when flexing her right wrist, random epigastric pain, bloating and irregular menses, all of which cannot be explained after medical examination. What is the diagnosis?**

Somatization disorder that is characterized by many unexplained medical symptoms involving multiple systems. In order to diagnose a patient with somatization disorder, one must have 4 or more unexplained pain symptoms. Symptoms generally begin in childhood and are fully developed by age 30. This is more common in women than men.

○ **Who is more successful at suicide, men or women?**

Males (3:1). However, women attempt suicide three times as often as men.

○ **Major depression and bipolar affective disorder account for what percentage of suicides?**

50%. Another 25% are because of substance abuse, and another 10% are attributed to schizophrenia.

○ **What psychiatric problems are associated with violence?**

Acute schizophrenia, paranoid ideation, catatonic excitation, mania, borderline, and antisocial personality disorders, delusional depression, posttraumatic stress disorder decompensating obsessive/compulsive disorder and substance abuse.

○ **What are the prodromes of violent behavior?**

Anxiety, defensiveness, volatility, and physical aggression.

○ **What are the potential side effects of naloxone administration?**

Tachycardia, ventricular arrhythmias, cardiac arrest, hypertension, pulmonary edema, reversal of analgesia, and precipitation of withdrawal syndrome.

○ **What are the characteristic withdrawal symptoms when opioids are discontinued?**

Nausea, vomiting, mydriasis, diarrhea, anorexia, piloerection, yawning, abdominal pain, muscle spasms, and leukocytosis.

○ **Explain the significant features of each "axis" in the DSM-III official diagnostic criteria and nomenclature for psychiatric illnesses.**

Axis I: Organic brain syndromes caused by intoxication or physical illness and major psychiatric disorders including psychosis, affective disorders, and disorders of substance use.

Axis II: Personality disorders including antisocial, schizoid, histrionic types and mental retardation.

Axis III: Medical problems such as heart disease and infections.

Axis IV: Life events that contribute to the patient's problems.

Axis V: Patient's adaptation to these problems. Global Assessment Functioning Scale

○ **According to Holmes and Rahe, what are life's top 10 most stressful events?**

(1) Death of spouse or child

(2) Divorce

(3) Separation

(4) Institutional detention

(5) Death of close family member

(6) Major personal injury or illness

(7) Marriage

(8) Job loss

(9) Marital reconciliation

(10) Retirement

○ **What are the four phases of the female sexual response cycle?**

- Excitement Phase
- Plateau
- Orgasmic phase
- Resolution phase

○ **Based on these phases, according to the DSM-IVTR what are the associated sexual dysfunctions:**

- Hypoactive sexual desire disorder
- Female sexual arousal disorder
- Female orgasmic disorder
- Postcoital dysphoria; postcoital headache.

○ **Describe the difference between dyspareunia and vaginismus:**

Dyspareunia is recurrent or persistent genital pain.

Vaginismus is an involuntary muscle constriction of the outer third-of-vagina that interferes with penile insertion and intercourse. They are often related.

○ **True or False: sexual trauma such as rape can cause vaginismus.**

True.

○ **Paraphilias are normal in some people.**

False. Paraphilias are abnormal expressions of sexuality. Some examples include exhibitionism, fetishism, frotteurism, pedophilia, masochism, sadism, voyeurism or transvestic fetishism.

○ **Diazepam is safe during pregnancy.**

False. Has been associated with cleft lip and cleft palate.

○ **Can lithium be used in pregnancy?**

No. It can produce cardiac anomalies (Ebstein anomaly).

○ **Can carbamazepine be used in pregnancy?**

No. carbamazepine is a class-D drug. Estimated 1% risk of spina bifida. A fetal carbamazepine syndrome has been described consisting of minor craniofacial defects and fingernail hypoplasia.

○ **What are the barriers to effective screening, detection, and referral of obstetric patients who abuse alcohol or illicit drugs?**

(1) Lack of physician knowledge about the physiology, risk factors, and sex differences of alcohol and drug abuse.

(2) Patient fear of being socially stigmatized or of losing legal custody of their children.

(3) Inadequate insurance reimbursement for the time consumed in counseling women, regarding substance abuse.

(4) Lack of physician familiarity with the available treatment resources and system of referral.

○ **Discuss the ethical principles as applied to the universal screening of women for alcohol and drug abuse.**

(1) *Beneficence:* Making the diagnosis of addiction and initiating treatment and counseling improves patient outcome

(2) *Nonmaleficence:* The physician must avoid stigmatizing the addicted patient, and must not use humiliation as a tool to force change because it is inappropriate, engenders resistance, and may act as a barrier to recovery.

(3) *Justice:* Physicians must screen all patients regardless of race, socioeconomic status, or pregnancy.

(4) *Autonomy:* Patients have the right to refuse to answer screening questions and must not be coerced into making medical decisions against their judgment.

(5) *Confidentiality:* Patients must be assured that their social status would not be threatened by their response to screening and treatment or referral.

○ **The use of 2D or 3D ultrasonography for solely nonmedical purposes, such as keepsake photographs or videos, has risen. Discuss the potential dangers of such use.**

(1) The possibility of adverse biological effects of ultrasonography cannot be totally ruled out; hence, such imaging should only be used in the context of a well-defined obstetric indication.

(2) A false reassurance of fetal well being may be implied by an aesthetically pleasing sonogram, and women may incorrectly believe that a limited nonmedical scan is diagnostic.

(3) Abnormalities, if detected, may create an undue sense of alarm if the personnel performing the scan are not trained to discuss their implications.

(4) Abnormalities detected may be lost to follow-up when the scan is performed outside an integrated prenatal-care delivery system.

○ **Discuss the ethical obligations of obstetricians when pregnant patients refuse to follow medical advice or make decisions that are deemed medically unsafe for their fetus?**

(1) To examine the sociocultural context of the patient's decision, and to question whether or not their own ethical judgments support racial, class, or gender inequalities.

(2) To clearly explain the reasons for the medical recommendations, examine the barriers to their acceptance, and continue to encourage healthy behavior.

(3) To present a balanced evaluation of expected outcomes for both the mother and the fetus, keeping in mind the limitations of medical knowledge.

(4) To respect patient's autonomy, continue to care for the pregnant woman, and not intervene against her wishes regardless of the expected consequences.

○ **Discuss the reasons why it would be ethically objectionable to legally coerce pregnant women to follow medical advice.**

(1) All competent adults are entitled to bodily integrity and informed consent, regardless of the impact of such a decision on others.

(2) The pregnant woman could best weigh for herself the risks and benefits of proposed medical intervention, in the context of her own values and concerns. Overriding this autonomy with a purely medical judgment could put the patient at risk, especially since medical judgments in obstetrics are fallible and imprecise.

(3) Coercing women to follow medical decisions would likely discourage prenatal care and undermine the physician–patient relationship.

(4) Coercing pregnant women to follow medical advice violates the principle of equality, since it tends to single out a vulnerable group of patients.

(5) Coercing pregnant women to follow medical advice violates the principle of justice, since it creates a potential for criminalizing otherwise legal patient behavior.

○ **Discuss the guidelines for ethical marketing of a medical practice.**

(1) A paid advertisement for a practice must be clearly identified as such, especially when delivered in the context of an infomercial.

(2) The information presented must be appropriate to the chosen communication medium, to avoid the potential for misleading patients. Special care must be exercised to avoid unduly influencing the decisions of vulnerable groups of patients, such as the elderly.

(3) Discriminatory statements about race, ethnicity, sexual orientation, or gender must be avoided. However, a neutral statement about the gender or the languages spoken by the physician is acceptable and is not usually construed as discriminatory.

(4) Advertisement that denigrates the competence of other physicians or practices should be avoided.

○ **When is partner consent needed for a woman to participate in a clinical research trial?**

(1) The partner is a subject of the trial himself.

(2) The partner will be exposed to an investigational agent, which has a potential for greater than minimal risks.

(3) The partner's acceptance of the treatment or the impact of his acceptance on the woman will be collected as data.

(4) If characteristics of the partner are listed as inclusion or exclusion criteria.

○ **What characteristic distinguishes innovative clinical practice from formal research?**

Innovative practice, like research, is driven by the desire to learn and improve treatment. However, research has the distinct purpose of producing knowledge that can be applied to other patients beyond the particular study group, which is not necessarily the case in innovative practice. The safety and comparative efficacy of such innovative practice might later be investigated under a formal research protocol. Conversely, innovative practice that is apparently safe and effective might be incorporated into accepted practice without the benefit of a formal research evaluation.

○ **What ethical issues may arise when innovative or experimental practices are adopted without the benefit of formal research?**

(1) Procedures that are not effective may incur unnecessary costs or undefined morbidity.

(2) Patients' right to accurate disclosure may be violated, when the risks have not been formally evaluated.

(3) A prior adoption of innovative practice may make it difficult to recruit patients for a formal research protocol to determine the safety or efficacy of such practice, since the control group would not receive the treatment.

○ **Discuss the ethical criteria for formalizing innovative treatment into a research protocol.**

(1) When there is significant departure from standard practice.

(2) When the risks are unknown and may be significant in proportion to the expected benefits.

(3) When the physician intends to produce knowledge that could be applied to the general population.

○ **What are the physician's duties to his patients when practicing clinical innovations?**

(1) Disclosing the experimental nature of the proposed treatment to the patient.

(2) Disclosing the purpose, benefits, and risks, including unquantified but plausible risks.

(3) Protect the patients from harm, by considering their own competence and familiarity with the innovative procedure.

○ **What are the physician's duties to his profession when practicing clinical innovations?**

(1) To structure the application of innovative practice in order to learn from it.

(2) Share what is learned, both positive and negative, with the medical community.

(3) Strive to move innovative practices into formal research trial to gauge safety and efficacy.

○ **Discuss the impact of lack of health insurance on women.**

(1) It limits contraceptive options.

(2) It leads women to come for prenatal care less frequently.

(3) It leads to a twofold increased rate of not receiving needed medical care.

(4) It is associated with increased likelihood of an adverse maternal outcome.

(5) It is associated with increased likelihood of an adverse neonatal outcome, including death.

(6) It is associated with a 35% to 50% increased risk of dying from breast cancer, because of a decreased frequency of screening.

(7) It is associated with a 60% increased risk of late-stage diagnosis of cervical cancer, because of a decreased frequency of Pap smears.

○ **How is a homeless woman defined?**

(1) Lacks a fixed, regular, or adequate nighttime residence.

(2) Has as primary nighttime residence, a supervised shelter, designed to provide temporary living accommodations.

(3) Has as primary nighttime residence, a public or private place not ordinarily used as regular sleeping accommodations for humans.

○ **What characteristics of homeless women have a direct impact on their health care?**

(1) Poor personal hygiene.

(2) Chronic recurrent diseases such as asthma, hepatitis, or tuberculosis.

(3) Multiple STD or HIV.

(4) Alcohol and drug abuse.

(5) Chronic mental illness, including suicide attempts.

(6) Repetitive nonspecific complaints, for which a diagnosis cannot be found.

(7) Poor nutritional state.

(8) Partner violence, including sexual abuse.

(9) Noncompliance with physician orders and directives.

○ **Discuss the guidelines for minimizing ethnic and racial disparities in clinical practice.**

(1) Advocating for a system of universal access to basic health care.

(2) Improving personal competency in cross-cultural communication skills.

(3) Using national best practice guidelines to reduce variation in health care outcomes.

(4) Actively encourage and recruit cultural minorities to the health professions.

(5) Conduct research and training regarding racial and ethnic disparities in health care.

○ **Describe the 5-A approach to smoking counseling for pregnant women**

(1) ASK about smoking status in multiple choice format: Never smoked? Smoked before pregnancy but not now? Smoked after discovering pregnancy but not now? Smokes now but less than before pregnancy? Smokes now with the same number of cigarettes as before pregnancy?

(2) ADVISE about the benefits of quitting and the impact of smoking on the woman and her fetus.

(3) ASSESS the willingness to quit within 30 days.

(4) ASSIST by providing skills and methods, as well as support groups, for smoking cessation.

(5) ARRANGE for follow-up evaluation of smoking status and the impact of the proposed interventions

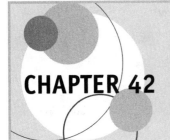

CHAPTER 42

Cervical Lesions and Cancer

Abby Gonik, MD

○ **When should Pap smear examinations be initiated?**

The American Cancer Society and the American College of Obstetricians and Gynecologists endorse the 2002 guidelines: Within 3 years after the onset of sexual activity and no later than age 21.

○ **Is HPV transmitted through vaginal intercourse alone?**

No. HPV can be acquired through same-sex and nonpenetrative sexual contact.

○ **Should all women who have not undergone hysterectomy have Pap smears performed annually?**

After initiation of screening, American Cancer Society recommends cervical screening be done annually with conventional cervical cytology smears or every 2 years using liquid-based cytology. The American College of Obstetricians and Gynecologists recommends annual screening regardless of the type of Pap performed. After age 30, women who have had three consecutive, technically satisfactory normal cytology results may be screened every 2 to 3 years (unless DES history, HIV positive, or are immunocompromised).

○ **How effective have Pap smears been in reducing the incidence of cervical cancer?**

Since the development of cytological screening in the 1940s, the incidence of cervical cancer in the United States has fallen by almost 80%. In contrast, cervical cancer remains the major cause of cancer-related deaths among women in many third world countries where Pap smears are not routinely performed.

○ **What is the false-negative rate for conventional Pap smears?**

Up to 40%.

○ **The quadrivalent HPV vaccine should be given to females in what age group?**

The FDA approved the vaccine for administration to girls and women between the age of 9 and 26 years.

○ **The HPV vaccine is effective against the oncogenic types 16 and 18. What percentage of cervical cancers is caused by these two types of HPV?**

HPV types 16 and 18 are responsible for about 70% of cervical cancers.

○ **What is the most common presenting symptom for patients with cervical cancer?**

Up to 80% of patients present with abnormal vaginal bleeding, most commonly postmenopausal. Only 10% note postcoital bleeding. Less frequent symptoms include vaginal discharge and pain.

○ **Is male circumcision thought to play a role in transmission of HPV?**

Yes. Circumcised males have a lower risk of HPV infection and therefore a reduced risk of cervical cancer in their female partners.

○ **What is the most appropriate management for a gross cervical lesion discovered during a routine examination?**

Biopsy. Specimens from ulcerated lesions should be obtained from their center.

○ **What is the next appropriate step in management of an ASC-US Pap test in a patient whose reflex HPV testing is positive for high-risk HPV subtypes?**

Colposcopy.

○ **If high-grade squamous intraepithelial lesions are left untreated over a period of several years, what percentage will progress to invasive cancer?**

Approximately 20%.

○ **What is the relative frequency of the two major histologic subtypes of cervical cancer?**

Approximately 80% of cervical cancers are squamous cell carcinoma, and 15% are adenocarcinomas.

○ **What is the most common stage at diagnosis of cervical cancer?**

Approximately half of the patients with cervical cancer present with stage I disease.

○ **What epidemiologic risk factors have been identified for the development of cervical cancer?**

Young age at first intercourse, multiple sexual partners, high parity, HIV infection, and history of other sexually transmitted infections.

○ **What other modifiable risk factor has been clearly linked to an increased risk of cervical cancer?**

Exposure to cigarette smoke. The relative risk of cervical cancer is increased two- to fourfold among cigarette smokers compared with nonsmokers.

○ **A carcinoma 5 cm in diameter and clinically confined to the cervix is assigned what FIGO stage?**

According to the 1995 FIGO staging modifications, lesions clinically confined to the cervix and less than or equal to 4 cm in diameter are designated stage IB1. Lesions greater than 4 cm are classified as stage IB2.

○ **How does para-aortic lymph node metastases detected by CT scan and confirmed by thin-needle sampling affect staging?**

This information helps to direct therapy, but it does not affect staging, which is clinically assigned.

○ **What radiographic study has the highest sensitivity to detect para-aortic lymph node metastases?**

Lymphangiogram, CT scan, and ultrasound were prospectively evaluated by the Gynecologic Oncology Group. Sensitivities were 79%, 34%, and 19%, respectively. Specificities were 96%, 73%, and 99%, respectively.

○ **Examination under anesthesia reveals a 3 cm in diameter cervical carcinoma with left parametrial involvement, not extending to the pelvic wall. The remainder of the staging evaluation is unremarkable. To what stage is this patient's tumor assigned?**

Stage IIB.

○ **For the above patient, if her IVP had revealed hydronephrosis, to what stage would her tumor be assigned?**

Stage IIIB classified as either tumor extension to the pelvic sidewall or hydronephrosis or a nonfunctioning kidney.

○ **If this patient's cystoscopy had identified bullous edema, what should her stage have been?**

It would remain stage IIIB. Bullous edema without pathologic confirmation of malignancy does not permit assignment to stage IVA.

○ **Are cystoscopy and proctoscopy necessary in the staging of all patients with cervical cancer?**

They may be omitted in the staging of asymptomatic patients with early disease (typically IIA or lower), for whom these studies are rarely abnormal.

○ **What is the incidence of pelvic and para-aortic lymph node metastasis for stage IB cervical cancer?**

Approximately 15% and 2%, respectively.

○ **For stage I cervical cancer, how does tumor size greater than 4 cm affect the incidence of pelvic lymph node metastasis?**

When compared to smaller lesions, an approximately threefold increase has been demonstrated.

○ **What lymph node group is most frequently involved with metastatic cervical cancer?**

In most series, the external iliac group is most commonly involved followed next by the obturator group.

○ **A colposcopically directed cervical biopsy from a 25-year-old G0P0 reveals a small focus of microinvasive squamous cell carcinoma. The resection margin is positive for carcinoma in situ. What is the next step in this patient's management?**

Cervical cone biopsy, to establish the full extent of invasion.

○ **For the above patient, final pathology shows invasion extending 2 mm below the basement membrane with a width of 4 mm. No lymph-vascular space invasion is present, and the margins are free of involvement. What is this patient's stage, and what are her therapeutic options?**

Stage IA1. The Society of Gynecologic Oncologists (SGO) defines microinvasion as stromal invasion of 3 mm or less below the basement membrane without lymph-vascular space involvement. For patients who desire preservation of fertility, most authorities agree that the risk of recurrence is very low, and that no additional therapy is necessary. If fertility is not desired, simple hysterectomy is recommended.

○   **What is the incidence of pelvic lymph node metastasis for squamous cell carcinoma of the cervix invading 1 mm to 3 mm and for lesions invading 3 to 5 mm?**

Less than 1% and 4%, respectively.

○   **For stage IB1 and early stage IIA disease, which therapy is more effective: Radical hysterectomy or radiation therapy?**

For these stages, the two modalities are considered equivalent therapeutically. Choice of therapy is dependent on a wide variety of factors.

○   **What is the 5-year survival for stage I cervical cancer?**

Approximately 90% overall. 5-year survival, when nodes are negative is often >90%. When nodes are involved, survival ranges from 20% to 75% depending on the number, size, and location of the positive nodes.

○   **The cardinal ligaments are exposed during a radical hysterectomy, when what two pelvic spaces are developed?**

The paravesicle space, anterior to the cardinal ligament, and the pararectal space posteriorly.

○   **Ureterovaginal and vesicovaginal fistulas occur in what percentage of patients undergoing radical hysterectomy?**

1% to 2% and <1%, respectively.

○   **Define the reference points A and B used in radiation treatment planning for cervical cancer.**

Point A: 2 cm lateral and 2 cm superior to the external cervical os, approximating the location where the uterine artery crosses the ureter.

Point B: 3 cm lateral to point A, corresponding to the pelvic wall.

○   **The standard unit for measuring absorbed radiation is the Gray (1 J/kg). How many rads are equivalent to one Gray?**

100 rads equal 1 Gray.

○   **What dosage of radiation is required to sterilize microscopic disease?**

4000 cGy to 5000 cGy will sterilize over 90% of occult tumor deposits.

○   **What dosage of radiation is required to sterilize clinically apparent disease?**

Greater than 6000 cGy.

○   **How many cGy given in 200 cGy fractions are required to produce ovarian failure?**

1000 cGy will cause ovarian failure in 50% of women.

○   **What organ is most radiosensitive in the pelvis?**

Rectum.

○ **What is the incidence of small-bowel obstruction following radiation used as primary therapy for cervical cancer?**

1% to 4%. The terminal ileum is most commonly involved because of its fixed position and limited blood supply. The majority of patients will present within 2 years of therapy. Recurrent disease must be ruled out.

○ **What radioisotopes are most commonly used in intracavitary radiation applicators?**

Cesium (Cs) for the traditional low dose rate brachytherapy, and Iridium (Ir) for high dose rate therapy.

○ **When radiation is used as primary therapy, what doses are delivered to points A and B?**

7000 cGy to 8500 cGy to point A and 6000 cGy to point B with individualization by lesion and treatment center.

○ **What are the radiation tolerances for the rectum and bladder?**

Approximately 6000 cGy and 7000 cGy, respectively.

○ **What are the advantages of radical hysterectomy relative to radiation therapy for stage I cervical cancer?**

- Ovarian preservation possible
- Unimpaired vaginal function
- Extent of disease established

○ **How does lesion size affect therapy for cervical carcinoma confined to the cervix?**

Though controversial, many consider lesion size greater than 4 cm to be a contraindication to radical hysterectomy. Radiation therapy is used with some recommending a simple hysterectomy following radiation.

○ **For locally advanced (stage IIB-IVA) cervical cancer, what treatment has become the standard of care?**

Concurrent cisplatin-based chemotherapy with radiation therapy.

○ **List pathologic findings following radical hysterectomy, which indicate a high risk for recurrence.**

- Lymph node metastasis
- Surgical margin involvement
- Parametrial invasion

○ **How does a modified radical hysterectomy differ from a radical hysterectomy?**

- The uterine artery is divided medial to the ureter rather than at its origin.
- The cardinal ligament is divided medial to the ureter rather than at the pelvic wall.
- Only the medial portion of uterosacral ligament is resected.
- Smaller vaginal margin.

○ **What is the incidence of para-aortic lymph node metastasis for stage IIB and III disease?**

Approximately 19% and 30%, respectively.

○ **What is the 5-year survival for stage IIB and III disease?**

Approximately 65% and 45%, respectively.

○ **What is the most common site of distant metastases of cervical cancer?**

Lung. 21% of distant metastases of cervical cancer are found in the lung.

○ **What are the usual borders used for whole pelvic external-beam radiation therapy?**

- Superiorly, the midvertebral level of L5.
- Inferiorly, the inferior aspect of the obturator foramina or at least 2 cm below the most distal vaginal tumor.
- Laterally, 1 cm lateral to the margins of the bony pelvis.

○ **How is the external-beam treatment field altered when the para-aortic nodes are included?**

A 10-cm wide portal extends from the pelvic field up to the T12-L1 interspace.

○ **Clinical staging of a 56-year-old with cervical cancer involving the left parametrium detects a 6 cm complex right adnexal mass. How is treatment affected by the mass?**

Surgical exploration is necessary to exclude a simultaneous ovarian cancer with staging or debulking, as indicated. Given the parametrial extension, a hysterectomy should not be performed.

○ **What percentage of cervical cancers occur in women during reproductive years?**

10% to 15%.

○ **What is the incidence of cervical cancer during pregnancy?**

Approximately, 1.2 per 10000 pregnancies.

○ **How does pregnancy affect survival for patients with cervical cancer?**

When prognostic factors are controlled, survival is not affected by pregnancy.

○ **What is the incidence of supraclavicular lymph node involvement when the para-aortic nodes contain metastatic disease?**

5% to 30%. The left side is more commonly involved (entry of portal for the thoracic duct).

○ **What percentage of cervical cancer recurrences will be detected within 1, 2, and 5 years of follow-up?**

50% of recurrences will be detected within 1 year, 75% within 2 years, and 95% within 5 years.

○ **How do survival rates for patients with adenocarcinoma of the cervix compare to those for squamous cell carcinoma?**

Controlling for prognostic factors, such as stage, volume of disease, and lymph node metastasis, survival appears to be similar.

○ **When invasive cervical cancer is incidentally discovered following a simple hysterectomy, what is the most common preoperative diagnosis?**

Cervical dysplasia.

○ **A simple hysterectomy is performed and invasive cervical cancer is incidentally discovered. What are the therapeutic options?**

Patients who are good candidates for radical surgery and who had small lesions with uninvolved surgical margins can be treated with radical parametrectomy, upper vaginectomy, and pelvic lymphadenectomy. All others should receive chemoradiation therapy.

○ **Is conservation of the ovaries appropriate for young patients undergoing radical hysterectomy for stage IB adenocarcinoma of the cervix?**

Yes, if the ovaries appear grossly normal. The incidence of ovarian metastasis is <2%.

○ **What is the incidence of vesicovaginal fistula formation following radiation therapy for cervical cancer with bladder invasion?**

4%, with 5-year survival of up to 30%.

○ **What procedure is often considered prior to initiating radiation therapy for locally advanced cervical cancer complicated by a rectovaginal fistula?**

A diverting colostomy is often recommended to avoid sepsis.

○ **What is the 1-year survival rate following cervical cancer recurrence?**

Approximately 15%.

○ **What is the therapy of choice for an isolated vaginal cuff recurrence following radical hysterectomy?**

External beam radiation therapy followed by brachytherapy. Exenteration is generally reserved for patients, who have previously received radiation.

○ **What criteria should be met prior to surgically exploring a patient for an exenteration?**

- Central pelvic disease, without evidence of extension to the pelvic wall.
- No evidence of distant disease.
- A physically and emotionally fit patient.

○ **What clinical triad is strongly indicative of surgically unresectable recurrent cervical cancer?**

- Unilateral leg edema
- Sciatic pain
- Ureteral obstruction

○ **What percentage of patients explored for an exenteration will be found to have unresectable disease?**

Approximately half. This is in part, due to the limitations of the pelvic examination, when radiation fibrosis of the parametria is present.

○ **What is the 5-year survival rate for patients undergoing pelvic exenteration for recurrent cervical cancer?**

With careful patient selection, up to 50%.

○ **What is the incidence of long-term response to cisplatin, when used for advanced or recurrent cervical cancer?**

Overall response to cisplatin is 25%. However, long-term response is generally not seen.

○ **Match the following characteristics to the appropriate histologic subtype of cervical cancer:**

(a) Histologically similar to oat cell cancer of the lung	Clear cell carcinoma
(b) Radiation may induce a more malignant transformation	Small cell neuroendocrine tumors
(c) Associated with DES exposure	Verrucous carcinoma
(d) Associated with Peutz-Jeghers syndrome	Minimal deviation adenocarcinoma (Adenoma malignum)

(a) Histologically similar to oat cell cancer of the lung	Clear cell carcinoma (c)
(b) Radiation may induce a more malignant transformation	Small cell neuroendocrine tumors (a)
(c) Associated with DES exposure	Verrucous carcinoma (b)
(d) Associated with Peutz-Jeghers syndrome	Minimal deviation adenocarcinoma (Adenoma malignum) (d)

CHAPTER 43

Endometrial Hyperplasia and Carcinoma

Abby M. Gonik, MD

○ **The World Health Organization classifies endometrial hyperplasia based on what two factors?**

1. Simple or complex glandular/stromal architecture.
2. The presence or absence of cytologic atypia.

○ **What is the best predictor that endometrial hyperplasia will progress to endometrial carcinoma?**

The presence or absence of cytologic atypia.

○ **What is the intent of the pathologist when he or she makes a diagnosis of endometrial hyperplasia?**

To communicate to the clinician his or her impression of the biologic potential of the endometrial proliferation to become cancer.

○ **What is the endocrinologic milieu for the development of endometrial hyperplasia?**

Unopposed estrogen.

○ **What other common risk factors have been correlated to the development of endometrial hyperplasia?**

- Polycystic ovary syndrome.
- Obesity.
- Diabetes mellitus.
- Late menopause (after age 55).
- Nulliparity.

○ **Which ovarian steroid hormone promotes growth of the endometrium?**

Estrogen.

○ **Which ovarian steroid hormone promotes differentiation of the endometrium?**

Progesterone.

○ **What percentage of women with atypical hyperplasia have coexistent endometrial cancer at the time of hysterectomy?**

Up to 43%.

○ **In the absence of cytologic atypia, what percentage of endometrial hyperplasia will progress to endometrial carcinoma?**

Approximately 1% to 3%.

○ **What percentage of complex atypical hyperplasia will progress to endometrial cancer?**

29%.

○ **Why is endometrial hyperplasia more common at the extremes of reproductive life, near puberty, and the perimenopause?**

At both extremes, anovulatory cycles are more common.

○ **In the postmenopausal woman, what is the main circulating estrogen and what is its source?**

Estrone. It arises from the peripheral conversion of adrenal and ovarian androstenedione. In a slender woman, this amounts to 40 μg/day. In an obese woman, it may exceed 200 μg/day.

○ **What are the most common presenting symptoms of endometrial hyperplasia in a woman of reproductive age?**

1. Metrorrhagia.
2. Menometrorrhagia.

○ **What is the most common presenting complaint in a postmenopausal woman with endometrial hyperplasia?**

Postmenopausal vaginal bleeding.

○ **Can endometrial hyperplasia be accurately diagnosed by transvaginal ultrasonography?**

No, endometrial hyperplasia is a histologic diagnosis. An endometrial sample is necessary to exclude adenocarcinoma. A thickened endometrial stripe in excess of 10 mm in a woman with abnormal uterine bleeding may suggest endometrial hyperplasia but is not diagnostic.

○ **What type of ovarian neoplasm is most commonly associated with endometrial hyperplasia?**

Granulosa cell tumor, because it secretes estradiol.

○ **In a postmenopausal woman, what sign on pelvic examination should suggest an elevated endogenous estrogen level?**

The absence of vaginal atrophy. The presence of a vagina with multiple rugal folds suggests an estrogen effect.

○ **What percentage of perimenopausal and postmenopausal women will have endometrial hyperplasia on an endometrial biopsy performed for abnormal or postmenopausal bleeding?**

8% to 9%. In women younger than 40 years, only 1% to 2% will have endometrial hyperplasia diagnosed on endometrial biopsy.

○ **What is the gland–stromal ratio in simple hyperplasia?**

The gland–stromal ratio in simple hyperplasia favors the glands. In a normal proliferative endometrium, the gland–stromal ratio favors the stroma.

○ **What are the earliest signs of cytologic atypia?**

- Enlarged, round nuclei.
- Fine and evenly dispersed chromatin.

○ **What differentiates complex atypical hyperplasia from well-differentiated adenocarcinoma?**

The presence of stromal invasion defined as a desmoplastic stromal response or a complex proliferation exceeding 1/2 a low power microscopic field, approximately 2.1 mm.

○ **In what type of hyperplasia is there back-to-back glandular crowding without cytologic atypia?**

This is the definition of complex hyperplasia.

○ **What is the value of mitotic activity in the diagnosis and prognosis of endometrial hyperplasia?**

It has none.

○ **What is the significance of squamous morules in the diagnosis and prognosis of endometrial hyperplasia?**

It is of no value. Squamous morules may be present in normal, hyperplastic, or neoplastic endometrium.

○ **Is there any difference between the biologic behavior of simple and complex hyperplasia?**

No, neither has cytologic atypia and both have a low incidence of progression to cancer.

○ **What characterizes the endometrial hyperplasia that is most likely to progress to endometrial carcinoma?**

A complex architectural pattern and a moderate degree of cytologic atypia.

○ **What factors influence the treatment of endometrial hyperplasia?**

- Age.
- Amount and duration of vaginal bleeding.
- Associated anemia.
- Desire for future childbearing.
- The presence or absence of cytologic atypia.
- The degree of cytologic atypia.

○ **What medical therapeutic options exist for treating endometrial hyperplasia in women who do not desire pregnancy at this time?**

- Progesterone.
- Oral contraceptive pills.
- Gonadotropin-releasing hormone analogs.
- A progesterone-containing IUD.

○ **What medical therapeutic options exist for the women who desire pregnancy at this time?**

Ovulation induction, typically with clomiphene citrate.

○ **What surgical options are currently available for the treatment of endometrial hyperplasia?**

- Curettage for acute bleeding.
- Hysteroscopy to exclude polyps and carcinoma.
- Hysterectomy, particularly if cytologic atypia is present.

○ **What nonmedical, nonsurgical life style changes are important in counseling the woman with endometrial hyperplasia?**

Dietary counseling and weight loss, screening for diabetes mellitus, discontinuing exogenous unopposed estrogen.

○ **What are the common side effects of depo-medroxyprogesterone therapy for endometrial hyperplasia?**

Spotting, breast soreness, weight gain, fluid retention, nervousness, irritability, bloating.

○ **What are common side effects of GnRH analog therapy for endometrial hyperplasia?**

Menopausal symptoms—hot flushes, vaginal dryness, changes in the serum lipid profile, effects on the coronary arteries, and bone loss.

○ **What is the recommended follow-up for a woman with a histologic diagnosis of simple or complex hyperplasia without cytologic atypia?**

In addition to medical therapy, follow-up endometrial sampling is recommended in 6 months.

○ **What is the failure rate of medical therapy for simple and complex hyperplasia?**

Approximately 20%.

○ **What is the recommended follow-up for a woman with a histologic diagnosis of atypical hyperplasia treated conservatively?**

In addition to medical treatment, repeat endometrial sampling in 3 months; however, more recent evidence suggests that intervals up to 6 months may be necessary to establish hormonal conversion.

○ **What is the incidence of simple and complex endometrial hyperplasia without atypia in postmenopausal women treated with unopposed estrogen?**

In the PEPI study, the incidence of hyperplasia without atypia was 27 of 170 women (16%).

○ **What is the incidence of complex atypical hyperplasia in postmenopausal women treated with unopposed estrogen?**

In the PEPI study, the incidence of complex hyperplasia with atypia was 14 of 170 women (8%).

○ **What is the most common gynecological malignancy in the United States?**

Endometrial cancer, of which 80% are the endometrioid adenocarcinoma type. Endometrial cancer accounts for 6% of all cancers in women.

○ **In 2007, approximately how many new cases and deaths from endometrial cancer occurred?**

Approximately 39,000 new cases and 7,400 deaths.

○ **What is the estimated prevalence of endometrial cancer in asymptomatic postmenopausal women?**

Approximately 7 per 100,000 for Caucasian women and 5.4 per 100,000 for other races.

○ **What is the 5-year survival rate for women with a diagnosis of endometrial carcinoma confined to the uterus at the time of surgical staging?**

Greater than 80%.

○ **What is the effect of cigarette smoking on the endometrium?**

Cigarette smoking significantly reduces the incidence of endometrial cancer. Endometrial atrophy, even in women on estrogen replacement therapy, is common in smokers, particularly if they are thin.

○ **Describe the screening test for endometrial cancer?**

There is no screening test for endometrial cancer; however, the American Cancer Society recommends annual endometrial biopsy starting at age 35 for all women at risk of HNPCC (hereditary nonpolyposis colorectal cancer).

○ **What percentage of women with endometrial cancer will have an abnormal Papanicolaou smear?**

Up to 50%.

○ **What are the risk factors associated with the development of endometrial carcinoma?**

Obesity, nulliparity, early menarche, and late menopause. Women weighing 21 to 50 pounds more than ideal body weight increase their risk of developing endometrial carcinomas threefold. Women in excess of 50 pounds more than ideal body weight increase their chance of developing endometrial carcinoma tenfold.

○ **What is hereditary nonpolyposis colorectal cancer (HNPCC) Lynch syndrome type II?**

A hereditary predisposition to the development of colon, breast, ovarian, and endometrial cancer. In approximately one-half of cases of affected women, endometrial and ovarian cancers precede colon cancer.

○ **Women who are at risk of HNPCC have what percent risk of developing endometrial and ovarian cancers?**

40% to 60% risk for developing endometrial cancer and 12% risk of ovarian cancer.

○ **What percentage of women who develop uterine malignancies have a history of prior pelvic radiation therapy?**

5% to 7% and typically develops 10 or more years after radiation therapy.

○ **Name four medical conditions that increase the risk for developing endometrial cancer because of excess endogenous estrogen?**

1. Women with chronic anovulation (PCO).
2. Women with estrogen secreting ovarian neoplasms, most commonly granulosa cell and theca cell tumors.

3. Obese postmenopausal women.

4. Women with severe liver disease.

○ **In whom should a diagnosis of endometrial cancer be excluded?**

1. All patients with postmenopausal bleeding.

2. Postmenopausal women with a pyometra.

3. Asymptomatic postmenopausal women with endometrial cells on a Papanicolaou smear.

4. Perimenopausal women with intermenstrual bleeding or increasingly heavy menses.

5. Premenopausal women with abnormal uterine bleeding, particularly if they are anovulatory.

○ **The background endometrium in a uterus with typical endometrioid endometrial adenocarcinoma histologically represents what process?**

Endometrial hyperplasia of varying types (asynchronous proliferative pattern).

○ **What effect does the prior use of oral contraceptive agents have on the development of endometrial cancer?**

Women who use combination oral contraceptive pills (OCP) for at least 12 months have a relative risk of endometrial cancer of 0.6. This protective effect persists for at least 15 years after cessation of OCP use.

○ **Epidemiologically, how many types of endometrial cancer are there?**

Two:

1. Type I is estrogen related and occurs on a background of endometrial hyperplasia. This type occurs in younger women and has a good prognosis.

2. Type II occurs predominantly in older women, appears to arise de novo, and is unassociated with estrogen excess. The histologic grade is high and histopathologic types associated with aggressive behavior (clear cell, papillary serous) are common. The prognosis is poor.

○ **What is the most common presenting complaint of a woman with endometrial cancer?**

Postmenopausal bleeding (or abnormal uterine bleeding in the premenopausal woman).

○ **What is the most common cause of postmenopausal bleeding?**

Atrophy.

○ **Describe the indicated office evaluation of a woman whose history is suspicious for endometrial cancer?**

Pelvic examination, PAP smear, biopsy of any abnormal cervical or vaginal lesion, and endometrial biopsy.

○ **What percentage of endometrial carcinomas will shed abnormal cells that can be seen on a cervico-vaginal cytology?**

25% to 35%.

○ **After which day of the menstrual cycle is the presence of endometrial cells a cause for concern?**

After day 14. Some authors would use day 10. During menses and immediately thereafter, the presence of endometrial cells in a PAP smear is normal.

○ **What histologic findings would be expected if atypical endometrial cells are identified on a routine PAP smear?**

- Adenocarcinoma 20%.
- Hyperplasia 11%.
- Polyps 11%.

  Thus, more than 40% of women with atypical endometrial cells identified on a PAP smear will have abnormal histology on an endometrial biopsy.

○ **In what clinical circumstances are pelvic and abdominal computed tomography (CT) scans helpful in evaluating patients with endometrial cancer on biopsy?**

1. Abnormal liver function tests.
2. Clinical hepatomegaly.
3. Palpable upper abdominal mass.
4. Palpable extrauterine pelvic disease.
5. Clinical ascites.

○ **How does endometrial carcinoma spread?**

1. Direct extension to adjacent structures.
2. Transtubal passage of exfoliated cells.
3. Lymphatic dissemination.
4. Hematogenous dissemination.

○ **Why do younger women have a better prognosis when they have endometrial carcinoma as compared to older women?**

Young women tend to have low-grade tumors with less myometrial invasion.

○ **Describe the gross appearance of deeply invasive endometrial cancer?**

Finger-like or broad based extensions beneath an exophytic endometrial growth. These extensions are firm, well demarcated, and lighter in color than adjacent myometrium.

○ **How is endometrial cancer staged?**

Surgically, and includes TAH/BSO, selective pelvic and para-aortic node sampling, and pelvic washings for cytology.

○ **What percent of women with endometrial cancer are diagnosed while in stage I?**

72%.

○ **Are postmenopausal women taking tamoxifen at higher risk of developing endometrial cancer than age-matched controls?**

Yes. The increased relative risk of developing endometrial cancer for postmenopausal women taking tamoxifen is two to three times higher than that of age-matched controls.

○ **A neoplasm that histologically has less than 5% solid area and invades approximately one-third of the myometrial thickness is what grade and stage? There is no other evidence of gross or microscopic disease.**

Grade 1, stage IB. Grade 1 has less than 5% solid area. Stage I disease is limited to the uterine corpus, and stage IB can have invasion of up to 50% of the myometrium.

○ **A neoplasm that histologically has more than 50% solid area and invades approximately three-fourths of the myometrial thickness is what grade and stage? There is no other evidence of gross or microscopic disease.**

Grade 3, stage IC. Grade 3 has more than 50% solid area. Stage I disease is limited to the uterine corpus, and stage IC has invasion of greater than 50% of the myometrial thickness.

○ **A neoplasm that histologically has more than 50% solid areas and invades for approximately three-fourths of the myometrial thickness is what grade and stage if the para-aortic nodes are positive for disease?**

Grade 3, stage IIIC. Grade 3 has more than 50% solid areas. Disease extension beyond the uterus is stage III. Involvement of the pelvic or para-aortic lymph nodes is stage IIIC. Stage II denotes cervical involvement.

○ **A woman has a diagnosis of well-differentiated adenocarcinoma (histologic grade 1) from a curettage specimen. If surgical staging is performed within one month, how often will the histologic grade be higher? Will there be deep myometrial invasion?**

1. Approximately one-third of neoplasms will be grade 2 or 3 (13%–50%).

2. Approximately 25% of uteri will have deep myometrial invasion.

○ **How does the presence of squamous change influence the prognosis of endometrial adenocarcinoma?**

Squamous change is typically nonmalignant and occurs in as many as 25% of endometrial adenocarcinomas. The overall prognosis is unchanged for those tumors known as adenocanthomas. The histologic grade is assigned based on the glandular element within the neoplasm.

○ **How does significant nuclear (cytologic) atypia affect the grading of an architectural grade 1 endometrial adenocarcinoma?**

Significant nuclear atypia, otherwise inappropriate for the architectural grade, increases the tumor grade by 1. This commonly occurs in papillary serous and clear cell endometrial carcinomas.

○ **What is the incidence of pelvic and para-aortic node involvement when the neoplasm appears grossly confined to the endometrium?**

Approximately 6% to 7% of patients will have pelvic node metastases and 2% to 3% will have para-aortic node metastases.

○ **What is the local and distant recurrence for typical endometrial adenocarcinoma?**

20% to 30% recur in the pelvis, 55% to 65% recur at distant sites, and 5% to 10% recur in both sites.

○ **What are the estrogen receptor status and the progesterone receptor status in papillary serous endometrial adenocarcinoma and clear cell endometrial adenocarcinoma?**

Papillary serous and clear cell endometrial carcinomas are usually negative for both estrogen and progesterone receptors.

○ **What is the effect of race on the prognosis of endometrial carcinoma?**

African-American women tend to have tumors of higher grade and higher stage. They have a poorer survival than Caucasian women. Also, a larger proportion of African-American women have unfavorable histologic types.

○ **What is the effect of gross cervical involvement in the prognosis of endometrial cancer?**

Gross cervical involvement is associated with a poor prognosis. When treated with intracavitary application of cesium followed by extrafascial hysterectomy, the mean survival time in women without gross cervical disease was 94.2 months, compared to 29.1 months for women with gross cervical disease.

○ **What are the two best prognostic indicators for endometrioid endometrial adenocarcinoma?**

Histologic grade and depth of myometrial invasion.

○ **What are the differences in frequency and 5-year survival between surgical stage I typical endometrioid adenocarcinoma and papillary serous carcinoma of the endometrium?**

Typical endometrioid adenocarcinoma accounts for approximately 80% of endometrial adenocarcinoma. Papillary serous carcinoma accounts for approximately 8% of all endometrial adenocarcinomas.

The 5-year survival for stage I typical endometrioid adenocarcinoma is 88% and that of stage I papillary serous carcinoma is 63%.

○ **Is the quantity of estrogen receptor (ER) and progesterone receptor (PR) higher or lower in endometrial carcinoma as compared to normal cycling endometrium?**

The concentration varies, but with adenocarcinoma the concentration is usually less than normal cycling endometrium.

○ **What is the significance of estrogen and progesterone receptor status in the prognosis of women with a diagnosis of endometrial carcinoma?**

ER status does not correlate well with prognosis. The absence of progesterone receptors is associated with a poor prognosis.

○ **What is the estrogen and progesterone receptor status in obese women with endometrial cancer?**

The majority of endometrial adenocarcinomas in obese women are ER+ and PR+.

○ **What is the correlation between visual inspection of the sectioned uterus for myometrial invasion and histologic measurement of myometrial invasion?**

Visual inspection of the uterus accurately determines the depth of invasion in 85% of cases.

○ **What percentage of women with endometrial carcinoma clinically confined to the uterus will develop recurrent disease?**

Approximately 16%.

○   **What is the average time from diagnosis to recurrence in endometrial carcinoma?**

2.2 years.

○   **When endometrial carcinoma recurs, what percentage of recurrence is detected within the first and second years?**

34% and 70%, respectively.

CHAPTER 44 Uterine Sarcomas

Mitchell I. Edelson, MD

○ **What is the incidence of uterine sarcomas?**

Sarcomas account for 2% to 4% of all uterine malignancies. The annual incidence is approximately 2 cases per 100,000 women.

○ **Define the following terms, which are used to classify uterine sarcomas according to cell type and origin: Pure, mixed, homologous, and heterologous.**

Pure—only one cell type present.

Mixed—more than one cell type present.

Homologous—cell types are indigenous to the uterus (i.e., leiomyosarcoma, stromal sarcoma, angiosarcoma).

Heterologous—cell types are foreign to the uterus (i.e., rhabdomyosarcoma, chondrosarcoma, osteosarcoma).

○ **List the four major groups of uterine sarcomas by decreasing incidence.**

Malignant mixed mesodermal tumors (MMMT, used here synonymously with carcinosarcoma)—50%.

Leiomyosarcoma—40%.

Endometrial stromal sarcoma—8%.

Adenosarcoma—<2%.

○ **Prior pelvic irradiation is associated with the development of which type of uterine sarcoma?**

Approximately 10% of patients with MMMT have a prior history of pelvic irradiation.

○ **What histologic criteria are used when diagnosing a benign endometrial stromal nodule?**

Endometrial stromal nodules are characterized by a proliferation of uniform, normal-appearing stromal cells with a well-circumscribed, noninfiltrative margin. Lymph-vascular space involvement is absent, and the mitotic count is usually less than 5 per 10 high power fields.

○ **How are endometrial stromal nodules treated?**

Hysterectomy is recommended. However, successful treatment using myomectomy has been reported.

○ **Worm-like extension of tumor into lymphatic and vascular channels, occasionally with extensive extrauterine extension, is seen in which type of sarcoma?**

Low-grade endometrial stromal sarcomas, formerly known as endolymphatic stromal myosis. A similar pattern has been described for intravenous leiomyomatosis.

○ **Why is the removal of ovaries recommended for patients undergoing surgery for a low-grade stromal sarcoma?**

These tumors often have high levels of estrogen and progesterone receptors, and their growth may be stimulated by estrogen. High-dose progesterone has been demonstrated to be therapeutically active.

○ **What percentage of stage I low-grade endometrial stromal sarcoma cases recur?**

Approximately 50% recur at a median of 3 years following diagnosis.

○ **What is the most common uterine neoplasm in reproductive women?**

Benign leiomyomata.

○ **What is the incidence of discovering a leiomyosarcoma following surgery for presumed benign leiomyomata?**

Approximately 0.2% to 0.3%.

○ **How does the origin of leiomyosarcomas differ from that of other uterine sarcomas?**

Leiomyosarcomas originate in the myometrium, all others originate in the endometrium.

○ **What histologic criteria are used to classify a leiomyosarcoma?**

Hypercellularity, nuclear atypia, mitotic index, and coagulative tumor cell necrosis.

○ **What is the average age for patients with leiomyosarcomas?**

53 years.

○ **What is the most frequent presenting symptom for patients with leiomyosarcomas?**

Vaginal bleeding, which occurs in more than three-quarters of patients.

○ **How reliable is the preoperative diagnosis of a rapidly enlarging uterus in predicting the presence of a leiomyosarcoma?**

A recent study found only one leiomyosarcoma among 371 patients undergoing hysterectomy for a rapidly enlarging uterus.

○ **A preoperative diagnosis of leiomyosarcoma is made in what percentage of cases?**

15%, despite up to one-third of the tumors being submucous.

○ **What therapy is recommended for disseminated peritoneal leiomyomatosis?**

This is a benign condition often associated with oral contraceptive use or pregnancy. No specific therapy is required, though discontinuation of oral contraceptives or resolution of a pregnancy often results in regression.

○ **How does the development of a leiomyosarcoma within a benign leiomyoma affect prognosis?**

This is considered to be a favorable prognostic feature.

○ **Are leiomyosarcomas generally solitary or multifocal lesions?**

Unlike leiomyomata, they are usually solitary lesions.

○ **What prognostic feature best predicts recurrence-free interval for early stage leiomyosarcomas?**

Mitotic index.

○ **What is the effect of adjuvant radiation therapy on early stage leiomyosarcomas?**

Although not demonstrated in all studies, pelvic recurrences are reduced by almost 50%.

○ **What is the most active chemotherapeutic agent in leiomyosarcomas?**

Adriamycin with an overall response rate of 25%.

○ **What two histologic components must be present to make the diagnosis of an MMMT?**

MMMTs are composed of an admixture of malignant epithelial and stromal components.

○ **How does an adenosarcoma differ histologically from an MMMT?**

The epithelial component of an adenosarcoma is benign.

○ **How does race affect the incidence of MMMT?**

The relative risk is greater for black women as compared to white women and rises at a disproportionately greater rate with advancing age.

○ **What is the most common epithelial histologic subtype in an MMMT?**

Approximately 60% are endometrioid followed in order of decreasing frequency by adenosquamous, serous, and clear cell histologies.

○ **What proportion of MMMTs contain heterologous stromal elements?**

Approximately 50% of cases.

○ **What is the most common heterologous stromal component in an MMMT?**

Rhabdomyosarcoma followed by chondrosarcoma and osteosarcoma.

○ **Are initial metastases from MMMTs usually of epithelial or stromal origin?**

Epithelial.

○ **How is the prognosis for patients with MMMT affected by the presence or absence of heterologous elements?**

Recent studies have shown no prognostic difference.

○ **The triad of pelvic pain, postmenopausal bleeding, and what physical finding is highly suggestive of an MMMT?**

Tissue protruding through the cervical os.

○ **Surgical staging will upstage what percentage of patients with MMMT clinically confined to the uterus?**

25% to 50%. Risk of extrauterine disease is related to depth of myometrial invasion, lymph-vascular space involvement, and cervical extension.

○ **What is the 5-year survival rate for surgical stage I MMMT?**

74%. Long-term survival for patients with extrauterine disease is rare.

○ **Which three chemotherapeutic agents have demonstrated the greatest activity in MMMTs?**

Cisplatin,ifosfamide, and paclitaxel.

○ **Which chemotherapeutic agent is recommended for leiomyosarcoma?**

Adriamycin.

○ **What is the frequency of pelvic lymph node metastases in uterine carcinosarcomas and leiomyosarcoma?**

15% for uterine carcinosarcoma and 3% for leiomyosarcoma.

CHAPTER 45 — Epithelial and Nonepithelial Ovarian Tumors

Mitchell I. Edelson, MD

○ **Epithelial tumors include what histologic types?**

1. Serous (75%).
2. Mucinous (20%).
3. Endometrioid (2%).
4. Clear cell.
5. Brenner carcinoma.
6. Undifferentiated carcinomas.

○ **The lifetime risk and mean age for developing epithelial ovarian cancers is:**

1.86% (1/70); 63 years.

○ **Characteristics of borderline tumors include:**

Tendency to remain confined to the ovary for long periods of time, occurrence predominantly in premenopausal women, associated with an excellent prognosis. There is no need for adjuvant treatment, even in those individuals with advanced disease.

○ **Criteria for diagnosis of borderline tumors are:**

1. Epithelial proliferation with papillary formation and pseudostratification.
2. Nuclear atypia and increased mitotic activity.
3. Absence of true stromal invasion.

○ **Percentage of invasive epithelial tumors that spread beyond the ovary:**

75% to 85%.

○ **Psammoma bodies are frequently associated with what types of ovarian tumors?**

Serous.

○ **Borderline serous tumors account for what percentage of all serous tumors?**

Approximately 15%.

○ **Well-differentiated serous adenocarcinoma is histologically defined by:**

A predominance of papillary and glandular cells, round to oval nuclei, and 0 to 2 mitoses per high power field.

○ **Poorly differentiated serous adenocarcinoma is histologically defined by:**

Solid sheets of cells, nuclear atypia, and 2 to 3 mitoses per high power field.

○ **Percentage of mucinous tumors of the ovary that are malignant:**

5%.

○ **Mucinous tumors histologically resemble what other cell type?**

Endocervical.

○ **What type of ovarian tumors is often associated with similar lesions in the endometrium?**

Endometrioid.

○ **Which ovarian tumors are associated with endometriosis and histologically are comprised of cells that project their nuclei to the apical cytoplasm, known as hobnail cells?**

Clear cell tumors.

○ **Clear cell tumors are often associated with which clinical/laboratory findings?**

Hypercalcemia and hyperpyrexia.

○ **A similar constellation of clinical symptoms seen in patients with ovarian cancer are also associated with:**

1. Mesothelioma.

2. Primary peritoneal carcinoma.

3. Tuberculous peritonitis.

○ **This solid tumor type is associated with epithelioid cells that show a coffee bean pattern caused by longitudinal grooving of the nuclei:**

Brenner tumors.

○ **What is the lifetime risk of developing ovarian cancer in BRCA1 and BRCA2 carriers?**

Women with BRCA1 mutations have a 20% to 40% risk of developing ovarian cancer while women with BRCA2 mutations have a 10% to 20% risk.

○ **List the hereditary syndromes of cancer that have been associated with an increased risk of ovarian cancer.**

1. Site-specific familial ovarian cancer.

2. Breast/ovarian familial cancer syndromes.

3. Hereditary nonpolyposis colorectal cancer (HNPCC) (formerly known as Lynch II syndrome).

○ **Surgical staging for ovarian cancer should involve what surgical steps?**

Submitting any free fluid for cytology (or peritoneal washings), a systematic exploration of all intra-abdominal surfaces and viscera, biopsy of multiple intraperitoneal sites, biopsy of the diaphragm, infracolic omentectomy, and pelvic and para-aortic lymph node dissection.

○ **The principal treatment for borderline ovarian tumors:**

Surgical resection alone.

○ **Chemotherapeutic treatment regimen of choice for patients with advanced epithelial ovarian cancer:**

A combination of platinum and taxane.

○ **Which chemotherapy regimen recently showed a significant survival benefit among women with optimally debulked epithelial ovarian cancer with a 65.6 months median survival?**

A regimen consisting of intraperitoneal cisplatin and paclitaxel and intravenous paclitaxel demonstrated the longest survival data from a randomized trial in advanced ovarian cancer.

○ **Nonepithelial tumors of the ovary account for what percentage of all ovarian cancers?**

10%.

○ **In the first two decades of life, what percentage of ovarian tumors are germ cell?**

70%.

○ **Germ cell tumors commonly secrete what two hormones?**

Alpha-fetoprotein and human chorionic gonadotropin.

○ **What are the different histologic types of germ cell tumors?**

1. Dysgerminoma.
2. Teratoma.
3. Endodermal sinus tumor.
4. Embryonal carcinoma.
5. Polyembryoma.
6. Choriocarcinoma.
7. Mixed forms.

○ **The most common malignant germ cell tumor:**

Dysgerminoma.

○ **Describe the histologic characteristics of dysgerminomas.**

Large round ovoid or polygonal cells with abundant clear, pale staining cytoplasm, large and irregular nuclei with prominent nucleoli.

○ **The most common chemotherapeutic regimens for germ cell tumors:**
1. BEP (bleomycin, etoposide, and cisplatin).
2. VBP (vinblastine, bleomycin, and cisplatin).
3. VAC (vincristine, actinomycin, and cyclophosphamide).

○ **What tumor markers may be elevated in a woman with a dysgerminoma?**
1. Lactic dehydrogenase.
2. Beta-hCG.

○ **Endodermal sinus tumors are derived from what structure?**
The primitive yolk sac.

○ **The majority of malignant ovarian germ cell tumors are unilateral except for which type?**
Dysgerminoma tumors can have bilateral involvement in 10% to 15% of cases.

○ **Which stage ovarian germ cell tumors do not require any further treatment following surgical resection and staging?**
The treatment of choice for a woman with a stage IA dysgerminoma and a stage IA grade 1 immature teratoma is observation.

○ **What is the characteristic microscopic finding of endodermal sinus tumors?**
Schiller–Duval body.

○ **What enzymes are secreted by endodermal sinus tumors?**
AFP and rarely, alpha-1-antitrypsin.

○ **What is the most common malignancy to develop in an initially benign teratoma?**
Squamous cell carcinoma.

○ **How do you distinguish an embryonal carcinoma of the ovary from choriocarcinoma of the ovary?**
There is an absence of syncytiotrophoblastic and cytotrophoblastic cells.

○ **What neoplasm closely resembles a similar carcinoma of the adult testes?**
Embryonal carcinoma.

○ **What do the tumors of embryonal carcinomas contain?**
hCG, syncytiotrophoblast-like cells, and AFP in large primitive cells.

○ **Name a rare germ cell neoplasm composed of numerous embryoid bodies resembling morphologically normal embryos.**
Polyembryonal tumors.

○ **Name the three ways choriocarcinomas can arise.**

1. As a primary gestational choriocarcinoma associated with ovarian pregnancy.
2. As a metastatic choriocarcinoma from a primary gestational choriocarcinoma arising in other parts of the genital tract.
3. As a germ cell tumor differentiating in a direction of trophoblastic structures and arising with other neoplastic germ cell elements.

○ **What do choriocarcinomas secrete?**

hCG.

○ **What percentage of choriocarcinomas arise in prepubescent children?**

50%.

○ **What is the most common component of a mixed germ cell tumor?**

Dysgerminoma.

○ **What is the most frequent complication of mature cystic teratomas and when does it most often occur?**

Torsion, most frequently occurring in pregnancy and the puerperium.

○ **What is contained in an immature teratoma?**

Immature neural elements.

○ **What is the most common tumor that secretes estrogen?**

Adult granulosa cell tumors.

○ **Describe the histologic appearance of granulosa cell tumors.**

Fibrothecomatous components with scant cytoplasm and coffee-bean grooved cells. Mature follicles and Call–Exner bodies are also common.

○ **What other malignancy is commonly associated with granulosa cell tumors of the ovary?**

Endometrioid adenocarcinoma of the uterus.

○ **Individuals with Peutz–Jeghers syndrome have increased:**

1. Sex cord stromal tumors of the ovary.
2. Adenoma malignum (minimal deviation) of the cervix.

○ **Which factors are protective against ovarian carcinomas?**

1. Pregnancy.
2. Bilateral tubal ligation.
3. Hysterectomy.
4. Use of oral contraceptives.

CHAPTER 46

Fallopian Tube Neoplasms

Mitchell I. Edelson, MD

○ **What embryologic layer gives rise to the majority of benign tumors of the fallopian tube?**

Mesoderm.

○ **What is a Walthard nest?**

A benign inclusion cyst created in the fallopian tube by invagination of the tubal serosa. It is filled with polygonal epithelial-like cells with distinctive, irregularly ovoid nuclei with longitudinal nuclear grooves that give them a coffee-bean appearance. They are common incidental findings of no clinical importance.

○ **What is the most common benign tubal tumor?**

Adenomatoid tumors (benign mesotheliomas). They appear as small (1–2 cm) nodular masses with multiple, spherical or slit-like channels lined by an attenuated layer of cells. There is no evidence of cytologic atypia.

○ **What histologic finding is associated with carcinoma in situ (CIS) of the fallopian tube?**

Cytologically malignant, mitotically active nuclei, with or without the formation of papillae by the endosalpingeal epithelial cells.

○ **What is salpingitis isthmica nodosa and how is it differentiated from primary carcinoma of the fallopian tube?**

Salpingitis isthmica nodosa is a localized diverticulosis of the isthmic portion of the fallopian tube. Grossly, it appears as a firm, nodular dilatation of the isthmus with a diameter of less than 2 cm. Microscopically, the glandular endosalpinx is seen extending from the lumen deep into the muscularis. It is differentiated from primary carcinoma of the fallopian tube by its lack of cytologic atypia.

○ **What is the most common carcinoma that involves the fallopian tube?**

Metastatic carcinomas from another site in the female genital tract. Almost 50% of women with ovarian cancer and up to 12% of women with uterine cancers will have spread to the fallopian tube.

○ **What percentage of primary malignancies of the female genital tract arises from the fallopian tubes?**

0.2% to 0.5%.

○   **What is the most common primary malignant neoplasm of the fallopian tube?**

Papillary serous adenocarcinoma, accounting for 90% of all fallopian tube malignancies.

○   **Describe the classic triad of symptoms associated with fallopian tube malignancies.**

Profuse clear or serosanguineous vaginal discharge (hydrops tubae profluens), pelvic pain, and a pelvic mass.

○   **What percentage of patients with fallopian tube malignancies presents with the classic triad of symptoms?**

Fewer than 15%; however, more than 50% present with vaginal discharge or bleeding and approximately 60% have a pelvic mass.

○   **How often is bilateral involvement found in adenocarcinoma of the fallopian tube?**

Dependent upon the stage of the tumor at the time of diagnosis. For stage I, II, and *in situ* lesions, the incidence is approximately 7%. In stage III and IV disease, however, bilateral involvement is seen in as many as 30%.

○   **Describe the staging system for fallopian tube tumors.**

Although there are several staging systems for tubal cancers, the most widely used is that of the International Federation of Gynecologists and Obstetricians (FIGO). It is similar to that used to stage ovarian malignancies.

Stage 0	Carcinoma in situ (limited to the tubal mucosa).
Stage I	Growth limited to the fallopian tubes.
Stage IA	Growth limited to one tube with extension into submucosa and/or muscularis, but not penetrating the serosal surface. No ascites.
Stage IB	Growth limited to both tubes with extension into submucosa and/or muscularis, but not penetrating the serosal surface. No ascites.
Stage IC	Tumor either IA or IB but with extension through or onto tubal serosa or ascites containing malignant cells or with positive peritoneal washings.
Stage II	Growth involving one or both fallopian tubes with pelvic extension.
Stage IIA	Extension and/or metastasis to uterus and/or ovaries.
Stage IIB	Extension to other pelvic tissues.
Stage IIC	Tumor either IIA or IIB but with ascites containing malignant cells or with positive peritoneal washings.
Stage III	Tumor involving one or both fallopian tubes with peritoneal implants outside pelvis and/or positive retroperitoneal or inguinal adenopathy. Superficial liver metastasis included.
Stage IIIA	Tumor grossly limited to true pelvis with negative nodes but with histologically confirmed microscopic seeding of abdominal peritoneal surfaces.
Stage IIIB	Tumor involving one or both tubes with negative nodes but histologically confirmed implants of 2 cm or less on abdominal peritoneal surfaces.
Stage IIIC	Abdominal implants of >2 cm in diameter and/or positive retroperitoneal or inguinal nodes.
Stage IV	Growth involving one or both fallopian tubes with distant metastases. Includes parenchymal liver metastasis and cytologically confirmed malignant pleural effusions.

○ **Based on the surgical findings at the time of laparotomy, how common are the four stages?**

Stage I disease accounts for approximately 20% to 33% of all fallopian tube malignancies, stage II for approximately 20% to 33%, and stage III or IV for 34% to 60%.

○ **What is the 5-year survival for patients with adenocarcinoma of the fallopian tube?**

Overall 5-year survival is approximately 40%, but is dependent upon the stage at the time of diagnosis. Carcinoma in situ is associated with a 5-year survival of 65% to 80%, stage I 65%, stage II 50% to 60%, and stage III–IV 10% to 20%.

○ **What tumor marker is useful in the follow-up of tubal serous carcinomas?**

CA-125.

○ **What is the standard treatment for tubal carcinoma?**

The standard method is similar to that used for ovarian or endometrial adenocarcinoma. Treatment for tubal carcinoma consists of total abdominal hysterectomy, bilateral salpingo-oophorectomy, and aggressive cytoreductive surgery, followed by chemotherapy.

○ **What is the role for cytoreductive surgery?**

Cytoreductive surgery has been demonstrated to have a beneficial effect in the treatment of fallopian tube carcinomas in a similar fashion to that of ovarian malignancies. Patients with a residual tumor mass of less than 1 cm have a significantly higher survival rate than do patients with larger residual tumors following primary surgery.

○ **Is there a role for radiation therapy in the treatment of tubal carcinoma?**

The role for radiation therapy in the treatment of tubal carcinoma is still unclear. Several studies suggest that pelvic irradiation can result in local control of disease, reducing the rates of local recurrence. Intra-abdominal and distance recurrences are common, however, and thus would likely require the addition of whole abdominal radiation therapy or chemotherapy.

○ **What are the most effective chemotherapeutic agents against tubal carcinoma?**

A combination of taxol and a platinum-based chemotherapeutic agent is currently used.

○ **Name the two most common metastatic tumors that involve the fallopian tube.**

Ovarian and endometrial carcinomas. Peritoneal spread often involves the serosal surface and lymphatic spread from adjacent primary sites may involve the mucosa or muscularis.

○ **What are the histologic criteria often employed in the diagnosis of a primary tubal carcinoma?**

(1) Grossly, the main bulk of tumor is confined to the fallopian tube and arises from the endosalpinx.

(2) Microscopically, the epithelium of the tubal mucosa is involved and shows a papillary pattern.

(3) A transition between benign and malignant tubal epithelium is identifiable.

(4) The ovaries and endometrium are either normal or contain less tumor than the tubes.

○ **A tubal lesion consisting primarily of trophoblastic proliferation in addition to hydropic villi represents what type of fallopian tube tumor?**

Ectopic molar pregnancy. Responsible for approximately 1 in 5000 ectopic pregnancies, they clinically present in a similar fashion to other ectopic gestations, but histologically demonstrate the appearance of either a complete or partial mole.

○ **Describe the methods of spread of tubal carcinomas.**

Tubal carcinomas spread in much the same manner as epithelial ovarian malignancies. Transcoelomic exfoliation of cells via the fallopian tube, direct extension, and lymphovascular invasion.

○ **Although transcoelomic exfoliation was initially suggested as the primary mechanism of spread of tubal carcinomas, why is this theory suspected?**

Typically, the gross appearance of a fallopian tube carcinoma is that of a hydrosalpinx, with a sealed distal end and a dilated tube.

○ **How does depth of invasion relate to survival in fallopian tube carcinomas?**

In a retrospective review, depth of invasion was inversely related to survival. Intramucosal lesions were associated with a crude 5-year survival of 91%, lesions with muscular wall involvement were associated with a 53% survival, and lesions penetrating the serosa with a 5-year survival of 25% or less.

○ **Describe the lymphatic drainage of the fallopian tube and its importance in predicting survival.**

The primary lymphatic drainage of the fallopian tube is via the para-aortic lymph nodes. Pelvic or para-aortic lymph node involvement has been found in 10% to 35% of patients at the time of their initial operation, in approximately 33% of patients at the time of surgery for recurrent disease, and in 75% of patients at autopsy. Survival of patients with positive retroperitoneal or inguinal lymph node involvement (stage IIIC) is lower than that for patients with earlier stages. Finally, the presence of lymphovascular space involvement in early tubal carcinomas is associated with a 5-year survival of only 29% compared to 83% for tumors without identifiable lymphatic or vascular invasion.

○ **What is the most common type of tubal sarcoma?**

Leiomyosarcoma.

○ **What is the prognosis for primary malignant mixed mesodermal tumors of the fallopian tube?**

The overall 5-year survival is 15%, with a mean survival of 17 months.

○ **What percentage of tubal carcinomas involve the ovary at the time of diagnosis?**

Approximately 13% of tubal carcinomas involve the ovary at the time of diagnosis, usually as a result of direct extension.

○ **What percentage of fallopian tube cancers will cause an abnormal cervical cytology specimen?**

Although some series report positive cervical cytology to be as common as 40% to 60%, most series show that only approximately 10% of patients with tubal carcinomas will have abnormal Papanicolaou smears.

○   **What is the lifetime risk of fallopian tube cancer in women with a BRCA mutation?**

0.6% to 3%.

○   **Which sites do fallopian tube cancers tend to recur?**

Retroperitoneal lymph nodes and extraperitoneal sites.

○   **What is hydrops tubae profluens?**

A sudden emptying of accumulated fluid in the distended fallopian tube, which causes a profuse watery serosanguineous discharge associated with a decrease in the size of a pelvic mass.

CHAPTER 47

Vulvar and Vaginal Carcinoma

Mitchell I. Edelson, MD

○ **What percentage of gynecologic malignancies originates on the vulva?**

3% to 5%.

○ **What is the average delay in diagnosis of vulva cancer?**

12 months (6 months patient delay, 6 months physician delay).

○ **What are the borders of the superficial inguinal nodes?**

Inguinal ligament superior.
Border of sartorius muscle laterally.
Border of adductor longus medially.

○ **What is the name of the fascia that is located above the deep inguinal nodes?**

The cribriform fascia, which makes up the covering of the femoral sheath.

○ **Observational association of what risk factors have been linked with vulvar cancer?**

Advancing postmenopausal age.
Hypertension.
Diabetes.
Obesity.
Smoking.

○ **What link does the human papilloma virus (HPV) have, if any, with vulvar cancer?**

HPV DNA can be identified in approximately 70% to 80% of intraepithelial lesions, but is seen in only 10% to 50% of invasive lesions. HPV type 16 seems to be the most common, but types 6 and 33 have also been identified.

○ **True or False: Lichen sclerosis has been proven to be a precursor of and leads to invasive vulvar cancer.**

False.

○ **What is the definition of a stage IA vulvar cancer according to the latest FIGO staging (1995)?**

Tumor confined to vulva or perineum, 2 cm or less in greatest dimension, no nodal metastasis with stromal invasion ≤1.0 mm.

○ **Name the three mechanisms of the spread of vulvar cancer.**

(1) Local growth and extension.

(2) Embolization to regional lymph nodes in groin.

(3) Hematogenous dissemination to distant sites.

○ **Name the three characteristics that describe the growth pattern of vulvar cancer as these growth patterns influence the rate of lymph node metastasis and survival.**

(1) Confluent.

(2) Compact.

(3) Finger like (or spray).

○ **What is the name and location of the last node of the deep femoral nodal group?**

The Cloquet node or node of Rosenmüller is located just beneath the Poupart ligament.

○ **Name, in order, the five most common histologic subtypes of vulvar neoplasms.**

(1) Epidermoid (squamous cell).

(2) Melanoma.

(3) Sarcoma.

(4) Basal cell.

(5) Bartholin gland.

○ **True or False: The deep pelvic nodes are essentially never involved with metastatic disease when the more superficial inguinal nodes are uninvolved, even with a clitoral lesion.**

True.

○ **Which vulvar lesion has the classic "cake-icing effect" appearance secondary to hyperemic areas associated with a superficial white coating?**

Paget disease of the vulva.

○ **What underlying malignancy must be ruled out when Paget disease of the vulva is diagnosed?**

Adenocarcinoma of the vulva.

○ **What is the treatment of Paget disease without an underlying adenocarcinoma?**

This is a true intraepithelial neoplasia and can be treated as such with wide local excision.

○ **What is the most frequent histologic subtype seen in Bartholin gland cancer?**

Adenocarcinoma and squamous cell carcinoma occur with equal frequency and comprise 80% of all primary malignant tumors at this site.

○ **How does the lymph node spread pattern of Bartholin gland cancer differ from typical squamous cell vulvar carcinoma?**

The lesion can have a tendency to spread into the ischiorectal fossa and can spread posteriorly directly to the deep pelvic nodes in addition to the typical inguinal lymph node spread pattern.

○ **What is the reported lymph node metastasis rate of stage I squamous carcinoma of the vulva with a thickness of 5 mm or more?**

At least 15%.

○ **Have squamous cell vulvar tumors with a depth of ≤1 mm shown any significant risk of lymph node metastasis?**

No, tumors of this depth or less carry little or no risk of lymph node metastasis.

○ **What is the name of the vulvar tumor that is a neuroendocrine tumor of the skin that morphologically resembles small-cell carcinomas of neuroendocrine type in other body sites and are associated with frequent lymph node metastasis and a poor prognosis?**

Merkel-cell tumor.

○ **What HPV subtype has been associated with verrucous carcinomas of the vulva?**

HPV type 6.

○ **Where is the most common site on the vulva to find an adenoid cystic carcinoma?**

The Bartholin gland. It comprises 15% of all Bartholin gland carcinomas.

○ **Name the most frequent primary vulvar sarcoma identified and its usual location.**

Leiomyosarcoma and it commonly arises in the labium majus or the Bartholin gland area.

○ **What is the single most important prognostic factor in women with vulvar cancer?**

Lymph node metastasis. The presence of inguinal node metastasis routinely results in a 50% reduction in long-term survival.

○ **What is the incidence of positive lymph node involvement in T1 and T2 lesions?**

The incidence of positive inguinal and pelvic lymph nodes varies considerably, however, in the largest study to date it was found that 20% of T1 lesions and 45% of T2 lesions had positive lymph node involvement (higher if adjuvant radiation therapy was administered).

○ **What are the two most common complications associated with radical vulvectomy?**

Wound breakdown occurs in approximately 50% of patients in most series and lymphedema following surgery has been reported in up to 70% of patients.

○ **What is the 5-year survival rate by stage in vulvar cancer?**

Stage I, 91%
Stage II, 81%

Stage III, 48%

Stage IV, 15%

○ **What is the effect of lymph node involvement on survival?**

If lymph node involvement is negative, overall survival is 90% regardless of stage; however, survival rate drops precipitously even if only one lymph node is positive for metastasis (57%).

○ **What is the survival rate with positive deep pelvic nodes in vulvar cancer regardless of stage?**

20%.

○ **How does the International Society for the Study of Vulvar Disease (ISSVD) define microinvasive carcinoma of the vulva?**

A squamous carcinoma having diameter of 2 cm or less, with depth of invasion ≤1 mm. The presence of vascular space involvement would exclude the lesion from this category.

○ **What parameters should be addressed in the pathology report in early superficial vulvar cancer?**

(1) Tumor thickness.

(2) Vascular invasion.

(3) Depth of invasion.

(4) Confluence of invasive neoplastic tongues.

(5) Grade of cell differentiation.

(6) Host response.

○ **What has the term "giant condyloma of Buschke–Löwenstein" been used to describe?**

Verrucous carcinoma of the cervix.

○ **What have postoperative spindle cell nodules on the vulva been confused with?**

Leiomyosarcomas.

○ **What are the most common metastatic tumors to the vulva?**

Squamous cell cancer of the cervix and adenocarcinomas of the endometrium. Other primary sites include the vagina, ovary, urethra, kidney, breast, melanoma, choriocarcinoma, rectum, and lung.

○ **Prior to treatment of Paget disease of the vulva, what screening should be performed?**

Because of the high incidence of associated carcinomas of the breast and genitalia, a thorough search for such tumors should be performed prior to any consideration of therapy. This should involve breast examination; mammography; cytologic and colposcopic evaluation of cervix, vagina, and vulva; and sigmoidoscopy/colonoscopy.

○ **What is the stage of a 3 cm vulvar cancer confined to the vulva with unilateral regional lymph node metastasis?**

Stage III—T_3 N_1 M_0.

○ **What is the stage of vulvar cancer that is 1 cm in size with adjacent spread to the lower urethra, nodes negative?**

Stage III—$T_3 N_0 M_0$.

○ **What alternatives to radical surgery are available for women with a locally advanced vulvar carcinoma?**

Preoperative chemoradiation has been utilized to reduce the size of many tumors, which may be initially invading structures such as the bladder and anus. This treatment plan may allow for limited surgical resection.

○ **Which vulvar cancer has a predilection for hematogenous spread?**

Vulvar sarcomas. In one series 50% had pulmonary metastases.

○ **What is the name of the vaginal tumor that presents as a mass of grape-like nodules most commonly in the first 2 years of life?**

Embryonal rhabdomyosarcoma (sarcoma botryoides).

○ **What is the current acceptable conservative surgical treatment for a vulvar cancer confined to one labia with no central involvement?**

Wide local excision or vulvectomy with ipsilateral groin node dissection, which should include all nodes and no attempt should be made to distinguish between superficial and deep inguinal lymph nodes. Groin node dissection cannot be totally dispensed of unless invasion is less than 1 mm.

○ **What is the overall rate of recurrence in treated vulvar cancer and where does it recur?**

Approximately 25% of patients will recur and 80% of these recurrences are in the first 2 years. Most recurrences are on the vulva, with a few in the groin.

○ **What is the treatment for node-positive vulvar cancer?**

Two factors appear to be important in the management of regional disease. Radiation therapy can have a significant impact on controlling or eradicating small volume nodal disease and surgical resection of bulky nodal disease also improves regional control and probably enhances the curative potential of radiation. Patients with positive nodes, particularly more than one positive node, are likely to benefit from postoperative irradiation to the groin and pelvis.

○ **Is surgical debulking of positive pelvic nodes in vulvar cancer superior to radiation for treatment?**

No, radiation therapy has been found to be superior in the management of patients with positive pelvic nodes.

○ **True or False: Primary cancer of the vagina is one of the rarest of the malignant processes in the human body.**

True.

○ **What is the most common type of vaginal cancer?**

Squamous cell carcinoma.

○ **If a malignant neoplasm involves both the cervix and the vagina and is histologically compatible with origin in either organ, is it classified vaginal or cervical?**

Cervical cancer.

○ **What is the spread pattern of vaginal cancer?**

If it occurs in the upper half of vagina, extension is similar to cervical cancer; if it occurs in the lower part of the vagina, extension is similar to carcinoma of the vulva.

○ **What is the cause of most vaginal tumors/cancer seen?**

Secondary carcinoma from extension of a cervical cancer; primary probably account for the greatest number of so-called vaginal cancers.

○ **What is the histologic distribution of primary vaginal cancers?**

Squamous, 85%

Adenocarcinoma, 6%

Melanoma, 3%

Sarcoma, 3%

Miscellaneous, 3%

○ **Where is the most frequent location of a primary vaginal carcinoma lesion?**

The predominance of lesions is in the upper third and posterior wall of the vagina.

○ **Have causes of chronic irritation of the vaginal wall (i.e., use of a vaginal pessary, prolapse of the vaginal wall, syphilis, leukoplakia) been proven to be a cause of vaginal cancer?**

No, the cause of squamous cell carcinoma of the vagina is unknown.

○ **What is the most frequent presenting symptom of vaginal cancer?**

Vaginal discharge, often bloody, is the most frequent symptom in most series. The signs and symptoms of invasive vaginal cancer are similar to that of cervical cancer.

○ **Are the course and destination of lymphatic channels from different areas in the vagina predictable and consistent?**

No, all lymph nodes in the pelvis may at one time or another serve as a primary site or regional drainage for vaginal lymph and its contents.

○ **How is vaginal cancer staged?**

Clinically similar to cervical cancer. All patients should have a physical examination, chest film, IVP, cystoscopy, and proctoscopy. Optional studies include lymph angiogram and barium enema.

○ **When should a barium enema be definitely included in patients with vaginal cancer?**

Patients with a history of recurrent diverticulitis since it may be important in planning radiation therapy.

○ **What is the primary mode of therapy for vaginal cancer?**

Radiation therapy.

○ **What is the typical radiation treatment plan for larger stage I vaginal cancers and above?**

4000 to 5000 cGy whole pelvis external radiation with an interstitial implant delivery approximately 3000 cGy locally.

○ **What is the stage of a vaginal cancer that has extended onto the pelvic sidewall?**

Stage III.

○ **What is typical treatment of a bulky stage I or II vaginal cancer?**

External radiation 4000 to 5000 cGy followed by (in some centers), vaginal ovoids and an intrauterine tandem (Fletcher–Suite) are used to deliver a surface dose of up to 6000 cGy in 72 hours or 8000 cGy in two applications of 48 hours each separated by 2 weeks, (depending on initial thickness and regression of the lesion). Many centers now administer high dose radiation (HDR) brachytherapy on an outpatient schedule.

○ **In addition to the standard radiation therapy, which additional treatments should be considered for a vaginal tumor occurring in the distal third of the vagina?**

Since these tumors frequently metastasize to the inguinal nodes, these nodes are best treated by radical inguinal dissection before radiation therapy.

○ **In clear cell adenocarcinoma of the vagina, what is the precursor lesion found?**

Adenosis.

○ **What has clear cell carcinoma of the vagina and cervix been thought to be associated with?**

DES exposure in utero. Sixty-five percent of clear cell carcinomas of the vagina and cervix have evidence of in-utero exposure to DES, however, data do not substantiate that DES intrauterine exposure is a carcinogenic event. It has been shown to be teratogenic with increased adenosis and other uterine anomalies.

○ **What is the treatment of clear cell adenocarcinoma confined to the upper vagina and/or cervix?**

Radical hysterectomy with upper vaginectomy and pelvic lymphadenectomy with retention of the ovaries.

○ **What is the overall survival rate of clear cell adenocarcinoma of the vagina/cervix?**

80%, this is better than 65% crude survival rate for squamous cell cancer of the cervix and much higher than 35% to 40% survival rate reported for squamous cell cancer of the vagina.

○ **Can primary adenocarcinoma of the vagina occur without intrauterine exposure to DES?**

Yes, in both pre- and postmenopausal women.

○ **What is the treatment of malignant melanoma of the vagina?**

Surgical excision (radical excision with nodal dissection). Radiation and chemotherapy have not been found to be effective in the upper two-third of the vagina. An exenterative procedure must be used.

○ **What is the overall survival rate of patients with vaginal melanomas?**

15%.

○ **What is the peak age at presentation of a DES exposure related clear cell adenocarcinoma of the vagina or cervix?**

19 years.

○ **What is the histologic finding associated with clear cell adenocarcinomas?**

Hobnails.

○ **Where are clear cell adenocarcinomas of the genital tract in the female most commonly located?**

These tumors appear to arise equally in the ectocervix and upper anterior wall of the vagina.

○ **What is the treatment of sarcoma botryoides in a young child?**

Surgery and adjuvant chemotherapy consisting of a combination of vincristine, actinomycin, and cyclophosphamide that can be used up front permitting more conservative surgery.

○ **What association has been described between the risk of developing vaginal cancer and the time of first exposure in utero to DES?**

The risk was greatest for those exposed the first 16 weeks in utero and declined for those whose exposure began in the 17th week or later.

○ **What is the incidence of clear-cell adenocarcinoma in women prenatally exposed to DES?**

0.14 to 1.4 per 1000.

○ **What is the frequency of recurrence in vaginal cancer by stage?**

Stage I—10%–20% pelvic recurrence.
Stage II—35% pelvic recurrence / 22% distant mets.
Stage III—35% pelvic recurrence / 23% distant mets.
Stage IV—58% pelvic recurrence / 30% distant mets.

○ **What is the classical gross appearance of adenosis of the vagina?**

Red, velvety grape like clusters in the vagina.

○ **Name the different types of vaginal cancers.**

Epithelial, squamous cell
Verrucous, small cell
Malignant melanoma, malignant lymphoma
Smooth muscle tumors, rhabdomyosarcoma
Clear cell adenocarcinoma

○ **Has chemotherapy been proven to be a useful adjuvant therapy in vaginal cancer?**

No, it has been used only as a salvage agent with poor results.

○ **What is the survival rate with locally recurrent vulvar cancer?**

Recurrence free survival can be obtained in up to 75% of cases when the recurrence is local and limited to the vulva and can be resected with a gross clinical margin.

○ **Does recurrence of vulvar cancer in the groin have a good prognosis?**

No, unanticipated recurrence in the groin is almost universally fatal.

○ **What are the major prognostic factors in vulvar cancer?**

Tumor size, depth of tumor invasion, nodal spread, and distant metastasis.

○ **When compared in a randomized prospective study, was radiation to the groin and deep pelvic nodes found to be superior compared to surgical debulking of the deep pelvic nodes in patients with clinically positive inguinal nodes of vulvar cancer?**

Yes, the 2-year survival rates were 59% compared to 31%.

○ **With a malignant melanoma, when can lymphadenectomy be avoided and is not necessary to complete?**

Superficial melanomas (Clark level I-II), as risk of metastatic disease is minimal. A poor prognosis is associated with Clark level IV-V, thickness >2 mm or mitotic count >10/mm^2.

Radiation Therapy, Chemotherapy, Immunotherapy, and Tumor Markers

CHAPTER 48

Mitchell I. Edelson, MD

○ **What is the dose limiting toxicity associated with cisplatin?**

Peripheral neuropathy. This is also the most common side effect usually involving the hands and feet.

○ **True or False: Cyclophosphamide is an appropriate drug for intraperitoneal administration.**

False. Cyclophosphamide must be metabolized in the liver to its active form and is thus not useful as directed chemotherapy.

○ **True or False: Anticancer drugs can kill a fixed number of tumor cells per dose.**

False. Anticancer drugs kill a fixed percentage of tumor cells per dose.

○ **What is the mechanism of action of methotrexate?**

Methotrexate binds dihydrofolate reductase, preventing reduction of folate to tetrahydrofolate, which is necessary for production of thymidine and purines.

○ **What side effects are seen with the use of serotonin antagonists (ondansetron/Zofran, granisetron/Kytril, dolasetron/Anzemet) as antiemetics?**

Headache and constipation.

○ **What is the maximum total cumulative dose of Adriamycin suggested to minimize the risk of cardiomyopathy?**

<500 mg/m^2.

○ **What immediate steps should be taken to minimize tissue damage following extravasation of Adriamycin?**

Stop the infusion, aspirate the drug from the site if possible, apply ice to the affected area, and apply dimethylsulfoxide (DMSO) topically and allow to air dry.

○ **While cold packs are recommended for the treatment of most extravasation injuries, with which class of chemotherapy agents should warm soaks be utilized?**

Vinca alkaloids such as vincristine and etoposide

○ **What is the mechanism of action of paclitaxel?**

Paclitaxel binds and stabilizes intracellular microtubules leading to abnormal spindle formations that lead to its cytotoxic effect.

○ **Serum albumin levels may be predictive of what toxicity associated with ifosfamide?**

Central nervous system toxicity may occur with serum albumin levels less than 3.0 mg/dL as a result of production of chloroacetaldehyde metabolite.

○ **What is the most common secondary malignancy associated with the use of chemotherapy?**

Acute nonlymphocytic leukemia.

○ **What antibiotics should be used initially in a febrile neutropenic patient?**

Drug combinations including gram-negative coverage (aminoglycosides or aztreonam) and an extended-spectrum penicillin (piperacillin). Alternatively, a third- (ceftazidime) or fourth-generation (cefepime) cephalosporin as a single agent may be used.

○ **How should chemotherapy-induced mucositis be treated?**

Topical solutions containing viscous Xylocaine, antacids, and antifungals may be used along with adequate pain relief.

○ **What drug is the hemolytic-uremic syndrome usually associated with?**

Mitomycin C.

○ **What is the dose-limiting toxicity of paclitaxel?**

Peripheral neuropathy.

○ **Describe steroid premedication for administration of paclitaxel vs docetaxel?**

Dexamethasone 20 mg is given 12 and 6 h prior to paclitaxel administration to prevent hypersensitivity reaction.
   Dexamethasone 8 mg is given bid for 3 to 5 days starting 24 h prior to docetaxel administration to prevent fluid retention.

○ **What is the best way to avoid cisplatin induced renal toxicity?**

Aggressive pretreatment hydration and possibly the addition of Ethyol/amifostine Ethyol (amifostine).

○ **What is the growth fraction of a tumor?**

The number of cells actively involved in cell division.

○ **Methotrexate is specific for what phase of the cell cycle?**

S phase.

○ **The chemotherapeutic combination with the most documented activity against recurrent squamous cell carcinoma of the cervix is:**

Cisplatin and topotecan.

○ **The use of chemotherapy concurrently with radiation for primary therapy of cervical cancer is termed:**

Radiosensitization.

○ **What are the most commonly used drugs for primary treatment of advanced ovarian cancer?**

Paclitaxel and carboplatin.

○ **What is the dose-limiting toxicity of topotecan?**

Myelosuppression.

○ **What is the most commonly used drug as a single agent for gestational trophoblastic neoplasia?**

Methotrexate.

○ **Pretreatment for prevention of hypersensitivity reactions associated with paclitaxel include the use of:**

Corticosteroids, H_1 and H_2 blockers.

○ **The etiology of the hypersensitivity reaction to paclitaxel is related to which component?**

Cremophor EL serves as a solvent to allow paclitaxel to be soluble and induces a histamine release leading the hypersensitivity reactions observed.

○ **What is the dose-limiting toxicity associated with vincristine?**

Neurotoxicity.

○ **What is the mechanism of action of 5-fluorouracil?**

Competitive inhibition of thymidylate synthetase.

○ **Cisplatin is associated with depletion of what electrolytes?**

Potassium, magnesium, and calcium.

○ **True or False: Fever is a frequent side effect of bleomycin.**

True. Bleomycin induced fever occurs within 24 hours of administration.

○ **The purpose of the use of the agent mesna in conjunction with ifosfamide is:**

Prevention of hemorrhagic cystitis.

○ **What is the mechanism of action of melphalan?**

It is an alkylating agent.

○ **Which chemotherapeutic drugs have the most activity against uterine sarcomas?**

Ifosfamide and cisplatin for carcinosarcomas (MMMT), Adriamycin for leiomyosarcoma.

○ **What is the mechanism of action of vinca alkaloid type drugs?**

Vinca alkaloids bind to tubulin to inhibit normal microtubular polymerization and lead to mitotic arrest.

○ **Ototoxicity associated with cisplatin typically involves what part of the audible range?**

High frequencies.

○ **What is the mechanism of action of topotecan?**

It is a topoisomerase I inhibitor.

○ **True or False: Cyclophosphamide is specific for the M phase.**

False. Cyclophosphamide is an alkylating agent, and is noncell-cycle specific, although it probably works best in the S phase. M phase specific agents include the vinca alkaloids.

○ **The diagnosis of syndrome of inappropriate antidiuretic hormone (SIADH) associated with cyclophosphamide is made by what laboratory findings?**

Hyponatremia with less than maximally dilute urine.

○ **True or False: Adriamycin is primarily excreted by the kidney.**

False. Adriamycin is primarily excreted by the liver.

○ **What is the mechanism of action of etoposide?**

It is an inhibitor of topoisomerase II.

○ **True or False: Methotrexate is primarily excreted by the kidney.**

True.

○ **What is Leucovorin?**

Folinic acid. It is used to prevent toxicity by rescuing normal cells from high-dose methotrexate.

○ **True or False: Alopecia is a frequent side effect of vinblastine.**

True.

○ **What is the dose-limiting toxicity of 5-fluorouracil?**

Stomatitis, often with nausea, vomiting, and diarrhea.

○ **Actinomycin D is frequently used as a single agent for therapy of what gynecologic malignancy?**

Gestational trophoblastic neoplasms.

○ **The most significant side effect associated with bleomycin is:**

Pulmonary fibrosis.

○ **What is the mechanism of action of bleomycin?**

It induces single-strand breaks in DNA by interacting with oxygen and a metal ion cofactor.

○ **Interstitial pneumonitis resulting from bleomycin can be measured by what parameter of pulmonary function testing?**

Decreased diffusing capacity of the lung for carbon monoxide (DLCO).

○ **What is the longest phase of the active cell cycle?**

G1 may last from 4 to 24 hours.

○ **True or False: Dermatitis and nail loss are frequent toxicities of bleomycin.**

True.

○ **What is the mechanism of action of actinomycin D?**

It blocks RNA synthesis by intercalating DNA nucleotide pairs.

○ **What is "radiation recall"?**

Skin erythema and irritation in a previously irradiated field following administration of chemotherapy. Adriamycin and actinomycin D are commonly reported.

○ **Cerebellar ataxia is associated with what chemotherapeutic agent?**

5-Fluorouracil.

○ **For what phase of the cell cycle is cisplatin specific?**

None, but it may be more effective in the S phase. The mechanism of action of cisplatin is poorly understood.

○ **Hexamethylmelamine is indicated as second-line therapy for what gynecologic malignancy?**

Ovarian cancer.

○ **Ifosfamide induced hemorrhagic cystitis may be treated initially by:**

Hydration and diuresis.

○ **If hemorrhagic cystitis persists despite hydration/diuresis, what is the most effective immediate topical treatment?**

Continuous bladder irrigation.

○   **The toxic metabolite of ifosfamide responsible for hemorrhagic cystitis is:**

Acrolein. Mesna, which is given before and after ifosfamide, binds this product to prevent cystitis.

○   **What is the dose-limiting toxicity of carboplatin?**

Myelosuppression (thrombocytopenia).

○   **For what phase of the cell cycle is paclitaxel specific?**

M phase, since it is an antimitotic.

○   **Retreatment of ovarian cancer with a platinum drug may be appropriate for which patients?**

Patients may be retreated with platinum if they have developed a recurrence at greater than or equal to 6 months after cessation of their last treatment (platinum sensitive).

○   **The use of a chemotherapeutic agent following definitive treatment of a tumor when a patient is clinically disease free is known as:**

Adjuvant therapy.

○   **Theoretical advantages of intraperitoneal administration of chemotherapy over intravenous administration for ovarian cancer include:**

High concentrations of the drug can be placed in immediate contact with the tumor for longer periods of time, and toxicities may be lessened by liver metabolism as the drug is absorbed into the portal system.

○   **Describe phase I, II, and III studies.**

Phase I studies determine the toxicities and maximally tolerated dose of a therapeutic agent in humans.

Phase II studies are used to obtain efficacy of an agent in order to determine whether further study is advised.

Phase III studies are randomized controlled trials with the purpose of comparing the efficacy of an investigational agent to a standard therapy.

○   **What is the purpose of maintaining the patient's urine pH below 7.0 when administering high-dose methotrexate?**

To minimize renal toxicity.

○   **When used as a radiosensitizer, 5-fluorouracil frequently exacerbates what side effect of radiation therapy?**

Diarrhea, which is a common side effect of both therapies.

○   **Why is intravenous etoposide administered slowly?**

To prevent hypotension.

○   **What agent can be used with ifosfamide to minimize the risk of hemorrhagic cystitis?**

Mesna (2-mercaptoethanesulfonate).

○ **What parameters are used to calculate body surface area?**

Height and weight. (BSA = SQRT [ht.wt/3600]).

○ **Why does tumor heterogeneity often result in drug resistance?**

Spontaneous mutations give rise to small numbers of resistant cells, which may rapidly reproduce when sensitive cells are killed.

○ **What is the MDR gene?**

The multi drug resistance (MDR) gene is normally present in some human tissues and may be activated in tumors by exposure to certain chemotherapeutic agents, resulting in resistance to many drugs.

○ **Adriamycin associated cardiotoxicity may be anticipated by the use of what imaging study?**

MUGA scan to estimate ejection fraction at baseline and after every two to three cycles of treatment.

○ **Tamoxifen is used to antagonize the effect of estrogen on breast cancer, yet may induce endometrial bleeding and cancer. Why?**

Tamoxifen is a mixed estrogen agonist/antagonist, depending on the target tissue.

○ **How long should high-dose progestins be used in patients with recurrent endometrial cancer to obtain maximum clinical response?**

At least 3 months.

○ **What is the most important factor for predicting the efficacy of progestin therapy in endometrial cancer?**

Progesterone receptor status of the tumor.

○ **Marinol (tetrahydrocannabinol) should be used as an antiemetic with caution in what age group?**

Elderly patients may experience dysphoria with the use of Marinol.

○ **5-Fluorouracil has been used in a topical form for the treatment of what condition?**

Multifocal vaginal intraepithelial neoplasia.

○ **What agent has the most documented activity in metastatic sex cord tumors of the ovary?**

Cisplatin. It is frequently used in combination with other agents.

○ **The combination of bleomycin, etoposide, and cisplatin (BEP) has been used successfully in what group of female genital tumors?**

Germ cell tumors of the ovary.

○ **Patients undergoing surgery after bleomycin treatment should avoid high inhaled oxygen concentrations. Why?**

Acute pulmonary decompensation can occur.

○ **In the palliation of primary tumors, what percentage of a curative dose is typically used?**

Relatively high doses, usually 75% to 80% of the curative dose.

○ **What determines the optimal dose of radiation used?**

It is determined by the anatomic location, histologic type, stage and other characteristics of the tumor and relationship of the cancer to other proximal organs.

○ **What are the six major classes of antiemetics used for prevention and treatment of chemotherapy induced nausea and vomiting?**

1. Phenothiazines (Compazine).
2. GI promotility agents (metoclopramide).
3. Benzodiazepines (lorazepam).
4. Steroids (dexamethasone).
5. Serotonin inhibitors (ondansetron, granisetron).
6. NK-1 receptor blocker (aprepitant/Emend).

○ **From the standpoint of cell burden, what represents a clinical tumor?**

A clinical tumor can be considered to encompass several compartments.

1. Macroscopic, visible or palpable.
2. Micro-extensions into adjacent tissues.
3. Subclinical disease, presumed to be present but not detectable even with the microscope.

○ **What constitutes "gross tumor volume (GTV)"?**

GTV is all known gross disease <u>including</u> enlarged regional lymph nodes.

○ **What constitutes the "clinical target volume (CTV)"?**

CTV encompasses the gross tumor volume and the regions proximal to the gross tumor, which are considered to harbor potential microscopic disease.

○ **What constitutes the "planning target volume (PTV)"?**

The region around the clinical target volume that allows for variation in treatment setup, breathing motion. It does <u>not</u>, however, include beam characteristics (penumbra).

○ **What are the most commonly used radiation in clinical radiation?**

X-rays and γ (gamma) rays. Electrons are also used and heavier particles have been employed in more experimental treatments.

○ **Where do x-rays and gamma rays arise from?**

Their names reflect their different origins. Gamma rays arise from within the nucleus (in practice, they are emitted from radioactive isotopes). X-rays arise from outside the nucleus, produced by bombardment of a target with high-speed electrons.

○ **As wavelengths become shorter, what occurs to their frequency and energy?**

The frequency and energy increases allowing them to break chemical bonds and produce biologic effect.

○ **What is the Compton effect?**

The Compton effect is the interaction of a photon with a loosely bound orbital electron in which part of the incident (incoming) photon's energy is transferred as kinetic energy to the electron and the remaining energy is transmitted to another photon. The energy of the incoming photon determines the probability of its interaction with a target atom's outer electrons; as the energy increases, the probability of interaction decreases.

○ **How does ionizing radiation affect damage at the intracellular level?**

Directly and indirectly. In the direct mechanism, the incoming photon displaces on electrons that directly ionizes a DNA strand causing a break in the indirect action, the displaced electron interacts with a water molecule to produce a hydroxyl radical (.OH), a highly reactive free radical that damages the DNA strand.

○ **What occurs following damage to the DNA following ionizing radiation?**

The initial DNA damage brings about a cascade of biologic events, which either interfere with mitosis or initiate programmed cell death (apoptosis).

○ **What is the principal target of ionizing radiation?**

DNA is the principal target within the nucleus of the cell.

○ **What type of DNA aberration caused by ionizing radiation is lethal to the cell?**

Most biologic effects of radiation are a result of incorrect joining of breaks in 2 chromosomes during the repair process. Specifically, 2 broken chromosomes may recombine to form dicentric (a chromosome with two centromeres) or a centric fragments (a chromosome with no centromeres). These are lethal lesions.

○ **What is the most likely mechanism for radiation-induced carcinogenesis?**

Radiation-induced carcinogenesis likely results from a translocation that moves one oncogene from a quiescent chromosome site to an active one.

○ **What is a cell survival curve?**

It is the relationship between the fraction of cells surviving and the dose of radiation delivered.

○ **In the treatment of malignancy, how is radiation therapy delivered?**

Radiation therapy is usually delivered in three ways:
1. Teletherapy (external beam).
2. Brachytherapy in which the source is placed within or close to the organ being treated (interstitial or intracavitary treatment).
3. Intracavitary radioisotopes (radioactive chromic phosphate 32 P).

○ **Define the term "growth delay".**

Growth delay refers to the amount of time following irradiation during which the tumor regrows to the size it was before it was exposed to radiation.

○ **At which point in the cell cycle are cells most sensitive to radiation?**

Cells are more sensitive to radiation during late G_1 and late G_2 phases and more resistant during early G_1 and late S.

○ **What defines "radiosensitivity"?**

The response both in terms of degree and speed of regression of the tumor to irradiation

○ **What four variables influence the differences in the radiosensitivity of tumors?**

1. The ability of cells to repair radiation damage (*Repair*), the degree of hypoxia a cell can tolerate (*Reoxygenation*), the proportion of clonogenic cells (*Repopulation*), and cellular (*Redistribution*).

2. The quality of radiation.

3. The temperature of tissues.

4. The presence of various drugs.

○ **Do higher doses of radiation produce better tumor control?**

Yes. Higher doses of radiation do produce better tumor control as demonstrated by numerous published dose–response curves. For every increment of radiation delivered, a certain fraction of cells will be killed. However, higher doses do result in greater toxicity to normal tissues.

○ **What radiation dose is typically used for subclinical disease in squamous cell carcinoma or adenocarcinoma of the cervix or endometrium?**

Doses of 4500 to 5000 cGy will result in control of local disease in more than 90% of patients.

○ **What doses of radiation are required for <u>microscopic</u> disease of the cervix and endometrium?**

Doses in the range of 6000 to 6500 cGy for epithelial tumors.

○ **What is meant by "subclinical disease"?**

Subclinical disease refers to deposits of tumor cells that are not microscopically detectable but which, if untreated, can progress to clinical disease.

○ **What are the acute effects of whole-body radiation?**

Three types of syndromes can develop depending on the dose:

1. Cerebrovascular, occurring at high doses (10000 cGy) with death occurring within 1 to 2 hours.

2. Gastrointestinal injury at moderate doses (500 to 1200 cGy) resulting in destruction of the gastrointestinal tract and death within several days.

3. Hematopoietic injury with doses of 250 to 500 cGy with death occurring within several weeks.

○ **What is the approximate mean lethal whole-body dose for humans?**

Approximately 400 cGy.

○ **Does radiation exposure lead to new mutations or does it just increase the incidence of those mutations that occur spontaneously in a population?**

It increases the incidence of the range of mutations that occur spontaneously.

○ **What is the approximate "doubling dose" of radiation, which is required to double the spontaneous mutation rate in humans?**

The best estimate based on mouse data is 100 cGy. The incidence of mutations is essentially a linear function of dose.

○ **What is meant by the "oxygen enhancement effect"?**

Well oxygenated cells are more sensitive to radiation because the oxygen molecules react with free radicals, which affect biologic damage. That is, a small amount of oxygen will potentiate the effect of radiation. Inadequately oxygenated cells have a significant impact on the radiosensitivity of a tumor, often necessitating higher doses of radiation.

○ **What is the latency period between exposure to radiation and the development of radiation-induced cancer and leukemia in humans?**

The latency period is usually long with leukemias typically occurring 5 to 7 years following exposure and solid lesions developing after 30 to 40 years.

○ **What concepts have been explored to potentiate radiation therapy and enhance tumor kill?**

1. Reoxygenation of hypoxic tumor cells between doses of radiation.
2. The use of radiation sensitizers that selectively increase the effect of ionizing radiation on a tumor.
3. Hypoxic cell-sensitizing compounds that, when administered, sensitize hypoxic cells to radiation.
4. Bioreductive drugs that specifically kill cells deficient in oxygen.

○ **What do actinomycin D, doxorubicin, mitomycin C, 5-fluorourasil, cyclophosphamide, methotrexate, bleomycin, and cisplatin have in common?**

They are all cytotoxic chemotherapeutic agents, which have been shown to interact with radiation to maximize tumor cell killing.

○ **What role does hyperthermia play in radiation therapy?**

Heat selectively kills cells that are hypoxic, nutritionally deficient and acidotic, all being hallmarks of tumor cells. Temperatures greater than 42.5°C have been demonstrated to enhance the effects of cytotoxic agents.

○ **Which phase in the cell cycle has been shown to be resistant to radiation?**

The S phase.

○ **What constitutes a rad. and a Gray (Gy)?**

The rad. is a unit, which is defined as the absorption of 0.01 joule per kilogram of the medium (1 rad. = 0.01 J/kg). One Gray (Gy) equals 100 rad.

○ **Define "maximum dose."**

The point of maximum dose for high energy x-rays and gamma-rays is several millimeters below the skin. The dose to the point for any given field is referred to as the maximum dose.

○   **The minimal tumor dose is the lowest delivered to the tumor/target volume. The maximum tumor dose should be what percentage above the minimal tumor dose?**

The maximum tumor dose should be no more than 10% to 15% over the minimum dose.

○   **What is the integral dose?**

It is the total dose delivered over the entire volume or to the body of the patient. It is defined in terms of rad-gram or megarad-gram.

○   **What is an isodose curve?**

An isodose curve represents points of equal distance and is used to provide a visual representation of the dose distribution within a single plane. A series of curves are drawn at 10% increments normalized to the dose at the reference depth. The shape of the isodose curve will be influenced by the type of radiation, the size of its source, its field, the filters employed, and integral dose.

○   **What is a dose profile?**

It is the representation of the dose in an irradiated volume as a function of spatial positions along a single line.

○   **What are three distinct types of radiation?**

1. An alpha (α) or helium nucleus, which has a positive charge.
2. A beta (β) particle or electron, which has a negative charge.
3. Gamma (γ) rays, which originate within the nucleus of the atom and have no charge.

○   **How does "intracavitary" differ from "surface-dose" and "interstitial" brachytherapy?**

"Intracavitary" brachytherapy consists of placing applicators with radioactive compounds within a body cavity so as to gain proximity to the target tissue. In contrast, "interstitial" brachytherapy consists of surgically implanting radioactive sources directly into the target tissue. "Surface-dose" brachytherapy consists of an applicator or mold containing radioactive sources designed to deliver a constant dose to a skin or mucosal surface.

○   **The vaginal cylinder, tandem, and colpostat applicators are used in what type of brachytherapy?**

They are used for intracavitary brachytherapy.

○   **How can radiation exposure to nursing and health care providers be reduced or eliminated?**

Radiation exposure can be greatly reduced by remote afterloading technology.

○   **How do high-dose rate and low-dose rate delivery systems differ from one another?**

Dose rates of 40 to 200 cGy/h are considered low-dose rates that, in order to deliver clinically useful doses of 1000 to 7000 cGy, must be administered to inpatients over 24 to 144 hours. In contrast, dose rates in excess of 1200 cGy/h are considered high-dose rates and may be given over several minutes as an outpatient procedure. In general, 2 to 8 high-dose rate fractions must be administered to approximate the therapeutic ratio of a single low-dose rate implant.

○ **What is the inverse square law?**

The absorbed dose at a given point is inversely proportional to the square of the distance from the source of radiation. This forms the basis for intracavitary treatment whereby a high dose can be delivered to local tissues (cervix) with the rapid falloff of dose sparing surrounding tissues (bladder and rectum).

○ **Intracavitary brachytherapy for carcinoma of the uterine cervix traditionally employs the use of an intrauterine tandem and vaginal colpostats. How are they typically positioned?**

The tandem should be in the midline equal distance from the lateral pelvic sidewalls and the vaginal colpostats symmetrically positioned against the cervix. The tandem should be equal distance from the pubis and sacral promontory.

○ **What determines the total milligram hours that are indicated for intracavitary brachytherapy for carcinoma of the uterine cervix?**

Several factors determine the total number of milligram hours to be delivered:

1. The tumor stage and volume, which in turn determine the total dose in cGy to be delivered at point A.

2. The strength of sources employed in the tandem and vaginal colpostats.

3. The number of insertions.

4. Whether whole pelvis radiation will be employed.

○ **Which two radionuclides are commonly used in brachytherapy for the treatment of cervical carcinoma?**

226 Radium (T1/2 = 30 days) and 137 Cesium (T1/2 = 30 years).

○ **What additional radiotherapy has been advocated to increase the parametrial dose after conventional external and intracavitary irradiation?**

Interstitial implantation transvaginally or transperineally into the parametrium or cervix with metallic needles containing ^{226}R, ^{60}Cc, or ^{137}Cs, or with Teflon catheters for insertion of ^{192}Ir wires or seeds.

○ **In treating carcinoma of the endometrium what three devices are commonly employed for delivery of intracavitary brachytherapy?**

Heyman–Simon capsules, afterloading tandem, and vaginal colpostats.

○ **What are typical doses for intracavitary brachytherapy for the treatment of carcinoma of the endometrium?**

For preoperative therapy, intracavitary doses of 3500 to 4000 mgh with 2000 mgh are given to the mucosal vaginal surface. In patients treated with radiation therapy alone, higher doses in the range of 8000 mgh combined with external radiation are given. In postoperative patients, irradiation doses of 1800 to 2000 mgh to the vaginal mucosa are given.

○ **What three main biologic processes are involved in the "dose-rate effect"?**

1. Repair of sublethal damage, which occurs when radiation is delivered slowly. As the dose rate diminishes, repair of sublethal damage occurs.

2. Cellular proliferation occurs during protracted radiation exposure if the dose rate is low enough.

3. Redistribution and accumulation of cells throughout the proliferative cycle. A low-dose rate limits cellular proliferation allowing cells to accumulate in the radiosensitive G_2 phase, ultimately leading to greater cell killing.

○   **What are some advantages of low-dose rate remote afterloading brachytherapy for interstitial and intracavitary applications?**

The advantages include reduced radiation exposure to hospital health care providers, improved control of isodose distributions, and no need for shielded rooms.

○   **In the treatment of carcinoma of the cervix with high-dose remote afterloading brachytherapy, what number of fractional doses are used on average and what is the approximate dose per fraction?**

On average, high-dose remote afterloading brachytherapy employs five fractional doses with the dose per fraction ranging between 500 and 800 cGy to point A.

○   **What are some advantages of high-dose rate remove afterloading brachytherapy for interstitial and intracavitary applications?**

1. The radiation exposure to hospital health care providers is essentially eliminated.

2. There are no complications from prolonged bedrest since patient mobilization time is significantly shortened.

3. Treatment is done on an outpatient basis, eliminating the need for general anesthesia.

4. Treatment planning and dosimetry are more exact.

○   **What factors predispose a patient to radiation injury?**

The patient's nutritional status, prior collagen-vascular disease, superimposed infection, and physical or chemical trauma.

○   **What doses of radiation will cause skin erythema?**

In general, single doses between 600 and 750 cGy will produce erythema. Dry desquamation appears with doses greater than 5000 cGy and skin ulceration with ulcers greater than 6500 cGy.

○   **What are some common gastrointestinal complaints following abdominal or pelvic irradiation?**

Adverse side effects include watery diarrhea, abdominal cramping, increased peristalsis, decreased absorption, and transit time. If the rectum is included in the radiation field, rectal discomfort and tenesmus and bleeding may be experienced.

○   **At what doses of radiation are bowel mucosal ulcerations, fibrosis, stenosis, and fistula formation encountered?**

These adverse changes are seen when the small and large bowel are exposed to doses of 6000 cGy or more.

○   **At what doses of radiation does radiation cystitis occur?**

Radiation cystitis occurs with moderate doses of radiation (more than 3000 cGy). With doses greater than 6000 cGy, chronic cystitis, fibrosis, and vesicovaginal fistula may occur.

○   **What doses of radiation will result in ovarian sterilization?**

The dose of radiation that will result in ovarian castration is age dependent, with younger woman requiring larger doses. In general, a single dose of 650 to 800 cGy or fractional doses of 1500 to 2000 cGy will bring about permanent sterilization.

○ **What is the rationale for preoperative radiation therapy?**

The rationale is based on its potential ability to eradicate subclinical disease beyond the anticipated margins of surgical resection, to reduce tumor volume, to sterilize lymph node metastases, to decrease the possibility for dissemination of clonogenic tumor cells.

○ **What is the rationale for postoperative radiation?**

The rationale for postoperative radiation is based on the assumption that subclinical foci of cancer cells will be destroyed along with any residual disease.

○ **How are the effects of combined radiation therapy and chemotherapy helpful?**

The effects of combined radiation therapy and chemotherapy can be independent, additive and/or interactive. Chemotherapy prior to radiation results in a diminished tumor load for radiation treatment. Concurrent use of chemotherapy with radiation therapy can bring about additive or supra-additive action, attenuating tumor kill. Chemotherapy after radiation has been used as an adjuvant to control subclinical disease.

○ **What radiation modality provides for the most optimal treatment of carcinoma of the cervix?**

The most optimal treatment combines external beam irradiation (teletherapy) with intracavity or interstitial brachytherapy.

○ **What is the survival rate for stage IA and IB (smaller than 1 cm) cervical carcinoma with radiation therapy?**

Intracavitary radiation alone results in a 96% survival. External radiation alone is much less successful, with survival rates two-third of those for combined intracavitary and external beam radiation.

○ **What is the prescribed dose for external beam radiation in the treatment of cervical carcinoma?**

The prescribed dose is dependent on tumor volume and the extent of combined brachytherapy. In general, the relative proportion of external beam radiation increases with tumor volume and stage; it usually precedes intracavitary brachytherapy with paracentral doses ranging between 70 and 85 cGy and pelvic sidewall doses between 45 and 50 Gy.

○ **What are points A and B?**

These are reference points in the pelvis that are used to describe the doses delivered. Point A is 2 cm lateral and 2 cm superior to the external cervical os and anatomically represents the area where the uterine artery crosses over the ureter. Point B is 3 cm lateral to point A and corresponds to the pelvic sidewall.

○ **What is the target "paracentral" or "point A" dose for the treatment of nonbulky stage IB, IIA, or IIB cervical carcinoma?**

The recommended "point A" dose is 75 to 80 Gy of combined external and low-dose rate brachytherapy. One approach would be to administer an initial 20 Gy of "whole pelvic" external beam irradiation in 2 Gy daily fractions followed by 55 to 60 Gy to be delivered by intracavitary means. For more advanced disease, "whole pelvic" external dose of 40 to 45 Gy and intracavitary contribution of 35 to 40 Gy is more appropriate.

○ **For which patients might extended field radiation therapy be indicated in the treatment of cervical cancer?**

The tendency of cervical carcinoma to spread via a stepwise lymphatic route selects for a subset of patients whose disease is contained within the pelvic and aortic lymph nodes outside the conventional pelvic radiation fields. Eradication of tumor in these sites by extended field radiation therapy produces cure rates of 10% to 50%.

○ **Brachytherapy is essential to the successful treatment of cervical cancer what doses are typically employed to achieve this success?**

The control of bulky pelvic tumor requires minimal doses of 75 to 85 Gy. These doses are not possible with external beam radiation, which would easily exceed the rectal and bladder tolerance of 60 to 70 Gy. The inverse square law allows brachytherapy to achieve the required dose gradient over a very short distance.

○ **What isotopes are used in brachytherapy?**

Radium-226 has been replaced by safer isotopes such as cesium-137 for low-dose rate intracavitary administration, iridium-192 for interstitial and high-dose rate administration, and cobalt-60 for some high-dose rate afterloading applications.

○ **What are three indications for interstitial therapy in the treatment of carcinoma of the cervix?**

The three indications for interstitial radiation therapy in cervical carcinoma are:

1. Centropelvic recurrence after radical surgery.

2. Distorted anatomy that makes intracavitary insertion difficult.

3. Bulky parametrial or sidewall disease.

○ **What are the common isotopes used for interstitial implantation?**

The commonly used isotopes are iridium-192 and iodine-125.

○ **Traditional low-dose rate (LDR) intracavitary brachytherapy is delivered at a dose rate of 0.4 to 0.8 Gy per hour. At what dose rate is high-dose rate (HDR) brachytherapy administered?**

High-dose rate irradiation is, by definition, greater than 0.2 Gy per minute. However, the dose rate is usually much higher in the 2 to 3 Gy per minute range.

○ **What is the role for palliative radiation therapy?**

Using external radiation, single doses of 10 Gy given 2 to 3 times per week can help palliate pelvic symptoms such as pelvic pain, vaginal bleeding and discharge, and edema.

○ **What percentage of severe complications occur following radiation therapy for carcinoma of the cervix?**

In general, severe complications occur in 5% to 10% of patients being treated with radiation therapy for cancer of the cervix. Specifically, 2% to 5% of stage IB and IIA, 5% to 10% of stage IIB, and 10% to 15% of stage III.

○ **How is radiation tolerance of an organ or tissue defined?**

It is defined as the dose required to produce a given risk of a life-threatening complication. Accepted nomenclature is expressed as the total dose, which produces a 5% incidence of a specified complication within 5 years of treatment or TD 5/5. Published values of TD 5/5 are based on external beam irradiation in fractions of 2 Gy given 5 days a week.

○ **Which two intracavitary brachytherapy techniques are used in the treatment of endometrial carcinoma?**

The two intracavitary brachytherapy techniques, which are employed either alone or combined with external pelvic irradiation, are the Heyman packing technique (here, the uterine cavity is packed with small capsules loaded usually with cesium-137) and the intrauterine tandem technique.

○ **Which part of the gastrointestinal tract is the most sensitive to radiation injury?**

The small bowel (TD 5/5 = 45 Gy) is the most susceptible, followed by increasing levels of tolerance in the transverse colon, sigmoid colon, and rectum, respectively. The most common site of chronic injury is the anterior rectum.

○ **What are the indications for postoperative radiation in the endometrial carcinoma patient?**

1. Deep myometrial invasion.
2. Invasion of the cervix or vaginal vault.
3. Metastases to the ovary, tubes, or other pelvic viscera.
4. High pathologic grade.
5. Lymph node metastases.
6. Positive peritoneal washings.
7. Unresectable tumor.

   At present, the role of adjuvant radiation therapy appears to be in reduction of pelvic recurrences in high-risk patients.

○ **What is the basis for preoperative radiation for adenocarcinoma of the endometrium?**

Radiation therapy can cure 25% of patients with nonresectable tumors confined to the pelvis and 50% of patients with resectable tumors who are medically inoperable.

○ **What is the standard dose for postoperative radiation in the patient with endometrial carcinoma with either deep myometrial invasion, metastases to the adnexa or lymph nodes or high pathologic grade?**

Whole-pelvis irradiation in a dose of at least 50 Gy given in fractionated doses over 6 to 7 weeks.

○ **What chemotherapy is utilized for neoadjuvant chemoradiation of unresectable vulvar cancer?**

Cisplatin, 5-FU, mitomycin.

CHAPTER 49 Gestational Trophoblastic Disease

Mitchell I. Edelson, MD

○ **What are the histologically distinct disease entities encompassed by the general terminology of gestational trophoblastic disease?**

1. Hydatidiform moles (complete and partial).

2. Invasive mole.

3. Gestational choriocarcinoma.

4. Placental site trophoblastic tumors.

○ **Describe the characteristics of trophoblastic cells (both normal and abnormal) that allow them to metastasize?**

Trophoblastic cells do not express transplantation antigens (HLA and ABO), allowing them to escape from maternal immunologic rejection. They are thus able to invade into maternal decidua, vessels, and myometrium. Embolization of trophoblastic cells from the endometrial sinuses into the maternal venous system occurs continuously. The maternal pulmonary circulation is responsible for filtering out these cells and thus preventing them access to the system circulation.

○ **What is gestational trophoblastic neoplasia (GTN)?**

This is the term used to describe the various diseases with the potential to invade normal tissue and metastasize. This would encompass choriocarcinoma, invasive mole, postmolar GTN, and placental trophoblastic tumors.

○ **What is the incidence of the various forms of gestational trophoblastic disease in the United States?**

Approximately 1 in 600 therapeutic abortions and 1 in 1500 pregnancies.

○ **What is the incidence of hydatidiform moles in the general population?**

The incidence of complete hydatidiform moles is estimated to be between 0.26 and 2.1 per 1000 pregnancies. Japanese and Saudi Arabian women share a twofold increase in risk compared to other populations.

○ **What are the features of complete hydatidiform moles?**

1. Complete hydatidiform moles lack identifiable embryonic of fetal tissues.

2. Most commonly results from an ovum that has been fertilized by haploid sperm, which then duplicates its own chromosomes.

3. The most common karyotype is 46XX followed by 46XY (5%).

4. Diffuse villous edema.

5. Postmolar malignant sequelae 6% to 32%.

○ **What are the features of a partial mole?**

1. Identifiable embryonic or fetal tissues.

2. Partial moles usually have a triploid karyotype (69XXX or 69XXY) with the extra haploid set of chromosomes derived from the father.

3. Focal villous edema.

4. Postmolar malignant sequelae <5%.

○ **How does age influence the incidence of hydatidiform moles?**

Compared to women 20 to 29 years of age, women older than 50 have a marked increase in risk, as well as women younger than 15. Similarly, increased paternal age (greater than 45 years of age) also confers an increased risk of a complete molar pregnancy, although the increase is only 4.9 times (2.9 when adjusted for maternal age).

○ **What are the signs and symptoms of an incomplete molar pregnancy?**

In general, these patients present with signs and symptoms of incomplete or missed abortion (amenorrhea, vaginal bleeding, absent fetal heart tones), and the diagnosis may only be possible after histologic review of curettings.

○ **What is the most common presenting symptom in a complete mole?**

Vaginal bleeding with abnormally elevated beta-hCG.

○ **Other symptoms of complete mole include:**

1. Excessive uterine size (50%).

2. Theca lutein cysts (because of increased serum levels of beta-hCG and prolactin)

3. Hyperemesis gravidarum (25%) (caused by markedly elevated beta-hCG).

4. Hyperthyroidism (7%).

5. Trophoblastic embolization.

6. The presence of gestational hypertension during the first-half of pregnancy should alert the possibility of molar gestation.

○ **What is the term used to describe the sonographic findings of molar pregnancy?**

Snowstorm pattern.

○ **How are patients with hydatidiform moles managed?**

The diagnosis of complete or partial moles is usually made after performing suction D and C for a suspected incomplete abortion. In these cases, patients should be monitored with serial determinations of quantitative hCG values. A baseline postevacuation chest x-ray should be considered.

○ **What is the phantom hCG?**

Is a false-positive test result caused by heterophilic antibodies cross-reacting with the hCG test.

○ **When should phantom hCG be suspected?**

When the hCG values plateau at relatively low levels and do not respond to therapeutic maneuvers. Heterophilic antibodies are not excreted in the urine; therefore, urinary hCG values will not be detectable. Also a false-positive hCG assay will not be affected by serial dilutions of the patient's sera.

○ **Which form of gestational trophoblastic disease is less sensitive to chemotherapy?**

Placental site trophoblastic tumors.

○ **How are patients monitored after evacuation of hydatidiform moles?**

Ideally, serum hCG should be obtained within 48 hours after evacuation then every week while elevated until normal for 3 weeks and then monthly until normal for 6 months.

True or False:

• **Patients with prior partial or complete moles have a 10-fold increased risk of a second hydatidiform mole in a subsequent pregnancy.**

True.

• **Pulmonary complications, such as the syndrome of trophoblastic embolization, are frequently observed around the time of molar evacuation among patients with uterine enlargement of more than 14 to 16 weeks gestational size.**

True.

• **IUD is the encouraged contraceptive during the entire interval of hCG follow-up.**

False. In fact, they have the potential risk for perforation.

• **Patients with hCG level greater than 100,000, excessive uterine enlargement, and theca lutein cysts larger than 6 cm in diameter are at high risk for postmolar persistent tumor.**

True.

• **The diagnosis of vaginal metastasis should be made with biopsy.**

False. Vaginal metastases are present in 30% of patients with metastatic disease. These lesions are highly vascular and can bleed vigorously if sampled for biopsy.

○ **The diagnosis of postmolar gestational trophoblastic neoplasia is made when one of the following occurs:**

1. Four values or more of plateauing hCG (+/− 10%) over at least 3 weeks.
2. Rise of hCG greater than 10% for 3 values or more over at least 2 weeks.
3. Choriocarcinoma confirmed by histology.
4. Persistence of hCG after 6 months following evacuation of a molar pregnancy.

○ **What pretreatment evaluation is required prior to beginning therapy for GTN?**

1. History and physical examination.
2. Laboratory evaluation including CBC, serum creatinine, liver function tests.
3. Radiographic studies including pelvic ultrasound, CT scan of abdomen and pelvis, chest x-ray or CT of chest, brain MRI or CT scan.

○ **What percentage of patients have metastatic disease when GTN is diagnosed?**

45%.

○ **What percentage of patients treated for nonmetastatic GTN with negative chest x-ray have pulmonary mets noted on chest CT?**

29% to 41%.

○ **What is the most common site of metastasis for gestational trophoblastic neoplasia?**

Lungs.

○ **Describe the management options by stage:**

A. Stage I disease (confined only to uterine corpus)
   (1) Patient no longer wishes to preserve fertility—hysterectomy with adjuvant single-agent chemotherapy.
   (2) Patient with placental site trophoblastic tumor—hysterectomy (because these tumors are resistant to chemotherapy).
   (3) Patient wishes to preserve fertility—single-agent chemotherapy.
   (4) Patient wishes to preserve fertility but tumor resistant to single agent chemotherapy—combination chemotherapy.
B. Stage II (metastasis to pelvis and vagina) and III (metastasis to lungs)
   (1) Low-risk patient (NCI classification system. See below)—single agent chemotherapy.
   (2) High-risk patient (NCI classification system. See below)—intensive combination chemotherapy.
C. Stage IV (distant metastasis)
   (1) All these patients should be treated with combination chemotherapy and the selective use of radiation therapy and surgery.

○ **What is the preferred single agent chemotherapy of choice?**

Methotrexate.

○ **Why is methotrexate the preferred agent?**

Less toxicity and greater ease of administration make methotrexate a more attractive agent. Dactinomycin is generally reserved for second-line therapy, although both single agent therapies yield similar response rates.

○ **What is an adequate response to chemotherapy?**

A fall in the hCG level by 1 log after a course of chemotherapy.

○ **Describe the characteristics of gestational choriocarcinoma.**

Gestational choriocarcinoma contain both cytotrophoblast and syncytiotrophoblast elements. Chorionic villi are absent, and if present represent an invasive molar pregnancy. Gestational choriocarcinoma readily invades the maternal venous system, producing metastasis by hematogenous dissemination. Metastases tend to outgrow their blood supply, resulting in central necrosis and often massive hemorrhage.

○ **Describe the characteristics of placental-site trophoblastic tumors (PSTT).**

Placental-site trophoblastic tumors are composed of a predominance of intermediate cytotrophoblast cells arising at the site of placental implantation. Because there is only a small proportion of syncytiotrophoblast cells, little beta-thCG is produced. In some patients, human placental lactogen (hPL) is a more reliable marker. These tumors are locally invasive, although a small percentage of patients will develop extrauterine metastasis.

○ **What is the treatment for PSTT?**

These are not sensitive to chemotherapy, therefore, surgery (hysterectomy) becomes the main treatment.

○ **What is the highest risk factor for having a choriocarcinoma?**

A hydatidiform mole in the previous pregnancy confers the greatest risk for the development of a subsequent gestational choriocarcinoma.

○ **Why is induction of labor with oxytocin or prostaglandins not recommended for the evacuation of molar pregnancies?**

Uterine contractions against an undilated cervix theoretically carries an increased risk for the dissemination of trophoblast throughout the systemic circulation.

○ **What type of ovarian cyst can be clinically evident (≥5 cm) in 25% to 35% of women with hydatidiform mole?**

Theca lutein cysts similar to those induced by gonadotropin/hCG ovarian hyperstimulation. These are generally detected preevacuation but can arise within the first week after evacuation and can take up to 8 weeks to disappear.

○ **List four possible etiologies for postevacuation associated respiratory distress.**

1. Trophoblastic deportation.
2. High output congestive heart failure secondary to anemia or hyperthyroidism.
3. Preeclampsia.
4. Iatrogenic fluid overload.

○ **Describe four important steps in the management of respiratory distress associated with molar evacuation.**

1. Ventilatory support with either supplemental oxygen or mechanical ventilation.
2. Central monitoring including Swan–Ganz catheter.
3. Diuresis as indicated by etiology.
4. Correction of anemia or hyperthyroid etiologies of high output CHF as indicated.

○ **What precaution should be taken prior to evacuation in patients diagnosed with hyperthyroidism as a result of a diagnosis of complete mole?**

Administration of a beta-adrenergic blocker such as propranolol helps to prevent thyroid storm at the time of evacuation or in the postevacuation period.

○ **List three other entities confused with twin gestation complicated by hydatidiform mole.**

Retroplacental hematoma, partial hydatidiform mole, and nonviable twin can have similar presentations.

○ **Of those patients diagnosed with postmolar GTN, what percentage represent patients with persistent or invasive moles vs those patients with choriocarcinomas?**

70% to 90% of these patients will have persistent or invasive moles, while 10% to 30% will have choriocarcinomas.

○   **Describe the NCI clinical classification system for malignant gestational trophoblastic disease.**

I. Nonmetastatic GTN: No evidence of disease outside of the uterus not assigned to prognostic category.

II. Metastatic GTN: Any metastases.

    A. Good prognosis metastatic GTN

        1. Short duration (<4 months)

        2. Low hCG level (<40,000 mIU/mL serum beta-hCG)

        3. No metastases to brain or liver

        4. No antecedent term pregnancy

        5. No prior chemotherapy

    B. Poor prognosis metastatic GTN: Any high risk factor

        1. Long duration (>4 months since last pregnancy)

        2. High pretreatment hCG level (>40,000 mIU/mL serum beta-hCG)

        3. Brain or liver metastases

        4. Antecedent term pregnancy

        5. Prior chemotherapy

○   **Describe the Revised FIGO 2000 prognostic index score for GTN.**

Prognostic Factor	0	1	2	4
Age (year)	≤39	>39		
Antecedent pregnancy	Hydatidiform mole	Abortion		Term pregnancy
Interval*	<4 months	4–6 months	6–12 months	>12 months
Pretreatment hCG (mIU/mL)	<1,000	1,000–10,000	10,000–100,000	>100,000
Largest tumor, including uterine (cm)		3–4 cm	5 cm	
Site of metastases		Spleen Kidney	GI tract	Brain Liver
Number of metastases	0	1–3	4–8	>8
Prior chemotherapy			Single drug	Two or more drugs

Total score 0–6 = low risk, 7 or higher = high risk.
*Interval: time in months from end of antecedent pregnancy to chemotherapy.

○   **Although most forms of metastatic cancers yield poor survival rates, malignant GTN is considered a curable form of cancer. Describe the life table survival rates for patients with nonmetastatic, metastatic good prognosis, and metastatic poor prognosis as defined by the clinical classification system.**

Approximately 100% of patients in the first two categories are cured of disease. However, this rate drops to approximately 80% in the metastatic poor prognosis group.

○ **What is considered to be the highest risk factor in the metastatic poor prognosis group in the clinical classification system?**

Failed prior chemotherapy is the most significant factor. Salvage rates of 14% and 70% have been reported for patients with poor-prognosis metastatic disease treated initially with single agent and multi-agent chemotherapy, respectively.

○ **High-risk/poor-prognosis metastatic GTN is generally treated with a multi-agent chemotherapy regimen called EMA-CO. What are the five drugs involved in this regimen?**

Etoposide, methotrexate, actinomycin D, cyclophosphamide, and vincristine are the five chemotherapeutic agents that make up the EMA-CO regimen.

○ **What percent remission rate is generally obtainable with the EMA-CO regimen in high-risk/poor-prognosis metastatic GTN patients?**

Approximately 80% of patients will have their disease put into remission by this treatment regimen.

○ **How long should a woman with non-metastatic GTN or low-risk metastatic GTN undergo chemotherapy?**

Treatment should continue one to two cycles after obtaining the first normal hCG value.

○ **How long should treatment continue for a patient with high-risk metastatic GTN?**

Chemotherapy should be continued for at least three additional courses after the hCG levels have normalized.

CHAPTER 50 Gynecologic Pathology

Mitchell I. Edelson, MD

○ **What is the sex-determining region Y gene?**

The SRY gene is found in the 1A1 region at the distal end of chromosome Yp. Its presence dictates development of testicles while its absence results in ovarian differentiation.

○ **What two substances are responsible for development of the Wolffian duct system and regression of the Müllerian ducts?**

Testosterone and Müllerian-inhibiting substance (MIS), which are produced by the testes.

○ **What is a hermaphrodite?**

The presence of both ovarian and testicular tissue in a single individual.

○ **What is the most common karyotype in Turner syndrome?**

45X.

○ **What is the most common cause of male pseudohermaphroditism?**

Androgen insensitivity syndrome (testicular feminization).

○ **What is the most common cause of ambiguous genitalia?**

Congenital adrenal hyperplasia.

○ **What are the causative agents of granuloma inguinale and lymphogranuloma venereum?**

Calymmatobacterium granulomatis and *Chlamydia*, respectively.

○ **What is the name of the cytology preparation whereby one scrapes the base of a fresh vesicle, spreads the material on a slide, and stains it in an attempt to diagnose herpes?**

Tzanck prep.

○ **What is the most common cause of a Bartholin cyst abscess?**

Gonorrhea.

○ **What happens to a large number of cases of lichen sclerosus et atrophicus of the vulva in children when they reach puberty?**

A large percentage of these cases involute or regress spontaneously.

○ **What is the most common age of development of lichen sclerosus et atrophicus?**

Postmenopausal women, but it can occur at any age and sex.

○ **What are some ectopic tissues that can occur in the labia?**

Breast (along the milk line), salivary gland tissue, and mesothelial cysts. In addition, various rests of embryonic tissues can occur.

○ **What benign lesion can occur in the vulva and is thought to arise from sweat glands?**

Papillary hidradenoma (hidradenoma papilliferum).

○ **Describe the typical patient who develops papillary hidradenoma.**

This tumor is rare overall, however, it tends to occur in Caucasian females after puberty. This correlates with the development of the apocrine sweat glands, which is the origin of this tumor.

○ **What types of human papillomavirus are typically recovered from condylomatous lesions of the vulva?**

As in other locations with HPV lesions, the benign appearing condyloma acuminata tend to have HPV types 6 and 11. While squamous cell carcinoma in situ and invasive squamous cell carcinoma of the vulva tend to be associated with types 16, 18, and 31.

○ **What tumor that most commonly occurs in the soft tissue of the vulva of young to middle-aged women, is characteristically well circumscribed, shows positive immunoreactivity for vimentin and desmin, and has been reported to occur in males?**

Angiomyofibroblastoma.

○ **What tumor typically occurs in women less than 40 and involves the genitalia, is poorly circumscribed, and has distinct myxoid and vascular areas histologically?**

Aggressive angiomyxoma.

○ **What is the most common type of HPV found in vulvar intraepithelial neoplasia (VIN) and invasive squamous cell carcinoma of the vulva?**

HPV type 16.

○ **What is the most common malignant tumor of the vulva?**

Squamous cell carcinoma.

○ **Name three of the features in the staging of vulvar carcinoma, which are important in determining prognosis?**

1. Diameter of the tumor.

2. Depth of invasion.

3. Status of regional lymph nodes.

○ **What is the classic presentation of bowenoid papulosis of the vulva?**

A pigmented papule in a young pregnant female.

○ **How common is the presence of an underlying, invasive adenocarcinoma in a patient with vulvar Paget disease?**

10% to 20% of the cases.

○ **What are the clinical features of Paget disease of the vulva?**

The lesions may have eczematoid appearance but can develop a raised and velvety appearance with more extensive lesions.

○ **Regarding depth of invasion of squamous cell carcinoma of the vulva, how much invasion is allowed before there is a significant risk of lymph node metastases?**

The so-called microinvasive carcinoma that invades 1 mm or less has almost no risk of lymph node metastases. Those that invade as little as 3 mm show metastatic lymph node involvement in more than 10% of the cases.

○ **What are some risk factors involved in the development of squamous cell carcinoma of the vulva?**

Cigarette smoking, diabetes mellitus, presence of HPV (particularly younger patients), and immunosuppression.

○ **What is the protein produced by HPV infected cells, which causes degradation of p53?**

Protein E6.

○ **How common is lymph node metastases in verrucous carcinoma of the vulva?**

While this tumor has a tendency to recur locally, it does not metastasize in the absence of altered, aggressive behavior secondary to radiation therapy. The treatment is local excision.

○ **What tumor, more characteristically found in the salivary glands, can occur in the vulva and is characterized by late hematogenous spread and perineural invasion?**

Adenoid cystic carcinoma.

○ **What percentage of vulvar malignancies are melanomas?**

Less than 5%.

○ **What is Sampson's theory regarding endometriosis?**

This hypothesis states that endometriosis (endometrial glands and stroma) occurs outside of the uterine mucosa via "reflux menstruation" through the fallopian tubes and into the abdominal cavity.

○ **What is Novak's theory regarding endometriosis?**

This theory, favored by many, states that tissue derived from the Müllerian system may undergo metaplasia to become endometrial tissue.

○ **What are the two most common causes of vaginitis?**

Candida albicans and *Trichomonas vaginalis*.

○ **What is the most common cause of bacterial vaginosis?**

Gardnerella vaginalis.

○ **What organism is occasionally seen in Pap smears classically in association with use of an intrauterine device (IUD)?**

Actinomyces israelii.

○ **What is the organism that, in association with the use of tampons, is associated with toxic shock syndrome?**

Staphylococcus aureus. Specifically, the enterotoxin F and exotoxin C produced by the organism and absorbed by the patient are the cause of this syndrome.

○ **What is the name of the rare simple vaginal cyst, which is typically found in the lateral or anterolateral wall of the vagina and is lined by a single layer of cuboidal-type cells?**

Gartner duct cyst (mesonephric cyst).

○ **What is the most common benign tumor of mesenchyme in the vagina?**

Leiomyoma.

○ **What is vaginal adenosis and what is it associated with?**

This is a collection of benign mucinous endocervical glands in the vagina and is associated with exposure to diethylstilbestrol (DES) in utero by the patient's mother. Specifically, the critical time of exposure is prior to the 18th week of gestation.

○ **What is the more serious complication associated with in utero exposure to DES?**

Development of clear cell adenocarcinoma of the vagina and cervix.

○ **What is the most common site in the vagina of adenosis and clear cell adenocarcinoma?**

The upper one-third of the vagina on the anterior wall.

○ **What benign polypoid lesion occurs in the vagina and tends to protrude from the introitus and can be confused with sarcoma botryoides?**

Fibroepithelial polyp.

○ **What is the most common malignant vaginal tumor found in children?**

Embryonal rhabdomyosarcoma, also known as sarcoma botryoides.

○ **What is the most common age of presentation of sarcoma botryoides?**

A diagnosis is made at age 5 or less in almost every case. The mean age is approximately 3 years. Tumors arising in the cervix occur at a somewhat older age. This tumor has a 90% or greater survival rate.

○ **What is the natural history of vaginal intraepithelial neoplasia?**

The vast majority of lesions will regress following biopsy only. Slightly more than 10% will persist and less than 10% will progress to an invasive squamous cell carcinoma.

○ **Q. What percentage of all vaginal malignancies are classified as primary tumors?**

10% to 20% are primary tumors.

○ **What is the most common malignant mesenchymal tumor of the vagina?**

Leiomyosarcoma.

○ **What is the term given to a subepithelial band of malignant cells in embryonal rhabdomyosarcoma?**

The cambium layer.

○ **What are some of the melanocytic lesions that occur in the vagina?**

Lentigo, blue nevus, cellular blue nevus, and melanoma.

○ **What type of herpes simplex virus is typically associated with genital infection?**

Type 2 (HSV-2).

○ **What are some of the potential complications of PID?**

Infertility, bacteremia, abdominal adhesions with resultant bowel obstruction, peritonitis, and chronic pain.

○ **What is the term given to describe the junction of the ectocervix and endocervix?**

The squamocolumnar junction is the point where the columnar epithelium of the endocervical canal meets with the squamous epithelium of the ectocervix. This squamocolumnar junction is constantly changing in relation to puberty, pregnancy, menopause, and hormonal stimulation. The transformation zone is the area between the original squamocolumnar junction and the new squamocolumnar junction that changes depending on the patient's age and hormonal status.

○ **What is the name of the process whereby columnar epithelium of the cervix is replaced by squamous epithelium?**

Squamous metaplasia.

○ **How can you tell where the original squamocolumnar junction was located?**

Identifying Nabothian cysts or cervical cleft openings will indicate the presence of columnar epithelium.

○ **What benign glandular proliferative lesion of the cervix is associated with the use of oral contraceptives in young females?**

Microglandular hyperplasia.

○ **What is the risk of subsequently developing an adenocarcinoma in an endocervical polyp?**

Essentially, no increased risk.

○ **What is the most common type of HPV associated with flat condylomas of the cervix?**

Types 6 and 11.

○ **What is the most common type of HPV found in high-grade squamous intraepithelial lesions and invasive carcinomas of the cervix?**

Type 16.

○ **What are some risk factors for development of cervical carcinoma?**

Smoking, oral contraceptives, multiple sexual partners, early age at initial sexual activity, and the presence of HSV and/or HPV.

○ **What is the classic colposcopic appearance of a high-grade squamous intraepithelial lesion of the cervix?**

A mosaic pattern.

○ **What is the classic colposcopic appearance of an invasive carcinoma of the cervix?**

Irregular, tortuous blood vessels extending across the cervix.

○ **What is the natural course or potential for progression to an invasive carcinoma in low-grade squamous intraepithelial lesions of the cervix?**

Approximately 20% in 5 years, 30% in 10 years, 33% in 15 years, and just less than 40% in 20 years.

○ **Is HPV found in association with adenocarcinoma in situ of the cervix?**

Yes, HPV types 16 and 18 have been found in adenocarcinoma in situ of the cervix indicating a possible causal factor in development of adenocarcinoma of the cervix.

○ **Briefly describe the staging system for carcinoma of the cervix?**

Stage I—Confined to cervix

Stage II—Beyond the cervix but not to the pelvic sidewall or limited to the upper two-third of the vagina

Stage III—Beyond the cervix extending to either the lateral pelvic sidewall or the lower one-third of the vagina or hydronephrosis/nonfunctioning kidney

Stage IV—Beyond the cervix extending to the bladder, rectum (A), or beyond the pelvis (B)

○ **What is the most common cause of death in patients with cervical carcinoma?**

Cervical carcinoma tends to spread locally and via lymphatics, not hematogenously. Thus, the ureters are frequently obstructed resulting in hydronephrosis, pyelonephritis, and renal failure, which is the most common cause of death.

○ **What types of human papillomavirus (HPV) have been isolated in verrucous carcinoma of the vagina/vulva?**

Types 6 and 16.

○ **Does one find HPV in adenocarcinomas of the cervix?**

Yes, at about the same rate (90%) as in squamous cell carcinoma.

○ **Describe the behavior of adenoid cystic carcinoma of the cervix.**

This is a rare cervical tumor, which is very aggressive and exhibits local recurrence with distant metastases. The prognosis is similar or worse than the more conventional squamous cell carcinoma of the cervix.

○ **Does the prognosis for adenoid cystic carcinoma of the cervix differ from adenoid basal carcinoma of the cervix?**

Yes, markedly, therefore it is critical to make the histologic distinction between the two tumors. Adenoid basal carcinomas exhibit a benign behavior with no metastases.

○ **What is the pattern of spread and prognosis in papillary villoglandular adenocarcinoma of the cervix?**

This unusual tumor is found in younger women and, although it can be deeply invasive, it does not appear to metastasize.

○ **What is the name of the benign lesion of the cervix that is composed of a nodular, circumscribed aggregate of dilated endocervical glands, which are superficially located beneath the epithelial surface?**

Tunnel clusters.

○ **How common is an associated squamous dysplastic lesion of the cervix found in association with adenocarcinoma in situ of the cervix?**

Very common, ranging from 50% to nearly 100% in a variety of studies.

○ **What is the definition of microinvasion in squamous cell carcinoma of the cervix?**

An invasive squamous cell carcinoma less than 3 mm in depth.

○ **In an endometrial biopsy, you see pronounced stromal edema, moderate glandular secretions, an absence of stromal/glandular mitoses, markedly tortuous glands and no significant decidual change. Approximately what day of the 28-day cycle is the biopsy obtained from?**

Approximately day 22. Day 22 is when stromal edema is maximal and glandular secretions are just beyond their peak (day 20 or 21) and predecidual change has not become evident yet.

○ **What is the most common site of endometriosis?**

The ovary.

○ **What is the name of the phenomenon that tends to occur in pregnancy and is characterized by a focus of tightly clustered endometrial glands, which appear hypertrophic and demonstrate nuclear pleomorphism and cytoplasmic vacuolization?**

Arias–Stella reaction, which can be confused with clear cell and adenocarcinoma in situ of the cervix.

○ **What substances are produced by the corpus luteum and are important in regulating the secretory phase of the endometrium?**

Estradiol and progesterone.

○ **What is the most common cause of dysfunctional uterine bleeding in reproductive age women?**

Anovulatory cycles.

○ **What is the term given to describe the presence of an inadequate corpus luteum resulting in dysfunctional uterine bleeding?**

Inadequate luteal phase.

○ **What is the most common cause of postmenopausal endometrial bleeding?**

Endometrial atrophy (60%). Endometrial carcinoma must be considered but is the cause in only 10% of the time.

○ **What is the most common etiology of chronic endometritis?**

It is most commonly an ascending infection by way of the cervix following such things as abortion or instrumentation.

○ **What are the most common etiologic agents of chronic endometritis?**

Chlamydia trachomatis and *Neisseria gonorrhoeae*.

○ **What is the name of the endometrial polypoid lesion, which has abundant smooth muscle, tends to occur in the lower uterine segment, and occurs in women of reproductive age?**

Atypical polypoid adenomyoma.

○ **What is the most common type of metaplasia seen in the endometrium?**

Tubal (ciliated) metaplasia.

○ **What is the relative risk of development of malignancy within the various types of endometrial hyperplasia?**

Simple hyperplasia without atypia—1%
Simple hyperplasia with atypia—8%
Complex hyperplasia without atypia—3%
Complex hyperplasia with atypia—29%

○ **What is the mechanism of development of endometrial hyperplasia in obese women?**

Androstenedione is converted to estrone in the adipose tissue, which serves as the stimulation for development of hyperplasia.

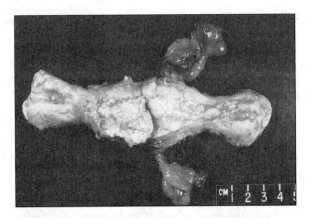

Gross Photo of Endometrial Carcinoma

○ **What is the nature of the endometrial carcinomas that develop in obese women secondary to peripheral conversion to estrogens?**

The tumors tend to be well differentiated, superficially invasive, and have a very good prognosis.

○ **What are some associations with development of adenocarcinoma of the endometrium?**

1. Obesity.
2. Diabetes mellitus.
3. Infertility.
4. Late menopause.
5. Any source of continuous unopposed estrogen.
6. Tamoxifen use.
7. Hypertension.

○ **What is the prognosis of clear cell carcinoma of the endometrium compared to typical endometrioid carcinoma?**

Clear cell carcinoma tends to occur in older women and carries a poor prognosis.

○ **What is the embryologic origin of the tumor cells in clear cell carcinoma?**

They are of Müllerian origin. Histologically, they are characterized by clear cells, frequently showing a "hobnail" pattern and focal papillary configuration.

○ **In general terms, what is the 5-year survival for endometrial carcinoma?**

Tumor Location	5-year Survival (%)
Limited to the endometrium	90%
Less than 1/2 of the myometrium	70%
Spread beyond the uterine corpus	15%

○ **Which is more important in the prognosis of endometrial carcinoma, the progesterone receptor status or estrogen receptor status?**

The progesterone receptor status.

○ **How does the presence of carcinoma in a focus of adenomyosis affect the prognosis?**

It does not alter the stage of prognosis.

○ **Is there a history of estrogen replacement in most patients with clear cell carcinoma of the endometrium?**

No, most patients are older and do not have that history.

○ **What tumor of the endometrium is characterized by a population of cells that are histologically similar to the stromal cells of a normal proliferative endometrium but exhibit an infiltrative pattern and extensive intravascular involvement by tumor?**

Low-grade endometrial stromal sarcoma.

○ **What is the prognosis in low-grade endometrial stromal sarcoma?**

It is excellent, although it can recur quite late (decades later). The most important factor is stage at presentation.

○ **What is an alternative term for mixed Müllerian tumors?**

Carcinosarcoma, which depicts the true nature of the neoplasm—a mixture of carcinoma and sarcoma.

○ **What is the classic clinical presentation for patients with mixed Müllerian tumor?**

They most commonly present with bleeding and on examination have a protuberant polypoid mass protruding through the cervical os.

○ **What do the designations homologous and heterologous elements mean in mixed Müllerian tumors?**

Homologous refers to the state of an undifferentiated sarcoma, while heterologous refers to the presence of differentiated sarcomatous elements, which are not derived from the normal uterus such as chondrosarcoma, osteosarcoma, or skeletal muscle differentiation (rhabdomyosarcoma).

○ **What is the prognosis of patients with mixed Müllerian tumor?**

It is very poor, and these tend to occur in older patients. It does not appear that the presence of homologous or heterologous elements markedly affects survival.

○ **What are some of the complications of acute salpingitis?**
- Infertility.
- Small bowel obstruction (secondary to adhesions).
- Pyosalpinx.
- Tubo-ovarian abscess.

○ **What is *Gardnerella* and what is its importance in the female genital tract?**

It is a small gram-negative rod, which can cause vaginitis and is associated with "clue cells" that are epithelial cells covered by bacteria.

○ **What is the best preparation by which one can demonstrate *Trichomonas vaginalis* at the time of pelvic examination?**

The use of a wet mount is ideal because one can see the flagellated and motile organism swimming in the saline after direct application to the slide from a sampling of the cervix.

○ **What is uterus didelphys?**

This is a congenital abnormality whereby the patient has a double uterus accompanied by a septate or double vagina as a result of lack of complete fusion of the Müllerian ducts.

○ **In a setting of chronic cervicitis, you note a prominent plasma cell infiltrate and distinct germinal center formation. What organism should you suspect most strongly as the etiologic agent?**

Chlamydia trachomatis.

○ **What organism should you suspect in a case of chronic cervicitis where there is significant epithelial spongiosis (intraepithelial edema)?**

T. vaginalis.

○ **In the pathogenesis of cervical cancer in relation to HPV, what does the E7 viral oncogene do?**

The E7 protein binds to the retinoblastoma gene and displaces some normal transcription factors. This affects normal cell cycle regulation and likely plays a role in the development of carcinoma.

○ **Is there a uniform progression in cervical squamous cell carcinoma from cervical intraepithelial neoplasia (CIN) I to CIN III and subsequent invasive squamous cell carcinoma?**

No, some lesions clearly do not arise from CIN I. As stated before, the majority of lesions never progress at all.

○ **How commonly do patients with CIN III that have been treated progress to invasive squamous cell carcinoma?**

Approximately 1 in 500.

○ **At what age are you most likely to find a patient with anovulatory cycles?**

They occur most commonly at menarche and in perimenopausal women.

○ **What are the most common sites of endometriosis?**

1. Ovaries.
2. Uterine ligaments.
3. Rectovaginal septum.
4. Pelvis.
5. Previous laparotomy scars.
6. Umbilicus, vagina, vulva, appendix.

○ **What are some of the typical clinical signs and symptoms of endometriosis?**

Dysmenorrhea, dyspareunia, pelvic pain, gastrointestinal abnormalities, and infertility. The disorder is most common in women in their 20s and 30s.

○ **What is the most common tumor in women?**

Leiomyoma (fibroids).

○ **What is the most reliable indicator of a leiomyosarcoma as opposed to a cellular leiomyoma?**

The mitotic rate is used to differentiate them. Leiomyosarcomas will typically have a mitotic rate exceeding 10 mitotic figures per 10 high-power fields.

○ **Do most leiomyosarcomas arise from a preexisting leiomyoma?**

No, most believe that leiomyosarcomas arise de novo and that if they do arise within a preexisting leiomyoma, that it is extremely rare (0.1%).

○ **How common is recurrence of leiomyosarcoma following resection?**

Quite common, greater than 50% of cases will metastasize hematogenously most commonly to the lungs.

○ **What is the typical histologic appearance of a benign endometrial polyp?**

These are polypoid portions of endometrial mucosa containing both glands and stroma with thick-walled vessels.

○ **What are the most common bacteria associated with acute salpingitis?**

Chlamydia trachomatis followed by *Neisseria gonorrhoeae*.

○ **How frequently are the fallopian tubes involved when there is tuberculosis involving the female genital tract?**

Essentially always.

○ **What are the histologic features of salpingitis isthmica nodosa?**

This represents bilateral nodules typically in the tubal isthmus, which are composed of tubal epithelial lined channels with admixed, prominent, smooth muscle bundles.

○ **What are some risk factors for a tubal ectopic pregnancy?**

A history of salpingitis isthmica nodosa, chronic salpingitis, and previous tubal pregnancy.

○ **What is the term given to describe small, simple cysts filled with clear serous fluid, which occur commonly next to the fallopian tubes?**

Paratubal cysts or, when larger and near the fimbria, they are called hydatids of Morgagni.

○ **What benign mesothelial-derived tumor can occur in the fallopian tubes?**

Adenomatoid tumor. This is the most common tumor of the epididymis.

○ **How often is primary adenocarcinoma of the tube bilateral?**

1 in 5 cases.

○ **What is the prognosis in tubal adenocarcinoma?**

It is quite poor with approximately 30% survival at 5 years.

○   **A patient has an ulcerative lesion on the vulva and you are told that microscopically there are Donovan bodies. What are those and what is the disease and organism?**

The disease is granuloma inguinale, which is caused by *Calymmatobacterium granulomatis*. The Donovan bodies are vacuolated macrophages, which are filled with the organism and are seen with the aid of Giemsa stain.

○   **By dark-field examination, you are able to detect spirochete organisms taken from a painless ulcer from the genitalia of a female. What is your diagnosis?**

Syphilis (*Treponema pallidum*).

○   **Where in the process of cell division are the oocytes of the ovary at the time of birth?**

They are in a resting stage of the first meiotic division. They will not complete that process until ovulation and fertilization occurs.

○   **In a primary follicle of an infant, what are the cells that lie around the oocyte?**

Granulosa cells.

○   **What is a Call–Exner body?**

This is a small, round collection of eosinophilic material, which is surrounded by a ring of granulosa cells. These are normal but can be seen in granulosa cell tumors of the ovary.

○   **What is the primary source of estrogen in the preovulatory stage of menses?**

The theca cells.

○   **What is the primary source of progesterone in the ovary, which is responsible for regulation of the secretory phase of menses?**

The corpus luteum.

○   **If fertilization occurs, when does primary production of progesterone no longer occur in the corpus luteum?**

After approximately 8 weeks the placenta begins taking over primary production of progesterone from the corpus luteum.

○   **How common is the resistant ovary syndrome?**

It accounts for approximately 20% of the cases of premature ovarian failure.

○   **What is the name of the benign, non-neoplastic cystic lesion of the ovary that occurs as a result of invagination of the cortex and surface epithelium?**

Epithelial inclusion cyst.

○   **At what age do solitary follicle cysts and corpus luteum cysts occur?**

The solitary follicle cysts occur in perimenopausal women and after menarche while corpus luteum cysts occur in women of childbearing age.

○ **What is the most common etiologic agent of vaginitis?**

Candida albicans.

○ **Why do leiomyomas often increase in size during pregnancy and decrease in postmenopausal women?**

They are estrogen sensitive, thus during the times of high estrogen (pregnancy) they get larger and in times of low estrogen they decrease in size.

○ **What is the most common benign tumor in the fallopian tubes?**

Adenomatoid tumor.

○ **What is the name of the condition whereby the patient has numerous follicle cysts in association with oligomenorrhea?**

Polycystic ovarian syndrome (Stein–Leventhal syndrome).

○ **In patients with polycystic ovarian disease, how common is true virilism?**

It is rare. They typically have persistent anovulation, hirsutism, and almost half are obese.

○ **What is the HAIR-AN syndrome?**

Hyperandrogenism (HA), insulin-resistance (IR), and acanthosis nigricans (AN).

○ **At what age does stromal hyperthecosis normally occur?**

Postmenopausal women, however, it can be a part of polycystic ovarian disease in younger women.

○ **What is the microscopic appearance of stromal hyperthecosis?**

It is characterized by nests and groups of luteinized stromal cells with vacuolated cytoplasm.

○ **In polycystic ovarian syndrome, what are the levels of follicle-stimulating hormone (FSH)?**

The level of FSH is normal as is 17-ketosteroid production. Androgens, on the other hand, are elevated in the cyst fluid and urine.

○ **Describe the typical clinical presentation in massive ovarian edema.**

The condition is usually unilateral and the patients are young with an average age of 20 years. They present with abdominal or pelvic pain and an associated palpable abdominal mass.

○ **How can you differentiate between fibromatosis and an ovarian fibroma?**

Fibromatosis occurs in younger patients (mean of 25 years) who sometimes have menstrual abnormalities and contains entrapped follicles and their derivatives. In contrast, fibromas are found in older patients, do not contain entrapped normal structures, and are not associated with menstrual abnormalities.

○ **What lesion of the ovary is related to hCG stimulation, and typically occurs in black multiparous females who are in their 20s or 30s?**

The pregnancy luteoma.

○   **How common is extraovarian spread by ovarian malignancies at the time of initial presentation?**

It is very common (70% of patients) thus the high mortality rate.

○   **What are some of the risk factors for development of ovarian carcinoma?**

Nulliparity, family history, early menarche and late menopause, white race, increasing age, and residence in North America and Northern Europe.

○   **What are three syndromes that have been described related to ovarian cancer?**

HNPCC (Lynch II syndrome) cancer of the ovary, endometrium, and colon; breast-ovary syndrome; and ovary-specific syndrome.

○   **Where are the genes located, which are responsible for the breast-ovary syndrome?**

The genes are: BRCA-1, which is found on chromosome 17 q21; and BRCA-2, which is found on 13 q12.

○   **What serum marker is useful in determining the efficacy of therapy and recurrence of ovarian carcinoma?**

CA-125.

○   **What is the most common cell of origin resulting in ovarian neoplasms (example germ cells, stromal cells, surface epithelium, etc.)?**

By far, the surface epithelium gives rise to the most ovarian neoplasms (more than 60% overall and more than 90% of malignant tumors).

○   **What is the most common malignant tumor of the ovary?**

Serous cystadenocarcinoma, and it is frequently bilateral (more than half the time).

○   **What are the three general categories, which surface epithelial tumors of the ovary are divided into?**

Benign, low malignant potential, and malignant.

○   **What are some of the histologic features that determine classification into the borderline category?**

These are tumors that are composed of the same cell type but generally lack "high grade" nuclear features, complex architecture, and destructive stromal invasion.

○   **Do ovarian low malignant potential tumors spread beyond the ovary?**

Yes. The majority (60% to 70%) present confined to the ovary while up to 40% will spread beyond the ovary, particularly as peritoneal implants. Overall, the prognosis is markedly better than the malignant counterpart with 100% 5-year survival when confined to the ovary and 90% when spread to the peritoneum.

○   **What are the two histologic types of mucinous tumors of the ovary based on histologic appearance?**

In addition to being divided into benign, borderline, and malignant varieties, the mucinous tumors may resemble endocervical mucosa or intestinal epithelium. Thus, the tumors are divided into endocervical-type and intestinal-type.

○ **What is pseudomyxoma peritonei?**

This is so-called mucinous or gelatinous ascites as a result of implantation of cells in the peritoneal cavity, which produce abundant mucus. This can be a result of a mucinous borderline tumor of the ovary or a mucinous tumor of the appendix. Although benign, death can occur as a result of extensive spreading and compression of abdominal viscera.

○ **Which has a better prognosis, borderline mucinous tumors of the endocervical or intestinal type?**

Endocervical type.

○ **What tumor is fairly commonly found concomitantly with an endometrioid carcinoma of the ovary?**

Approximately one-third of patients with an endometrioid carcinoma of the ovary have a coexistent adenocarcinoma of the endometrium. These are thought to be separate primaries.

○ **What ovarian epithelial tumor is characterized by large epithelial cells with abundant intracytoplasmic glycogen and form a so-called "hobnail" appearance as they protrude into the lumen of small tubules/cysts?**

Clear cell carcinoma.

○ **How are most Brenner tumors discovered?**

Incidentally, as approximately half are microscopic in nature. The vast majority are less than 2 cm.

○ **How common is bilaterality in endometrioid carcinoma of the ovary?**

It is quite common, up to 50% of patients have bilateral tumors at the time of surgery.

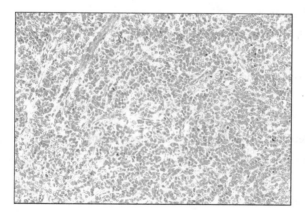

Ovary

○ **The tumor shown above occurred in the ovary of a 20-year-old female with hypercalcemia, which resolved following resection of her ovary. What is the diagnosis?**

Small cell carcinoma.

○ **What is the most common benign tumor of the ovary?**

Dermoid cyst or mature cystic teratoma.

○   **What is the term given to a benign ovarian teratoma where almost all of the tissue is composed of benign thyroid elements?**

Struma ovarii.

○   **Do mature teratomas undergo malignant change?**

The vast majority (99%) do not; however, it can occur and has been well described and is most commonly a squamous cell carcinoma.

○   **What is Meigs syndrome?**

This is the presence of a large ovarian fibroma with associated ascites and pleural effusion both of which resolve upon resection of the fibroma.

○   **What is produced by the majority of granulosa cell tumors, which result in "feminizing" signs and symptoms?**

Estrogenic hormones.

○   **What is the characteristic shape of the nuclei of granulosa cells?**

They are round to oval, haphazardly arranged, and frequently contain a longitudinal groove imparting a "coffee bean" appearance.

○   **What ovarian tumor is associated with the basal cell nevus syndrome?**

Fibromas. These tumors are almost universally bilateral, multinodular, and at least focally calcified in these patients.

○   **What is the typical age of presentation in patients with a thecoma?**

They are almost always postmenopausal with a mean age of approximately 60.

○   **Although this can be true in several ovarian tumors, which sex cord-stromal tumor is associated with the classic yellow gross tumor appearance?**

Thecoma.

○   **In contrast to thecomas, what is the typical age of patients with Sertoli–Leydig cell tumors?**

They occur during reproductive years with a mean age of 25 years.

○   **What syndrome is found in approximately a third of patients with the sex cord tumor called "sex cord tumor with annular tubules"?**

Peutz–Jeghers syndrome.

○   **What is a so-called Krukenberg's tumor?**

This is a gastric carcinoma, which is metastatic to the ovary, although it can be of any site of gastrointestinal origin.

○   **What is the ovarian counterpart of the testicular seminoma?**

Dysgerminoma.

○ **In general, what is the prognosis for dysgerminoma?**

It is excellent as the tumor is quite radiosensitive and responsive to chemotherapy. Thus, for a stage I tumor, the 5-year survival is almost 95%. Overall, the 5-year survival is between 70% and 90% for all tumors.

○ **A 17-year-old female has an ovarian tumor, which has resulted in an elevated serum alpha-fetoprotein. What is your diagnosis?**

Endodermal sinus tumor.

○ **In an ovarian endodermal sinus tumor, what are some of the characteristic histologic features you would expect to see?**

Schiller–Duval bodies and eosinophilic globules, which are PAS positive and diastase resistant.

○ **What is the typical genotype and phenotype in patients with gonadoblastoma?**

They are usually phenotypic females and genotypic males (have a Y chromosome).

○ **What are some conditions, which increase the incidence of hydatidiform mole?**

Poverty, poor nutrition, extreme ends of reproductive life, and consanguinity.

○ **What is the most common karyotype in complete hydatidiform mole (CHM) compared to partial hydatidiform mole (PHM)?**

In CHM, they are almost always 46XX and both "X"s are paternally derived (diandrogenic dispermy); while in PHM, the majority are 69XXY with 69XXX representing up to 40% of cases.

○ **Which is at a greater risk for development of choriocarcinoma—CHM or PHM?**

CHM results in choriocarcinoma in approximately 5% of cases.

○ **Which type of mole is associated with a higher level of beta-hCG?**

The beta-hCG in CHM is usually twice that of PHM.

CHAPTER 51

Hypothalamic-Pituitary-Ovarian-Uterine Axis

Dana Shanis, MD

○ **What is the blood supply to the posterior lobe of the pituitary gland?**

The inferior hypophyseal artery, a branch from the carotid artery.

○ **What is the blood supply to the anterior pituitary?**

Branches of the superior, middle, and inferior hypophyseal arteries.

○ **Which vessels drain into the "primary plexus" of veins of the hypophyseal portal system?**

Capillary portions of the superior hypophyseal arteries drain from the hypothalamus, the median eminence, and the superior portions of the pituitary stalk.

○ **Long hypophyseal portal veins originate from the primary plexus and travel to the anterior pituitary lobe to from a secondary plexus, which drains to what?**

The cavernous sinus.

○ **Who has the larger pituitary gland, men or women?**

The average adult female gland in approximately 20% larger than the average adult male.

○ **Why does the female pituitary gland increase in size by approximately 10% during pregnancy?**

Because of the hypertrophy of prolactin secreting cells.

○ **What does the posterior lobe of the pituitary, the pituitary stalk, and the median eminence form?**

The neurohypophysis.

○ **Where do axons from the supraoptic and paraventricular nuclei of the hypothalamus terminate?**

The posterior pituitary, or neural lobe.

○ **What hormones are synthesized from the supraoptic and paraventricular nuclei?**

Antidiuretic hormone (ADH) and oxytocin precursors.

○ **What is the anterior pituitary gland composed of?**

The pars distalis, pars intermedius (vestigial in man), and the pars tuberalis.

○ **Where is the hypophysis (pituitary gland) located?**

Within the sella turcica.

○ **The roof of the sphenoid sinus is formed by what structure?**

The floor of the sella turcica.

○ **Just lateral to the sella turcica is the cavernous sinus, which contains what structures?**

The carotid arteries and cranial nerves III, IV, and VI.

○ **What forms the roof of the sella turcica?**

The diaphragma sella, a thick reflection of the dura mater.

○ **In what percentage of individuals does the diaphragma sella closely encircle the pituitary stalk, thus acting as an anatomic barrier?**

50%.

○ **What is the possible problem for those individuals in which the diaphragma sella does not closely surround the pituitary stalk?**

Pituitary tumors may extend superiorly.

○ **What is a concern in these patients?**

Residual secretion of adenohypophyseal hormone may be observed after hypophysectomy.

○ **What is the function of gonadotropes and where are they located?**

These cells synthesize and secrete FSH and LH, and are located in the adenohypophysis.

○ **What percentage of cells in the pituitary gland are gonadotropes?**

Approximately 10%.

○ **What six hormones are secreted by the anterior pituitary?**

Growth hormone (GH).
Adrenocorticotropic hormone (ACTH).
Thyroid-stimulating hormone (TSH).
Prolactin (PRL).
Luteinizing hormone (LH).
Follicle-stimulating hormone (FSH).

○ **What is the action of oxytocin?**

It stimulates uterine contraction during labor and elicits milk ejection by myoepithelial cells of the mammary ducts.

○ **What stimuli cause release of ADH (Vasopressin)?**

Plasma osmolality >285 mOsm/L.

Decreases in circulating blood volume by >5%.

Catecholamines.

Renin-angiotensin system.

Opiates.

○ **What is the action of ADH?**

It causes increased rates of Na^+ and Cl^- reabsorption and enhances permeability within the collecting ducts of the renal medulla.

○ **What are the functions of testosterone?**

Stimulates growth of the penis and scrotum.

Stimulates development of facial, axillary, and pubic hair.

Influences appetitive states of libido and aggressiveness.

○ **What is the source of a majority of the circulating testosterone in a woman?**

Peripheral conversion of androstenedione by 17β-hydroxysteroid dehydrogenase. Only 30% to 40% is directly secreted.

○ **What limits peripheral conversion of testosterone to dihydrotestosterone in females?**

Higher levels of sex hormone-binding globulin.

Peripheral conversion of testosterone to estrogen by aromatase.

○ **In the adult female, what is the function of FSH?**

It stimulates maturation of the Graafian follicle and its production of estradiol.

○ **In the adult female, what is the function of LH?**

It causes follicular rupture, ovulation, and establishment of the corpus luteum.

○ **Accumulation of what substance leads to up-regulation of LH receptors?**

FSH-induced cAMP.

○ **Activation of LH receptors in theca cells leads to production of what substance?**

Androstenedione (weak androgen).

○ **What inhibits the release of TSH?**

Elevated circulating levels of T3 and T4 and somatostatin.

○ **What are the functions of TSH?**

Stimulates increased rates of iodide transport.

Stimulates thyroglobulin synthesis.

Stimulates triiodothyronine (T3) and thyroxin (T4) formation.
Stimulates release of T3 and T4.
It elicits increases in size and vascularity of the thyroid gland.

○   **What stimulates the release of ACTH?**

Hypothalamic corticotropin-releasing factor (CRF) and circulating glucocorticoids.

○   **What limits the secretion of ACTH and CRF?**

Circulating levels of ACTH.

○   **Where are ACTH receptors located?**

In the adrenal cortex.

○   **What is the result of ACTH binding to receptors on the adrenal cortex?**

Activation of membrane bound adenyl cyclase.

○   **What potentiates the conversion of cholesterol to androgen, estrogen, and corticosteroid precursor?**

Increased cellular levels of cAMP.

○   **Under normal circumstances, when are plasma ACTH and serum cortisol at their lowest, and when are they at their highest?**

Lowest between 10:00 PM and 2:00 AM.
Highest at approximately 8:00 AM.

○   **What factors can alter the diurnal pattern of secretion of ACTH and serum cortisol?**

Periods of stress such as acute illness, trauma, fever, and hypoglycemia.

○   **Where do the endogenous opioids, beta-endorphin, and met-enkephalin bind?**

To receptors in the brain and spinal cord.

○   **What are the actions of the enkephalins and endorphins?**

They have potent analgesic properties and influence release of pituitary hormones such as LH, PRL, and vasopressin.

○   **What stimulates release of the endogenous opioids?**

Periods of stress, shock, or hypoglycemia.

○   **What are the effects of growth hormone (GH)?**

Elicits longitudinal growth of the skeleton.
Antagonizes the effects of insulin in peripheral tissues.

Stimulates insulin secretion from the pancreas.

Directly stimulates liver cell growth.

Directly stimulates adipocyte metabolism and increased serum levels of free fatty acids.

○ **Where are somatomedins synthesized?**

In the liver.

○ **GH is released in bursts at what specific times?**

3 to 4 hours after mealtime and during stage III and IV sleep.

○ **What stimulates the release of GH?**

Stress, exercise, hypoglycemia, protein depletion, and administration of glucagon and L-dopa.

○ **How does GH secretion change with the onset of puberty?**

Increase in pulse amplitude, but no increase in frequency of secretion.

○ **What inhibits release of GH?**

GH-releasing factor (GH-RH) and glucocorticoids.

○ **What cells within the pituitary secrete prolactin?**

Lactotrophs.

○ **What is the function of prolactin?**

It initiates and sustains lactation by the breast glands and it may influence synthesis and release of progesterone by the ovary and testosterone by the testes.

○ **What inhibits the release of prolactin?**

Dopamine.

○ **What is the main physiological stimulus for prolactin release?**

Suckling of the breast.

○ **How do drugs such as metoclopramide, haloperidol, chlorpromazine, and reserpine enhance prolactin secretion?**

By interfering with release of dopamine into the pituitary portal circulation.

○ **What are the signs and symptoms of a pituitary neoplasm related to enlargement of the gland?**

Visual field defects (characteristically bitemporal hemianopsia), abnormal extraocular muscle movements, and occasionally spontaneous CSF rhinorrhea.

○ **What are the characteristics of pituitary apoplexy caused by hemorrhage?**

Severe headache, sudden visual loss, meningismus, decreased sensorium, bloody CSF, and ocular palsy.

○ **What are the characteristic radiological findings indicative of a pituitary tumor?**

Asymmetrical enlargement in one dimension, focal bony erosion, and a double floor.

○ **What pathology is demonstrated in this H&E stain of the pituitary?**

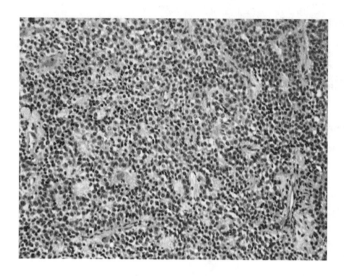

Pituitary adenoma.

○ **On radiological examination for a pituitary tumor, what does elevation of the anterior clinoids and posterior displacement of the posterior clinoids indicate?**

Suprasellar extension of the tumor.

○ **What is the imaging modality of choice when a pituitary lesion is suspected?**

MRI.

○ **On CT scan, what is the most characteristic appearance of a pituitary microadenoma?**

A well-circumscribed, focal, non-midline lesion that may be hyper- or hypodense.

○ **What is included in the differential diagnosis of a sellar or parasellar tumor?**

Pituitary adenoma, craniopharyngioma, parasellar meningioma, sarcoidosis, metastatic lesions, and gliomas.

○ **Thyroid stimulating hormone deficiency can be diagnosed by measurement of:**

Basal serum TSH and thyroid hormones, simultaneously.

○ **What would a low serum T4 in the presence of an inappropriately low TSH level suggest?**

A central cause of hypothyroidism.

○ **In a patient with hypothyroidism, what test would distinguish a hypothalamic defect from a pituitary defect?**

TRH stimulation test (normally, TSH, prolactin, and GH would increase in response to TRH stimulation). If there is an increase, then it suggests a hypothalamic process; if there is no response, then it suggests pituitary insufficiency.

○ **In diagnosing ACTH deficiency, what test will identify a hypothalamic CRH deficiency versus a pituitary ACTH deficiency?**

CRH stimulation test.

○ **What would be the result of the CRH stimulation test in a patient with a pituitary corticotrope deficiency?**

Absence of ACTH response to CRH.

○ **What is the ACTH stimulation test used to evaluate?**

The capacity of the adrenals to secrete cortisol.

○ **What tests are used to determine gonadotropin deficiency?**

Simultaneous measurement of FSH, LH, and gonadal steroids.

○ **What two tests will stimulate the entire hypothalamo-hypophyseal adrenal axis?**

The insulin-induced hypoglycemia test and the glucagon test.

○ **What does low circulating gonadal steroid levels associated with an inappropriately low gonadotropin level suggest?**

A hypothalamic or pituitary disturbance.

○ **What is diabetes insipidus?**

Insufficient secretion of vasopressin from the posterior pituitary.

○ **When the kidney fails to respond to an appropriate elevation in serum vasopressin, this is known as?**

Renal diabetes insipidus.

○ **How is the diagnosis of central diabetes insipidus established?**

By the water deprivation test. The diagnosis is based on the development of abnormally concentrated plasma (osmolality greater than 300 mOs/kg) and of urine that remains dilute (osmolality less than 270 mOs/kg).

○ **What is the treatment of choice for central diabetes insipidus?**

Administration of exogenous vasopressin.

○ **What is the response to vasopressin in a patient with renal diabetes insipidus?**

No change. The kidney is resistant to vasopressin.

○ **What is Sheehan syndrome?**

Postpartum infarction and necrosis of the pituitary.

○ **What are the main clinical features of Sheehan syndrome?**

1. Postpartum failure to lactate.
2. Postpartum amenorrhea.
3. Progressive signs and symptoms of adrenal insufficiency and hypothyroidism.

○ **What are the two most common types of pituitary adenomas?**

Prolactin-secreting and null-cell adenomas.

○ **What is the most common functional pituitary tumor?**

Prolactinoma.

○ **Do prolactinomas occur more frequently in men or women?**

Women.

○ **What is the most common presenting symptom of a prolactinoma in a woman?**

Secondary amenorrhea.

○ **In patients with a prolactinoma and secondary amenorrhea, what percentage have an associated galactorrhea?**

50%.

○ **What is the primary symptom of a prolactin-secreting tumor in males?**

Decrease in libido.

○ **How is the diagnosis of a prolactin-secreting tumor confirmed?**

Radiographic evidence of a pituitary lesion with an elevation of serum prolactin.

○ **What pharmaceutical agent has been shown effective in reducing serum prolactin, reducing tumor, and inhibiting tumor growth?**

Bromocriptine (a dopaminergic agonist).

○ **What is hypersecretion of ACTH by the pituitary referred to as?**

Cushing disease.

○ **Is Cushing disease more common in men or women?**

It is eight times more common in women.

○ **How is the diagnosis of Cushing disease confirmed?**

Increased basal plasma cortisol levels with loss of diurnal variation.

Failure of serum cortisol suppression with the low-dose dexamethasone suppression test.

Increased 24 hour urinary free cortisol excretion (>100 μg/24 h).

○ **What is the most likely diagnosis in a patient with Cushing syndrome with low plasma ACTH levels?**

An adrenal tumor.

○ **What is the most likely diagnosis in a patient with Cushing syndrome with elevated plasma ACTH levels (>200 pg/mL)?**

An ectopic ACTH-secreting tumor.

○ **What does an abnormal high-dose dexamethasone suppression test suggest?**

An autonomous adrenal adenoma.

○ **True or False: Most patients with Cushing disease harbor microadenomas that lend themselves to complete surgical resection.**

True. 90% are microadenomas.

○ **Acromegaly is caused by what process?**

Excess GH secretion in adults.

○ **What is the result if excess secretion of GH occurs before the epiphysis of long bones have fused?**

Gigantism.

○ **What is the most common cause of excess GH secretion?**

GH-secreting pituitary adenomas.

○ **What are the metabolic manifestations associated with acromegaly?**

1. Hypertension.
2. Diabetes mellitus.
3. Goiter.
4. Hyperhidrosis.

○ **What would you expect the basal fasting GH level to be in a patient with acromegaly?**

Less than 10 ng/mL.

○ **What test is used to confirm the diagnosis of acromegaly?**

The glucose suppression test. (Oral administration of 100 g of glucose fails to suppress the GH level to less than 5 ng/mL at 60 minutes.)

○ **What is the treatment of choice of a GH-producing pituitary adenoma?**

Surgical excision.

○ **What is the next best option for a patient with a GH-producing pituitary adenoma who cannot withstand the surgical procedure?**

Long-term treatment with octreotide.

○ **What are the two most important hormones to evaluate prior to surgical intervention in order to avoid possible perioperative catastrophe?**

Cortisol and thyroid levels.

○ **Which surgical approach to the pituitary is considered the procedure of choice?**

The transnasal transsphenoidal approach.

○ **What is the most common cause of surgical death with the transnasal transsphenoidal approach?**

Direct injury to the hypothalamus with delayed mortality attributed to CSF leaks and possible septic complications or to vascular injury.

○ **What are the contraindications to the transsphenoidal approach?**

Extensive lateral tumor herniating into the middle fossa with minimal midline mass.
Ectatic carotid arteries projecting toward the midline.
Acute sinusitis.

○ **What is the standard dosing regimen of glucocorticoids given to all patients undergoing surgical excision of a pituitary tumor?**

Methylprednisolone 40 mg IV (or 10 mg dexamethasone) every six hours, usually starting the day prior to surgery and continuing for 1 to 2 days postoperatively, followed by a tapering dose regimen.

○ **A patient in the ICU 1 day postoperative from a pituitary tumor resection suddenly develops loss of vision. What is the likely diagnosis and treatment?**

The patient probably has an evolving hemorrhagic complication. If CT confirms this, the patient should be taken for an emergent transsphenoidal reexploration.

○ **In a patient with a pituitary tumor who is a poor surgical candidate, what is the treatment of choice?**

4000 cGy radiation therapy. (50% recurrence rate.)

○ **What is the most common location of a craniopharyngioma?**

In the suprasellar cistern.

○ **What is hypersecretion of vasopressin known as?**

Syndrome of inappropriate secretion of antidiuretic hormone (SIADH).

○ **What pathology is demonstrated in this MRI?**

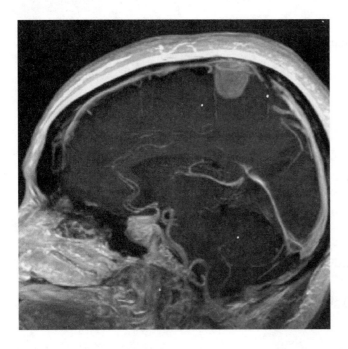

Meningioma.

○ **What are common presenting symptoms in a patient with a meningioma?**
   1. Asymmetric visual field defects.
   2. Optic atrophy.
   3. Facial sensory deficits.

○ **What is the embryologic origin of the adrenal cortex?**
Coelomic mesothelial cells.

○ **What is the embryologic origin of the adrenal medulla?**
Ectodermal neural crest cells.

○ **What hormones are synthesized and secreted by the adrenal cortex?**
Cortisol, aldosterone, adrenal androgens, and estrogen.

○ **In a premenopausal woman, what percentage of estradiol is directly secreted from the ovary?**
95%.

○ **What hormones are synthesized and secreted by the adrenal medulla?**
Epinephrine, norepinephrine, enkephalins, neuropeptide Y, and corticotropin-releasing hormone.

○ **What is the pathophysiological mechanism of Cushing syndrome?**

Hypersecretion of adrenal corticosteroids.

○ **What are the common presenting symptoms in a patient with pheochromocytoma?**

1. Palpitations.
2. Headaches.
3. Emesis.
4. Pounding pulse.
5. Retinitis.

○ **What is the primary neurotransmitter of sympathetic postganglionic fibers?**

Norepinephrine.

○ **What are the glands of Zuckerkandl?**

Ectopic adrenal medullary cells located lateral to the aorta, near the origin of the inferior mesenteric artery.

○ **What is the arterial supply to the adrenal glands?**

1. Superior suprarenal artery.
2. Inferior suprarenal artery.
3. Branch from inferior phrenic artery.

○ **What does the right adrenal vein empty into?**

The posterior inferior vena cava.

○ **What does the left adrenal vein empty into?**

The left renal vein.

○ **What is the innervation of the adrenal medulla?**

Preganglionic sympathetic neurons from the celiac and renal plexi via splanchnic nerves.

○ **What is the basic precursor of all adrenal steroids?**

Cholesterol.

○ **What is the major site of cortisol metabolism?**

The liver.

○ **Most circulating plasma cortisol is bound to what protein?**

Cortisol binding globulin (CBG), though small amounts are bound to albumin and other plasma proteins.

○ **What percentage of circulating plasma cortisol is bound to plasma proteins?**

>90%.

○ **What conditions cause low levels of plasma CBG?**

Liver disease, multiple myeloma, obesity, and the nephrotic syndrome.

○ **What conditions increase the level of plasma CBG?**

Pregnancy, estrogen supplements, oral contraceptives, and hyperthyroidism.

○ **What is the physiologic active form of plasma cortisol?**

Free cortisol.

○ **What physiologic stimuli cause the adrenal gland to secrete cortisol?**

Decrease in blood volume, tissue damage, hypoxia, deviations in body temperature, and hypoglycemia.

○ **What is the effect of glucocorticoids on insulin and glucagon?**

It stimulates the production of glucagon and inhibits secretion of insulin.

○ **What are the metabolic effects of glucocorticoids?**

Hyperglycemia, negative nitrogen balance, and lipolysis.

○ **What is the mechanism of these metabolic effects of glucocorticoids?**

1. Stimulate release of glucose from peripheral tissues.
2. Stimulate liver gluconeogenesis and glycogen deposition.
3. Inhibit protein synthesis in peripheral tissues.
4. Stimulate degradations of proteins in peripheral tissues.
5. Stimulate protein synthesis in the liver.

○ **In which tissues/organs is glucose uptake not affected by glucocorticoids?**

The liver, brain, and erythrocytes.

○ **What are the effects of glucocorticoids on the immune system?**

They block interleukins, leukotrienes, histamine, and bradykinin.
They block the release of arachidonic acid and thromboxane.
They inhibit the local increase in vascular permeability caused by serotonin.
They inhibit macrophage and neutrophil chemotaxis.
They decrease complement levels.
They suppress natural killer cell activity.
Thus, patients treated with high doses of corticosteroids demonstrate more frequent infectious complications.

○ **From what part of the adrenal gland is aldosterone produced?**

The zona glomerulosa of the cortex.

○ **What physiologic stimuli cause release of aldosterone?**

Decreased circulating blood volume and increased serum potassium concentration.

○   **Where is aldosterone primarily metabolized?**

The liver.

○   **What physiologic stimuli cause secretion of renin?**

Decrease in arterial pressure in the renal afferent arteries.

Decrease in chloride concentration in the renal tubules (sensed by the macula densa).

Stimulation of the renal sympathetic nerves via a beta-adrenergic mechanism.

○   **What cells secrete renin?**

The juxtaglomerular cells of the kidney.

○   **What is the function of renin?**

It cleaves angiotensinogen to form angiotensin I (subsequently cleaved to form angiotensin II).

○   **What enzyme converts angiotensin I to angiotensin II, and where does this occur?**

Angiotensin converting enzyme, which is located in the lung.

○   **What is the function of angiotensin II?**

It is a potent vasoconstrictor that plays an important role in blood pressure maintenance.

○   **What are the physiologic actions of aldosterone?**

1. Stimulates renal tubular reabsorption of sodium.

2. Stimulates renal tubular excretion of potassium, hydrogen ions, and ammonia.

3. Stimulates active sodium and potassium transport in other epithelial tissues such as sweat glands, gastrointestinal mucosa, and salivary glands.

○   **What is the most common cause of Cushing syndrome?**

Pituitary microadenoma.

○   **What is the most common tumor causing ectopic ACTH secretion?**

Small cell carcinoma of the lung.

○   **What is the most common tumor of the pituitary gland?**

Chromophobe adenoma.

○   **In what part of the adrenal cortex are the sex steroids produced?**

The zona reticularis.

○   **What should be the initial evaluation of a patient suspected of having Cushing syndrome?**

Urinary free cortisol level (would be markedly elevated).

Low-dose dexamethasone suppression test (no suppression of cortisol).

○ **What is the most likely diagnosis of a patient with elevated free cortisol levels, elevated plasma ACTH, persistent elevation of free cortisol after both low-dose and high-dose dexamethasone administration?**

An ectopic source of ACTH production.

○ **What tests are useful in differentiating hypercortisolism caused by pituitary sources of ACTH from those caused by ectopic sources of ACTH?**

The dexamethasone suppression test and the metyrapone test.

○ **What is the most common cause of primary hyperaldosteronism?**

A solitary adrenal adenoma.

○ **What enzymatic deficiency is associated with most cases of the adrenogenital syndrome (congenital adrenal hyperplasia)?**

21-hydroxylase.

○ **Are virilizing adrenal tumors more common in females or males?**

They are twice as common in females.

○ **What is the major catecholamine produced in the adrenal medulla?**

Epinephrine.

○ **What is the rate-limiting step in catecholamine synthesis?**

Hydroxylation of tyrosine to dihydroxy-phenylalanine (DOPA) by tyrosine hydroxylase.

○ **What is the cause of Nelson syndrome?**

Continued growth of untreated ACTH-secreting pituitary microadenomas.

○ **What are the characteristics of Nelson syndrome?**

1. Marked hyperpigmentation of the skin.
2. Visual disturbances.

○ **What is the only chemotherapeutic agent that has been proven to be of some value in the treatment of adrenal carcinoma?**

Mitotane.

○ **What is the most common cause of acute adrenocortical insufficiency?**

Withdrawal of chronic steroid therapy.

○ **What is the most common cause of spontaneous adrenal insufficiency?**

Autoimmune destruction of the adrenals (>80%).

○ **What is the most common associated disorder in patients with autoimmune adrenocortical insufficiency?**

Hashimoto's thyroiditis.

○ **What is Waterhouse–Friderichsen syndrome?**

Acute adrenal hemorrhage secondary to sepsis.

○ **What are the classic signs of adrenal crisis?**

Hypotension, hypoglycemia, and hyperkalemia.

○ **What is the treatment for a patient suspected of having an adrenal crisis?**

200 mg of a water-soluble corticosteroid.

○ **What is the most useful test to evaluate a patient suspected of having adrenocortical insufficiency?**

The rapid ACTH stimulation test.

○ **What is the treatment for acute adrenocortical insufficiency?**

Hydrocortisone, 100 mg IV every six hours for 24 hours.
Correction of volume depletion, dehydration, hypotension, and hypoglycemia.
Correct precipitating factors, especially infection.

○ **What is the etiology of primary hyperaldosteronism?**

Adrenocortical adenoma (85%), adrenal carcinoma, bilateral cortical nodular hyperplasia.

○ **What are the classic clinical manifestations of primary hyperaldosteronism?**

Diastolic hypertension with spontaneous hypokalemia.

○ **What is the biochemical test of choice to differentiate between hyperplasia and adenoma as the cause of primary hyperaldosteronism?**

Measurement of plasma aldosterone concentration after change in posture. Only patients with an adenoma experience a postural decrease in aldosterone.

○ **What is the best noninvasive test to localize an aldosteronoma?**

CT scan.

○ **What percentage of aldosteronomas can be localized by CT?**

75%.

○ **What is the most accurate test for localizing an aldosteronoma?**

Selective catheterization of the adrenal veins with sampling for aldosterone levels.

○ **What is the treatment of choice for an adrenaloma?**

Adrenalectomy.

○ **What is the treatment of choice for idiopathic hyperaldosteronism?**

Medical management with spironolactone, a competitive antagonist of aldosterone. (200–400 mg/d in divided doses.)

○ **What is the treatment of choice for idiopathic hyperaldosteronism refractory to medical management?**

Total or subtotal adrenalectomy.

○ **What is the etiology of the adrenogenital syndrome?**

Adrenal androgen hypersecretion.

○ **What is the most common enzymatic defect seen in congenital adrenal hyperplasia?**

A deficiency in C-21 hydroxylation.

○ **What is the effect of a C-21 deficiency in females? In males?**

It causes pseudohermaphrodites in females and macrogenitosomia praecox (enlarged external genitalia) in males.

○ **What is the most classic symptom of androgen excess?**

Hirsutism.

○ **What test would rule out congenital adrenal hyperplasia?**

Failure of the dexamethasone suppression test.

○ **What is the treatment for congenital adrenal hyperplasia?**

Glucocorticoid administration to suppress ACTH.

○ **What hormones are synthesized and secreted by the adrenal medulla?**

Epinephrine, norepinephrine, and small amounts of dopamine.

○ **What is the precursor of all catecholamines?**

Tyrosine.

○ **What are the two major enzymes that metabolize catecholamines?**

Monoamine oxidase (MAO) and catechol-o-methyl transferase (COMT).

○ **What stimuli cause adrenal secretion of catecholamines?**

1. Hypoxemia and hypoglycemia.
2. Changes in temperature, pain, and shock.
3. CNS injury.
4. Local wound factors and endotoxin.
5. Severe respiratory acidosis.

○ **Pheochromocytomas are tumors derived from what cells?**

Chromaffin cells that secrete catecholamines.

○ **What percentage of pheochromocytomas are bilateral? What percent are malignant?**

10% are bilateral and 10% are malignant.

○ **In which gender are malignant pheochromocytomas more common?**

They are three times more common in females.

○ **What is the test of choice to confirm the clinical suspicion of pheochromocytoma?**

Measurement of free epinephrine, norepinephrine, or their metabolites.

○ **Under what conditions should a patient who is undergoing resection of a pheochromocytoma be given preoperative alpha blockers?**

1. Blood pressure greater than 200/130.
2. Frequent and severe uncontrolled hypertensive attacks.
3. Pronounced decrease in plasma volume.

○ **Under what conditions should a patient who is undergoing resection of a pheochromocytoma be given preoperative beta blockers?**

1. Heart rate >130.
2. History of cardiac arrhythmia.
3. Persistent ventricular extra systoles.
4. Tumors, which secrete predominately epinephrine.

○ **What is the incidence of neuroblastomas in children?**

7% of all childhood cancers. It is the third most common malignancy in childhood (behind brain tumors and hematopoietic-reticular endothelial cell malignancies).

○ **What is the most common location of a neuroblastoma?**

Intra-abdominal or retroperitoneal (60%–70%).

○ **What percentage of neuroblastomas are intra-adrenal?**

40% to 50%.

○ **How do neuroblastomas most commonly present?**

In an asymptomatic patient with an irregular, firm intra-abdominal mass.

○ **What is considered a stage III neuroblastoma?**

One that extends in continuity beyond the midline with bilateral lymph node involvement.

○ **Complete cures with surgical resection can be obtained for neuroblastomas of what stages?**

Stage I, II, and IV-S.

○ **What is the treatment of choice for stage III neuroblastoma?**

Radiation and chemotherapy followed by delayed resection.

○ **What are the classic electrolyte findings of hyperaldosteronism?**

Hypernatremia and hypokalemia.

○ **What are the characteristic signs and symptoms of adrenal insufficiency?**

Hyperkalemia and hyperpigmentation.

○ **In what syndromes are pheochromocytomas associated?**

MEN-IIa, MEN-IIb, von Recklinghausen disease, tuberous sclerosis, and Sturge–Weber disease.

○ **What stimulates Leydig cells to produce testosterone in the adult male?**

LH.

○ **What stimulates Sertoli cells to enhance spermatogenesis in adult males?**

FSH.

○ **In the adult male, what stimulates secretion of LH and FSH?**

Hypothalamic release of gonadotropin-releasing hormone (LH-RH, FSH-RH).

○ **What cells release inhibin in adult males?**

Sertoli cells.

○ **In the adult male, what inhibits release of LH?**

Androgens synthesized by the testes.

○ **What is the function of inhibin in adult males?**

Inhibits release of FSH.

○ **What other substance inhibits FSH release in the adult male?**

Androgens synthesized by the testes.

○ **What is the physiologic effect of follicle-stimulating hormone (FSH) in males?**

It promotes spermatogenesis.

○ **What is the physiologic effect of luteinizing hormone (LH) in males?**

It stimulates testosterone production.

○ **What hormones are secreted by the posterior pituitary?**

Oxytocin and vasopressin.

○ **What hormones are using cAMP intracellular messenger?**
FSH, LH, hCG, TSH, ACTH.

○ **What hormones do not use cAMP as an intracellular messenger?**
Oxytocin, insulin growth hormone, prolactin cytokines, GnRH.

○ **What is the rate-limiting factor in synthesis of all the glycopeptides?**
Availability of β subunits.

○ **What is the half-life of FSH?**
3 to 4 hours.

○ **What is the half-life of LH?**
20 minutes.

○ **How long are the FSH vs LH β-chains?**
118 aa vs 121 aa.

○ **What condition results from a G protein mutation that autonomously activates the LH receptor?**
Precocious puberty in males.

○ **What condition results from a G protein mutation that autonomously inactivates the LH receptor?**
Male pseudohermaphroditism.

○ **G protein mutation with resultant inactivation of FSH receptor results in?**
Premature ovarian failure.

○ **What is the location of the GnRH gene?**
Short arm of chromosome 8.

○ **What syndrome results from absence of the axonal and GnRH neuronal migration from the olfactory placode?**
Kallmann syndrome.

○ **What are the modes of transmission of Kallmann syndrome?**
X-linked, autosomal dominant, and autosomal recessive.

○ **Characteristics of Kallmann syndrome?**
Absence of secondary sexual development, amenorrhea, lack of GnRH, and anosmia.

○ **What is the half-life of GnRH?**
2 to 4 minutes.

○ **What is the effect of norepinephrine on GnRH release?**

Stimulatory effect.

○ **What are the effects of dopamine and serotonin on GnRH release?**

They inhibit GnRH release.

○ **What part of the cell is the site of gonadotropin synthesis?**

Gonadotropin synthesis occurs on the rough endoplasmatic reticulum.

○ **What is the main effect and source of inhibin?**

Inhibits FSH but not LH, secreted by granulosa cells.

○ **What are inhibin A and inhibin B markers of?**

Inhibin A—corpus luteum function, under control of LH.
Inhibin B—granulosa cell function, under control of FSH.

○ **What are the effects of activin?**

Upregulates FSH receptor expression, increases pituitary FSH synthesis and secretion. Also, a physiologic antagonist to inhibin.

○ **What is the main effect and source of follistatin?**

Inhibits FSH and FSH response to GnRH. Product of granulosa cells.

○ **What is the time of the peak in oxytocin levels?**

Peak oxytocin levels are present during the LH surge.

○ **What fold increase in oxytocin receptors occurs throughout pregnancy and labor?**

Number of oxytocin receptors increases 80-fold throughout the pregnancy and doubles during the labor.

○ **What is necessary for midcycle LH surge?**

Increase in estradiol levels above critical concentration and duration (200 pg/mL for 48 hours).

○ **What are the effects of high levels of progesterone?**

Inhibits GnRH pulses at hypothalamus level and subsequently inhibits secretion of gonadotropins.

○ **What are the non-endocrine functions of the hypothalamus?**

Temperature regulation, the activity of the autonomic nervous system, and control of appetite.

○ **What are the possible sites of ectopic production of hypothalamic peptides?**

Normal white blood cells and chromaffin cell tumors.

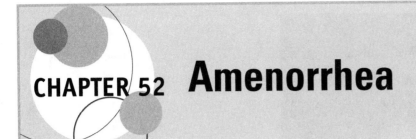

CHAPTER 52 Amenorrhea

Stephanie J. Estes, MD

○ **Define primary amenorrhea.**

- No menses by age 14 in the absence of growth or development of secondary sexual characteristics.
  <u>Or</u>
- No menses by age 16 with the appearance of secondary sexual characteristics.

○ **Define secondary amenorrhea.**

In a menstruating women, the absence of menstruation for three previous cycle intervals or 6 months.

○ **What is the maximum number of oogonia reached in a female's life cycle?**

6 to 7 million at 16 to 20 weeks gestation.

○ **What general compartments are evaluated for diagnosis in cases of amenorrhea?**

Compartment I: Disorders of the outflow tract or uterus.
Compartment II: Disorders of the ovary.
Compartment III: Disorders of the anterior pituitary.
Compartment IV: Disorders of the hypothalamus (CNS factors).

○ **What is the number one cause of secondary amenorrhea after pregnancy?**

Anovulation (28%).

○ **The absence of secondary sexual characteristics indicates that a woman has never been exposed to what?**

Estrogen stimulation.

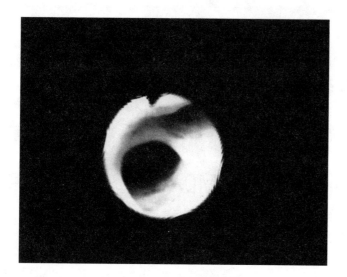

○ **32-year-old patient develops amenorrhea status post D&E for a septic abortion. Her hysteroscopy revealed the findings as shown above. What is the diagnosis?**

Asherman syndrome. Thick intrauterine adhesion shown. (Figure courtesy of Dr Elizabeth Ginsburg, Brigham and Women's Hospital, Boston, MA.)

○ **What laboratory tests should you consider in a patient with primary amenorrhea who does not have a uterus?**

Karyotype, serum testosterone (Müllerian abnormality with 46XX karyotype with normal testosterone versus androgen insensitivity syndrome with 46XY karyotype and male serum testosterone levels).

○ **What laboratory tests should you consider in a patient with primary amenorrhea who DOES have a uterus?**

hCG, TSH, PRL, progestin challenge, FSH, LH.

○ **When should an MRI be ordered in cases of primary amenorrhea?**

For symptoms of visual changes, headache, or hypogonadotropic hypogonadism.

○ **What is the differential diagnosis of vaginal agenesis?**

Congenital absence of the vagina (with or without uterine structures).
Androgen insensitivity.
Transverse septum.
Imperforate hymen.
17α-hydroxylase deficiency (46,XY with complete male pseudohermaphroditism).

○ **In primary amenorrhea, if FSH is elevated and no breast development is present, what is the diagnosis?**

Gonadal dysgenesis (50% of primary amenorrhea cases). Check karyotype next.

○ **What is the first test that should be ordered in a patient with second-degree amenorrhea?**

Pregnancy test.

○ **When should you order a karyotype in patients with second-degree amenorrhea?**

In all patients younger than 30 years or shorter than 60 inches with ovarian failure.

○ **Why are chromosomes important?**

If the patient is mosaic for the Y chromosome, the gonads must be removed surgically because of increased malignant tumor transformation.

○ **What is the most common chromosomal abnormality causing gonadal failure and primary amenorrhea?**

45,X (Turner syndrome—50%).

○ **Partial deletions of the X chromosome can also cause amenorrhea. What is the characteristic of patients who have the deletion in part of the long arm of the X chromosome (Xq-)?**

Sexual infantilism, normal stature, no somatic abnormalities, and streak gonads.

○ **What is the characteristic of patients with Xp- (deletion of the short arm of the X chromosome)?**

Phenotypically similar to Turner syndrome.

○ **Primary amenorrhea is associated with various mosaic states 25% of the time, the most common of which is:**

45,X/46,XX (mixed gonadal dysgenesis).

○ **How does "pure gonadal dysgenesis" differ from "gonadal dysgenesis"?**

Gonadal dysgenesis is absent ovarian function associated with abnormalities in the sex chromosomes. In pure gonadal dysgenesis individuals have primary amenorrhea, with normal stature and no chromosomal abnormalities. Hence, the gonads are usually streaks.

○ **What enzyme deficiency may be associated with either 46,XX or 46,XY and cause primary amenorrhea?**

17α-hydroxylase deficiency. Patients with this deficiency have primordial follicles, but gonadotropin levels are elevated because the enzyme deficiency prevents synthesis of sex steroids.

○ **What distinguishes a patient with 46,XX 17α-hydroxylase deficiency from one with the same deficiency but an XY karyotype?**

Patients with 46,XY karyotype lack a uterus. Both of these patients have primary amenorrhea, no secondary sexual characteristics, female phenotypes, hypertension, and hypokalemia.

○ **Name two other enzyme deficiencies that result in a female phenotype with an XY karyotype?**

5α-reductase deficiency and 17–20 desmolase deficiency.

○ **What is the diagnosis of a patient with normal FSH & LH but with a negative progestational challenge test (assuming normal outflow tract)?**

Pituitary-CNS failure (patient needs sella turcica imaging).

○ **What is the term for amenorrhea caused by inadequate amounts of GnRH or pituitary gonadotropins?**

Hypogonadotropic hypogonadism.

○ **What is the most common manifestation of hypogonadotropic hypogonadism?**

Constitutional delay of puberty.

○ **What is the treatment for this?**

Reassurance.

○ **What is Kallmann syndrome?**

Hypogonadotropic hypogonadism because of a lack of GnRH as a result of failure of migration of the GnRH neuron from the olfactory bulb. These patients are anosmic and have primary amenorrhea.

○ **The most common central nervous system tumor that can lead to primary amenorrhea is:**

Craniopharyngioma. It is an extracellular mass that interferes with the production and secretion of GnRH or the stimulation of pituitary gonadotropins. Usually, these patients have disorders of other pituitary hormones.

○ **What one test can distinguish hypergonadotropic and hypogonadotropic forms of hypogonadism?**

FSH.

○ **If FSH is elevated, the next appropriate test would be:**

A karyotype.

○ **Is an elevated FSH an absolute indicator of infertility?**

No.

○ **Why does FSH rise prior to menopause?**

Because of decreased inhibin.

○ **In amenorrhea, what are the causes of high gonadotropins?**

- Tumors producing gonadotropins (often lung cancer, but rare).
- Single gonadotropin deficiencies, homozygous mutations in gonadotropin genes.
- Gonadotropin-secreting pituitary adenoma (not associated with amenorrhea).
- Perimenopause, menopause, premature ovarian failure.
- Resistant or insensitive ovary syndrome, mutations in gonadotropin receptor genes.
- Galactosemia, direct toxic effect of galactose metabolites on germ cell migration.
- 17α-hydroxylase deficiency.

○ **What three tests are helpful in diagnosing 17α-hydroxylase deficiency?**

Serum progesterone—elevated (>3 ng/mL).

17α-hydroxyprogesterone—low (<0.2 ng/mL).

Serum deoxycorticosterone (DOC)—low.

○ **What is the confirmatory test and what is the response in a patient with 17α-hydroxylase deficiency?**

ACTH stimulation test. These patients will have an increase in serum progesterone and no change in 17α-hydroxyprogesterone.

○ **At what age is premature ovarian failure diagnosed?**

<40 years.

○ **What other testing should be considered in a patient with premature ovarian failure?**

This is often associated with autoimmune diseases. Check thyroid and adrenal antibodies, TSH, T4, calcium, phosphorus, fasting glucose. Also, consider fragile X testing and genetic counseling.

○ **What other rare conditions are associated with premature ovarian failure?**

Hypoparathyroidism.
Moniliasis.
Myasthenia gravis.
Idiopathic thrombocytopenic purpura.
Rheumatoid arthritis.
Vitiligo.
Autoimmune hemolytic anemia.

○ **What is the treatment for hypergonadotropic hypogonadism?**

Cyclic estrogen and progestin therapy.

○ **In addition to estrogen and progesterone, individuals with 17α-hydroxylase deficiency need what?**

Corticosteroid replacement.

○ **What is the cause of premature ovarian failure?**

The cause is probably accelerated follicular atresia. However, the etiology of this accelerated atresia is unknown. In addition, it can result from an autoimmune process, infections, or a physical insult such as radiation or chemotherapy.

○ **What infection is a cause of premature ovarian failure?**

Mumps oophoritis.

○ **What bad habit is associated with ovarian failure?**

Cigarette smoking.

○ **What radiation dose will permanently sterilize 100% of women?**

More than 800 rads. 150 rads will give some risk to women older than 40. Using 200 to 500 rads 60% of women ages 15 to 40 will be sterilized. With 500 to 800 rads 70% of women ages 15 to 40 will be sterilized (younger age = increased resistance to radiation).

○ **Which chemotherapeutic agents are most toxic to the ovaries?**

Alkylating agents.

○ **Genetic disorders (i.e., mosaicism, deletions) account for a number of patients with premature ovarian failure. What region of the X chromosome is critical to prevent ovarian failure prematurely?**

Xq26-28.

○ **Name the causes of obstructive amenorrhea?**

Imperforate hymen; transverse vaginal septum; hypoplasia; or absence of the uterus, cervix and/or vagina.

○ **What test can help delineate the female anatomy the best?**

MRI.

○ **How does one differentiate a transverse vaginal septum from an imperforate hymen?**

A transverse vaginal septum lacks distention at the introitus with Valsalva's maneuver.

○ **What is the treatment for a vaginal septum?**

Surgical removal followed by Frank dilators to distend the vagina and prevent vaginal stenosis.

○ **The majority of vaginal septums occur in what two areas of the vagina?**

The upper one-third (46%) and the middle one-third (40%).

○ **What is the karyotype of a patient with Müllerian agenesis?**

46,XX.

○ **In a patient with known Müllerian agenesis, what other systems need to be evaluated and why?**

The renal tract because approximately one-third of patients will have urinary tract abnormalities; the skeletal system since 12% have skeletal abnormalities including spinal deformities, absent digits, and syndactyly.

○ **Aside from surgical construction of a neovagina what other method is available?**

Vaginal dilators. 80% of women are able to achieve satisfactory intercourse.

○ **What is the diagnosis of a patient with primary amenorrhea, an absent uterus, and little to absent body hair?**

Complete androgen insensitivity syndrome (AIS is the third most common cause of first-degree amenorrhea).

○ **What is the karyotype of a patient with complete androgen insensitivity?**

46,XY.

○ **Why is there no uterus, tubes, and upper vagina in AIS?**

Anti-Müllerian hormone is present.

○ **How is AIS inherited?**

It is an X-linked recessive gene responsible for the intracellular androgen receptor.

○ **Given that AIS patients have testes and the high incidence of neoplasia if left in situ, when should the testes be removed?**

After puberty (exception to the rule), at approximately 16 to 18 years of age. This is because the development of secondary sexual characteristics achieved with hormone therapy does not match that with endogenous hormones. In addition, the incidence of gonadal tumors in these patients is rare before puberty.

○ **Do AIS patients have normal female levels of testosterone?**

No. The levels of testosterone in these phenotypic females are in the normal to slightly elevated male range. Thus, they produce testosterone but are not able to respond to those androgens.

○ **How can one differentiate a patient with androgen insensitivity from one with 5α-reductase deficiency?**

The patient with 5α-reductase deficiency does not develop breasts at puberty. This is because of the levels of testosterone that are present in sufficient amounts to suppress breast development.

○ **What is 5α-reductase responsible for?**

Converting testosterone to its more potent form dihydrotestosterone.

○ **A very rare cause of amenorrhea in which both male and female gonadal tissue is present is known as what?**

True hermaphrodite.

○ **What is the diagnosis of a female patient with XY karyotype and palpable Müllerian structures but lack of sexual development?**

Swyer syndrome (remove gonads as has a high incidence of malignancy).

○ **What is the most common cause of secondary amenorrhea?**

Pregnancy.

○ **Describe the initial laboratory evaluation for secondary amenorrhea.**

hCG, TSH, prolactin, progestin withdrawal, FSH. Consider testosterone, DHEAS, and pelvic ultrasound for investigating polycystic ovarian disease.

○ **What are the Rotterdam criteria for diagnosing PCOS?**

Need two out of three of the following:

- Clinical and/or biochemical hyperandrogenism.
- Oligo- and/or anovulation.
- Polycystic ovaries (presence of 12 or more follicles in each ovary measuring 2–9 mm in diameter, and/or increased ovarian volume >10 mL).

○ **How is a patient's estrogen status and competence of the outflow tract assessed?**

Administer medroxyprogesterone acetate 5 or 10 mg for 5 to 10 days, to determine whether the patient bleeds after withdrawal of the medication. Alternatively, can use 200 mg IM progesterone in oil or micronized progesterone 300 mg qd.

○ **How much bleeding is needed for a positive withdrawal response in a progestational challenge?**

Any amount of bleeding no matter how scant.

○ **If no withdrawal bleed occurs, what is the next step?**

To add estrogen prior to the progestin withdrawal (1.25 mg conjugated estrogen or 2 mg of estradiol daily for 21 days with 10 mg of Provera added for the last 5 days).

○ **A patient fails to bleed with the aforementioned regimen and a hysterogram reveals a typical pattern of synechiae, this is indicative of what cause of amenorrhea?**

Asherman syndrome.

O   **What is the treatment for Asherman syndrome?**

Hysteroscopy with lysis of adhesions, +/− method to keep the uterine cavity open and high-dose estrogen for 2 months (add MPA 10 mg daily after the third week) and broad-spectrum antibiotics preoperatively and 10 days afterward.

O   **Name the methods often used to keep the uterine cavity open?**

IUD or pediatric Foley filled with 3 mL of fluid left in for 7 days.

O   **What percentage of patients with Asherman syndrome have achieved a successful pregnancy after surgical lysis of the intrauterine adhesions?**

70% to 80%.

O   **What complications may these patients then experience with their pregnancy?**

Preterm labor; placenta accreta, previa; postpartum hemorrhage.

O   **How does hyperthyroidism cause amenorrhea?**

It inhibits gonadotropin release.

O   **How does hypothyroidism cause amenorrhea?**

TRH stimulates prolactin secretion. It works by acting directly on prolactin secreting cells. In addition, the deficiency of thyroid hormones (in hypothyroidism) affects dopamine's inhibitory control of prolactin resulting in hyperprolactinemia.

O   **If elevated TSH and prolactin levels are found in an amenorrhea work-up what do you treat?**

Only the hypothyroidism. The prolactin will normalize with the treatment of the hypothyroidism based on its mechanism of causing amenorrhea.

O   **Hyperprolactinemia causes amenorrhea by what mechanisms?**

Prolactin suppresses the GnRH pulsatile release necessary for ovulation and menstruation and increases opioid activity. It may also act to reduce the granulosa cell number and FSH binding.

O   **What proportion of women with both galactorrhea and amenorrhea will have hyperprolactinemia?**

Two-thirds.

O   **What test is necessary in women with amenorrhea and hyperprolactinemia once drug induced and physiologic causes of the elevated prolactin have been ruled out?**

MRI of the sella turcica.

O   **In patients with galactorrhea and second-degree amenorrhea, how many will have an abnormal sella turcica?**

50%.

○ **What two diseases can cause endometritis and uterine scarring as a result?**

Tuberculosis endometritis, schistosomiasis.

○ **A patient with amenorrhea because of absent FSH receptors or postreceptor defects has what syndrome?**

The resistant ovary syndrome or *Savage syndrome.* These patients have unstimulated ovarian follicles in their ovaries. In addition, there is no evidence of autoimmune disease (i.e., lymphocytic invasion) yet the ovaries are nonfunctional.

○ **Postpartum amenorrhea can be due to what?**

Sheehan syndrome. It is postpartum necrosis of the pituitary from a hypotensive episode also causing failure to lactate and loss of pubic and axillary hair.

○ **Which hormone deficiencies are most common in Sheehan syndrome?**

Growth hormone.
Gonadotropins.

○ **What percentage of body fat is necessary for the initiation of menses and then for the maintenance of menses?**

Approximately 17% and 22%, respectively. It is thought that decreasing weight can affect GnRH pulsatile secretion.

○ **What three items comprise the female athlete triad?**

Amenorrhea.
Disordered eating.
Osteoporosis/osteopenia.

○ **Name three causes of amenorrhea that are thought to be caused by abnormalities in neuromodulation in hypothalamic GnRH secretion.**

Anorexia, stress, and exercise.

○ **What is hypothalamic amenorrhea?**

Defect in GnRH pulsatility frequently associated with stressful situations, probably secondary to elevated CRH/cortiso,l which inhibits gonadal secretion.

○ **How does one diagnose hypothalamic amenorrhea?**

All studies are normal—diagnosis of exclusion (gonadotropin may be low or normal), and failure to demonstrate withdrawal bleeding.

○ **What are three other causes of secondary amenorrhea because of affected pituitary function?**

Lymphocytic hypophysitis—often occurring during pregnancy or 6 months postpartum.
Carotid artery aneurysm.
Obstruction of aqueduct of Sylvius.

○   **Are leptin levels in anorectic and bulimic patients increased or decreased?**

Decreased.

○   **If a patient has Turner syndrome clinically, what other things must you evaluate or consider?**

Autoimmune disorders are common.

Cardiovascular abnormalities.

Renal abnormalities.

Karyotype—since 40% are mosaic and may have XY aberrations.

○   **When should evaluation of a patient begin if a patient is amenorrheic after discontinuing oral contraceptive pills? After discontinuing Depo-Provera?**

• 6 months after discontinuation of OCPs.
• 12 months after the last injection of Depo-Provera.

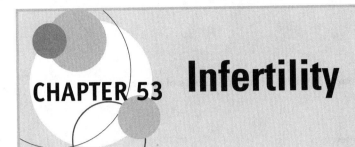

CHAPTER 53 Infertility

Vasiliki A. Moragianni, MD

○ **What is infertility?**

Infertility is synonymous to subfertility and is defined as either 1 year of unprotected coitus without conception in a female younger than 35 years or 6 months in a female older than 35 years.

○ **What is the difference between primary and secondary infertility?**

Primary infertility refers to patients who have never conceived, whereas secondary infertility refers to those who have a history of pregnancy, regardless of outcome.

○ **What is sterility?**

An intrinsic inability to achieve pregnancy.

○ **What are the rates of infertility and sterility?**

Infertility: 10% to 15%
Sterility: 1% to 2%

○ **What is fecundability?**

The probability of achieving a "pregnancy" within one menstrual cycle (20%–25% in normal couples).

○ **What is fecundity?**

The probability of achieving a "live birth" within one menstrual cycle.

○ **In each ovulatory cycle, what is the probability of becoming pregnant?**

30%.

○ **What is the percentage of couples that will attain pregnancy at 3 months, 6 months, 1 year, and 2 years?**

3 months: 57%
6 months: 72%
1 year: 85%
2 years: 93%

○ **The age range of optimal fertility is?**

20 to 24 years.

○ **Which lifestyle modifications have been proven to improve a couple's chances of conception?**

Smoking cessation.

Weight loss to achieve a BMI of 20 to 25.

Decrease alcohol intake to four or fewer drinks per week.

Limit caffeine intake to <250 mg/d.

○ **How does smoking affect fertility?**

Women who smoke are 20% to 30% more likely to have 1 year of unprotected coitus prior to conception. Women who smoke, have a 20% decreased pregnancy rate with assisted reproductive techniques.

○ **What are the primary diagnoses in the infertile couple? What percentage of all infertile couples has each diagnosis?**

Ovulation defect (27%)

Semen abnormality (25%)

Tubal defect (22%)

Unexplained (17%)

Endometriosis (5%)

Other (4%)

○ **What are the primary diagnoses in the infertile woman? What percentage of all infertile women has each diagnosis?**

Ovulatory dysfunction (40%)

Tubal and pelvic pathology (40%)

Unexplained (10%)

Unusual problems, i.e., anatomic abnormalities, thyroid disease (10%)

○ **How many oocytes are present in each stage of reproductive development?**

16 to 20 weeks gestation: 6 to 7 million oogonia

Birth: 1 to 2 million oocytes

Onset of puberty: 300,000 to 500,000 oocytes

Age 37 to 38: 25,000 oocytes

Menopause: 1000 oocytes

○ **What is the average age of menopause in the United States?**

51 years.

○ **How many years prior to menopause does follicular loss occur?**

10 to 15 years.

○ **What are the means of documenting ovulation?**

Basal body temperature (BBT) rises in response to progesterone.

Elevated progesterone levels.

Endometrial biopsy.

○ **How much does BBT rise during the luteal phase?**

0.4°F to 0.8°F higher. (97.0°F–98.0°F during follicular phase.)

○ **When does the thermogenic shift in BBT occur?**

When progesterone levels rise 1 to 5 days after the midcycle LH surge and up to 4 days after ovulation.

○ **When should coitus be encouraged in relationship to BBT?**

Alternate-day coitus beginning 7 days before the earliest observed rise and ending on the day before the latest observed shift in BBT.

○ **When should serum progesterone be measured to document ovulation?**

Approximately, 1 week before the expected menses.

○ **A serum progesterone greater than what level is diagnostic of ovulation?**

3 ng/mL.

○ **What are the causes of adult-onset anovulation?**

Hypothalamic dysfunction (38%)

Pituitary disease (17%)

Ovarian dysfunction (45%)

○ **Hypothalamic dysfunction may result in anovulation. Name 3 causes.**

Stress, weight and body composition, and strenuous exercise.

○ **The most common pituitary disorder that causes anovulation is:**

Prolactinoma (then empty sella, Sheehan, and Cushing syndromes).

○ **The most common ovarian causes of anovulation are:**

Ovarian failure and polycystic ovary syndrome (PCOS).

○ **What is the estimated, fertilizable lifespan of the oocyte?**

12 to 24 hours.

○ **What is the estimated, fertilizable lifespan of the sperm?**

48 to 72 hours.

○ **When is the endometrial biopsy performed during an infertility evaluation?**

2 to 3 days prior to expected menses. Alternatively, a biopsy may be timed to LH surge plus 7 to 8 days.

○ **What is a luteal phase defect?**

Defined as a lag of more that 2 days in histologic development of endometrium compared to the day of the cycle (3%–4% of women will be diagnosed as having luteal phase defect). Others consider a midluteal progesterone of less than 10 ng/mL to be a good indication of a luteal phase defect. This diagnosis has fallen into disfavor.

○ **What is clomiphene citrate (CC)?**

A nonsteroidal estrogen agonist/antagonist.

○ **What is the initial dose of CC?**

50 mg for 5 days starting on day 3, 4, or 5 of the cycle.
50% of the women will ovulate at the 50 mg dose.

○ **What are the most common symptoms experienced by women taking CC?**

Vasomotor (20%)

Adnexal tenderness (5%)

Nausea (3%)

Headache (1%)

Scotoma or vision changes (rare)

○ **Most CC-induced pregnancies in patients with ovulatory dysfunction occur within how many months?**

Within the first three menstrual cycles.

○ **What is the percentage of twin and triplet gestations after CC?**

7% and 0.3%, respectively.

○ **What is the WHO classification for anovulation?**

WHO group I: Anovulation with low-endogenous gonadotropins and little endogenous estrogen production.
WHO group II: Anovulation or oligo-ovulation with a normal (or elevated) gonadotropin level and evidence for significant endogenous estrogen production.
WHO group III: Ovarian failure.

○ **CC is most effective at inducing ovulation in which WHO group?**

WHO group II. CC is unlikely to induce ovulation in women with FSH >20 mIU/mL.

○ **If DHEAS is higher than 2 μg/mL, what medication can be combined with CC to induce ovulation?**

Glucocorticoids.

○ **What is metformin?**

Biguanide antihyperglycemic agent, which decreases blood glucose levels by inhibiting hepatic glucose production and by improving peripheral glucose uptake.

○ **Does metformin cause hypoglycemia?**

No. It does not increase insulin secretion.

○ **What is the most common side effect of metformin?**

Gastrointestinal disturbances such as diarrhea, nausea, vomiting, and bloating.

○ **Can metformin be used alone or in combination with CC to induce ovulation in infertile women with oligoovulation, hyperandrogenism, and insulin resistance?**

Yes.

○ **Should metformin be discontinued when pregnancy is achieved?**

Controversial. Metformin is category B and may decrease risk of spontaneous abortions.

○ **What are the main indications to use gonadotropins for induction of ovulation?**

WHO I patients.
PCOS patients in whom CC fails.
Empirical ovarian hyperstimulation for treatment of unexplained infertility or early-stage endometriosis.
Assisted reproduction techniques, such as IVF.

○ **In WHO group I patients, what is the pregnancy rate after treatment with gonadotropins for six cycles?**

91%.

○ **How is ovulation induction with gonadotropins performed?**

Start FSH or LH/FSH at 75 IU or 150 IU daily, starting day 2 or 3 of a cycle. Measure estradiol at day 6 or 7, and if adequate, (500 to 1500 pg/mL) perform transvaginal ultrasound until diameter of largest follicle is 16 to –18 mm. Then administer 5000 to 10000 IU of hCG and time intercourse or insemination.

○ **What are the findings of ovarian hyperstimulation syndrome on TVUS (OHSS)?**

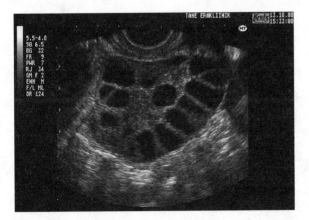

Multiple ovarian follicles and ovarian enlargement. OHSS then results in weight gain, hemoconcentration, electrolyte imbalance that could lead to ascites, renal dysfunction, thrombosis, pleural effusion, ovarian torsion, ARDS, and even death in severe cases.

○ **What is the treatment of OHSS?**

Bedrest, maintain intravascular volume, prophylaxis against thrombosis, culdocentesis for symptomatic relief of shortness of breath.

○ **Mild OHSS occurs in what percentage of women, receiving gonadotropin treatment?**

3% to 5%.

○ **What percentage of gonadotropin stimulated cycles result in multiple birth pregnancies?**

15%.

○ **True or False: Pulsatile GnRH administration has been used to induce ovulation ?**

True.

○ **How is pulsatile GnRH treatment performed?**

A computerized pump delivers pulse of GnRH every 90 minutes at a dose of 75 to 100 ng/kg per pulse.

○ **Which is more effective at ovulation: Induction; gonadotropins, or pulsatile GnRH?**

They have equivalent rates of ovulation and pregnancy. However, at the present, pulsatile GnRH (Lutrepulse) is no longer available in the United States.

○ **Name the two most common causes of hyperprolactinemia.**

Prolactin-secreting pituitary gland tumors and psychiatric medications.

○ **What is the treatment of infertile women with hyperprolactinemia and anovulation?**

Bromocriptine 2.5 to 7.5 mg daily or Cabergoline 0.25 to –1 mg twice a week.

○ **When should prolactin levels be retested after beginning dopamine agonist therapy?**

4 weeks after initiating therapy or changing the dosage.

○ **What test is used for the diagnosis of a prolactinoma?**

MRI of the sella turcica.

○ **Should one begin ovulation induction in women with large pituitary gland tumors?**

No. Large tumors are associated with an increased risk of neurosurgical complications during pregnancy.

○ **In women with microadenomas that secrete prolactin, what is the risk of pituitary insufficiency or neurosurgical complications during pregnancy?**

Less than 1%.

○ **What percentage of microadenomas increase in size over 4 to 6 years of observation?**

Less than 5%.

○ **What percentage of women will ovulate after establishment of euprolactinemia?**

80%.

○ **What is the treatment of women with inhibited ovulation because of adrenal hyperplasia?**

Glucocorticoids or CC with glucocorticoids.

○ **Should women with premature ovarian failure (POF) undergo testing of adrenal reserve?**

Yes, up to 10% of women with POF are at risk for developing adrenal failure, and a random morning cortisol is the most cost effective test.

○ **What BMI is associated with an increased risk of ovulatory infertility?**

Greater than 27.

○ **What is the mechanism by which anorexia nervosa causes anovulation?**

Hypothalamic amenorrhea, decreased FSH and LH with apulsatile or low-amplitude, low-frequency pulsatile hormone secretion.

○ **What are the criteria for initiating ovarian reserve testing?**

Age >35.
Longstanding duration of infertility.
Unexplained infertility, regardless of age.
Family history of early menopause.
Previous ovarian surgery, chemotherapy, or radiation.
Smoking.
Poor response to exogenous gonadotropin stimulation.

○ **What laboratory test is a good predictor of follicular and oocyte competence?**

Day 3 FSH.

○ **What ultrasound measurement(s) has been used to predict ovarian reserve?**

Basal antral follicle counts and ovarian volume.

○ **What is an abnormal value for day 3 FSH?**

In most laboratories, it is >10 to 15 IU/L.

○ **What FSH concentration is associated with a <5% pregnancy rate?**

25 mIU/mL.

○ **What is a more sensitive test than day 3 FSH to identify women with diminished ovarian reserve?**

The clomiphene citrate challenge test (CCCT).

○ **How does the CCCT detect women with diminished follicular reserve?**

CC blocks the negative feedback of estrogen leaving only inhibin to suppress FSH. Inhibin levels in women with diminished ovarian reserve are low and cannot suppress FSH.

○ **Describe the CCCT.**

Measure day 3 FSH and estradiol. Administer 100 mg daily of CC on cycle days 5 to 9. Measure day 10 FSH. An elevated FSH on either day is associated with diminished ovarian reserve.

○ **True or False: In a patient with normal day 3 FSH, an elevated day 10 FSH carries the same poor prognosis as an elevated day 3 FSH.**

True.

○ **What is the prevalence of abnormal CCCT in the general population?**

10% in women of all ages.

○ **What is the treatment of ovarian failure?**

Donor egg.

○ **What percentage of women with ovarian failure have multiglandular failure?**

Up to 10%; screen yearly for thyroid, adrenal, and parathyroid function.

○ **What factors contribute to tubal disease?**

Pelvic inflammatory disease (PID), appendicitis with rupture, septic abortion, previous tubal or abdominal surgery.

○ **What is the rate of tubal infertility after one-, two-, and three episodes of PID?**

12%, 23%, and 55%, respectively.

○ **What are the tests used to evaluate the uterine cavity?**

Hysterosalpingogram (HSG)
Transvaginal ultrasound
Sonohysterogram
Hysteroscopy

○ **When is sonohysterography used instead of a HSG?**

Sonohysterography provides superior visualization of the uterine cavity especially in regard to endometrial polyps and submucous leiomyomata, which is useful in a patient with abnormal bleeding evaluation. HSG is still the test of choice in infertility patients because it allows one to investigate tubal patency.

○ **What are the tests used to determine tubal patency?**

HSG
Laparoscopy with chromotubation

○ **What are the sensitivity, specificity, positive and negative predictive values of the HSG as compared to hysteroscopy for determining intrauterine pathology?**

Sensitivity-98%; Specificity-35%; PPV-70%; NPV-8%.

○ **When is the HSG performed in the cycle?**

Days 6 to 12. Prefer not to perform after ovulation, as thickened endometrial lining may obscure image and the possibility of conception.

○ **When is antibiotic prophylaxis recommended for an HSG?**

Only if dilated fallopian tubes are demonstrated.

○ **What is the recommended regimen?**

Doxycycline 100 mg PO, twice daily for 5 days.

○ **Why should the contrast be injected slowly into the uterine cavity?**

To assess filling and to minimize pain and avoid tubal spasm.

○ **What types of contrast are used?**

Water soluble and oil soluble (rarely).

○ **Can an HSG be diagnostic or therapeutic?**

Both, there is a suggestion that in women with endometriosis a slight increase in pregnancy rate occurs in the cycle of the HSG.

○ **By what mechanisms may an HSG increase pregnancy rates?**

It can dislodge mucus plugs, break adhesions, stimulate cilia, or inhibit phagocytosis of sperm by peritoneal macrophages.

○ **What are the complications of an HSG?**

Contrast embolization (patient has blurry vision), allergic reaction (abdominal pain and respiratory distress), salpingitis (abdominal pain).

○ **What dye is used to examine tubal patency on laparoscopy?**

Indigo carmine.

○ **What is the appropriate fertility treatment of salpingitis isthmica nodosa?**

IVF-ET.

○ **Surgery is most successful for tubal disease, if the disease is located in which portion of the tube (proximal, middle, or distal)?**

Distal portion.

○ **What are the factors associated with a high success rate for tubal surgical reanastomosis?**

Age <40 years

Tubal length >5 cm after anastamosis

Absence of associated pelvic disease

○ **Ectopic pregnancy rate after PID is increased by:**

6- to 7-fold.

○ **Intrauterine and ectopic pregnancy rates after tubal reanastamosis are:**

50% to 80% and 5%, respectively.

○ **What are the poor prognostic factors for successful pregnancy in regards to tubal disease?**

Tubal diameter >20 mm

Absence of visible fimbriae

Dense pelvic adhesions

Ovarian adhesions

Advanced age of male partner

Duration of infertility problem

○ **What is the treatment of tubal factor infertility?**

Surgery (reanastamosis, salpingoplasty, lysis of adhesions) or IVF for irreparable or absent tubes.

○ **True or False: Laparoscopic fimbrioplasty may increase pregnancy rates.**

True, in selected patients, where fimbriae are present (mild/moderate/severe hydrosalpinges) pregnancy rates may be 80%, 30%, and 15%, respectively, following surgery.

○ **True or False: IVF success in women with communicating hydrosalpinges is decreased .**

True. It may be reduced by up to 50% in some women.

○ **What procedure would be indicated for proximal tubal occlusion and otherwise normal anatomy?**

Hysteroscopic tubal cannulation

Up to 40% pregnancy rates after successful tubal cannulation

○ **Name the test used to examine cervical factor infertility.**

The postcoital test (PCT or Sims-Hühner test). This test has been evaluated in multiple studies and found not to be predictive of any fertility outcome and should no longer be a part of routine fertility evaluation.

○ **Describe the PCT.**

Collection of the specimen of cervical mucus, shortly before the expected time of ovulation (as determined by BBT or urine LH secretion in previous cycles) 2 to 12 hours after intercourse.

○ **What is spinnbarkeit?**

The stretchability of the cervical mucus.

○ **What organism is found at increased levels in cervical mucus and in semen of infertile couples compared with fertile controls and how is it treated?**

Organism: Mycoplasma
Treatment: Doxycycline

○ **What is the treatment of endometriosis in the infertile patient?**

Surgical removal/ablation of endometrial implants.

○ **Fecundability is highest up to how many months after the first surgery?**

6 to 12 months.

○ **Which empiric treatments of unexplained infertility are successful?**

IVF (35 to 40%)
Gonadotropin-IUI (17.1%)
Gonadotropin (7.7%)
CC-IUI (8.3%)
CC (5.6%)
IUI (3.8%)
Observation alone (1.3%–4.1%)

○ **What percentage of couples with unexplained infertility for <3 years duration will become pregnant with 3 years of expectant management?**

60%.

○ **Is dilatation and curettage a part of routine infertility work-up?**

No.

○ **What uterine anomalies are associated with in utero exposure to DES (diethylstilbestrol)?**

Hypoplastic T-shaped uterus with cornual bands and pretubal bulges, lower segment dilatation, and small cavities with irregular borders.

○ **How much more likely is it to have an ectopic pregnancy in women exposed to DES in utero?**

Five to six times.

○ **What effective therapy has been described for treatment of the hypoplastic T-shaped uterus?**

None, some reports of surgical resection or use of exogenous estrogen exist.

○ **How may submucous myomas cause infertility?**

Impaired endometrial blood flow and poor implantation environment.

○ **How may intramural myomas cause infertility?**

Enlarged endometrial cavity, which may result in poor sperm transport or occlusion of the tube.

○ **What are common presentations of intrauterine adhesions?**

Menstrual disorders/amenorrhea/hypomenorrhea, infertility, recurrent pregnancy loss and abnormal placentation.

○ **What is Asherman's syndrome?**

Disorder of amenorrhea and infertility that results from intrauterine adhesion and synechiae formation after uterine instrumentation.

○ **What indications for curettage lead to the most frequent development of intrauterine adhesions?**

Missed abortion (30.9%)
Late postpartum hemorrhage (23.4%)
Elective abortion (22.9%)
Incomplete abortion (6.4%)
Any postpartum hemorrhage (3.7%)

○ **Damage to which layer of the endometrium is related to the development of intrauterine adhesions?**

The basalis layer.

○ **What is the most common test used to diagnose intrauterine adhesions?**

HSG.

○ **What is the treatment of intrauterine adhesions?**

Hysteroscopic lysis of the adhesions.

○ **The overall pregnancy rate following treatment of intrauterine adhesions is?**

60% to 75%.

○ **After lysis of adhesions, what medical therapy is initiated to inhibit further development of adhesions?**

Placement of IUD or sequential 5-mg conjugated estrogen daily with medroxyprogesterone acetate, 10 mg during the last 5 days of estrogen therapy. Hormone therapy assists the endometrium in re-epithelializing.

○ **What are the WHO parameters of a normal semen analysis?**

Volume: >2 mL
Count: >20 million/mL
Motility: >50% with forward progression
Morphology: >30% normal form
WBC: <1 million/mL
Liquification: 30 minutes
pH: 7.2 to 7.8

○ **Semen morphology may be graded using what "strict" criteria?**

Kruger strict morphology. This assessment results in a more rigorous systematic evaluation of sperm morphology. Normal is defined as >14% normal forms and is associated with highest fertility rates. Less than 4% is associated with poor fertility and may require IVF and intracytoplasmic sperm injection (ICSI) or donor sperm.

○ **Semen analysis sample should be collected after _____ day period of abstinence and be received in the lab within _____ hour(s) of collection.**

2 to 3 days and 1 hour, respectively.

○ **The best rates using insemination are achieved using sperm concentrations of:**

Greater than 10 to 15 million total motile sperm; pregnancy rates are minimal, if the total number of motile sperm is less than 1 million for insemination.

○ **What are the causes of male factor infertility?**

Varicocele (37%)

Idiopathic (26%)

Testicular failure (9%)

Obstruction (6%)

Cryptorchidism (6%)

Low semen volume (5%)

Sperm agglutination (3%)

Semen viscosity (2%)

Genetic (<5%; microdeletion of the Y chromosome; translocations, aneuploidy, i.e., 47 XXY)

Infection (3% to 4%)

Environmental toxins (5%)

Other (5%)

○ **What is a varicocele?**

Dilation of the pampiniform plexus of the scrotal veins.

○ **What is the treatment of clinically evident varicoceles?**

Surgical repair may improve semen parameters and fertility rates in up to 40% of cases.

○ **Azoospermia and a negative fructose test suggest what diagnosis?**

Obstruction. Causes include infection, surgery and congenital absence of the vas deferens as is seen in up to 80% of males with cystic fibrosis. Fructose is produced in the seminal vesicle and would be present in the semen, if at least one tract is patent.

○ **What is the pregnancy rate after vasovasostomy (vasectomy reversal)?**

Within 3 years of vasectomy: 70% to 97%

Within >3 or <15 years of vasectomy: 30%

○   **What is the treatment for gonadal failure associated with Klinefelter syndrome (47,XXY)?**

Typically donor sperm. However, there are reports of healthy deliveries now, using IVF, testicular sperm aspiration, and preimplantation genetic diagnosis to identify euploid embryos.

○   **A male with low testosterone and serum gonadotropin values less than 5 IU/L or lower would have what diagnosis?**

Hypogonadotropic hypogonadism.

○   **What is the treatment for hypogonadotropic hypogonadism in men?**

hCG 2000 IU IM three times per week for 6 months followed by 37.5 IU of FSH IM three times per week, or pulsatile administrations of GnRH 4 μg q 3 h by an infusion pump.

○   **What is the most common cause of retrograde ejaculation? How is it diagnosed?**

The most common cause is prostatectomy. The second most common cause is testicular carcinoma. Diagnosis is made by finding ejaculate of low volume with azoospermia or severe oligospermia and multiple sperm in urine specimen postejaculation.

○   **How do you treat retrograde ejaculation?**

Phenylpropramide 75 mg BID or ephedrine sulfate 25 mg QID or urine can be collected and sperm can be harvested from the urine for insemination.

○   **Exposure to which drug toxins are hypothesized to produce disorders of sperm production?**

Chemotherapeutic agents
Sulfasalazine
Alcohol
Cimetidine
Lead, cadmium, mercury
Carbon disulfide industrial solvent
Nematocide (DBCP)
B-blockers

○   **Does radiation therapy cause gonadal failure more commonly in males, or females?**

Males. Almost all males at any age will have testicular failure.

Females in early reproductive years treated with less than 700 rads usually do not have ovarian dysfunction. Greater than 2000 rads cause ovarian failure in most women.

○   **How does chemotherapy affect gonadal function in males and females?**

In postpubertal males, approximately 90% will have azoospermia while women with the same treatment have 50% to 75% chance of ovarian failure. In prepubertal boys, 83% had azoospermia, while 13% of prepubertal girls had ovarian failure.

CHAPTER 54

Assisted Reproductive Technology

Annette Lee, MD

○ **What are assisted reproductive technologies (ART)?**

Treatments that involve obtaining the eggs (oocytes) from the ovaries in order to facilitate conception in couples experiencing infertility.

○ **What are the types of ART?**

IVF or in vitro fertilization—the eggs are aspirated from the ovary, mixed with the sperm in a dish, and the fertilized eggs (embryos) are transferred to the uterus 3 to 5 days later. In recent years, more than 99% of ART procedures are now IVF. "In vitro" is Latin for "in glass"—in the first IVF procedures, the eggs were fertilized with sperm in glass Petri dishes.

GIFT or gamete intrafallopian transfer—the eggs are aspirated from the ovary and deposited with the sperm in the fallopian tube via laparoscopy (GIFT and ZIFT are much less commonly performed recently because of relative invasiveness of these procedure as compared to IVF).

ZIFT or zygote intrafallopian transfer—eggs are aspirated from the ovary, mixed with the sperm in a dish, and the fertilized eggs (embryos) are transferred to the uterus the next day.

○ **What are the indications for IVF?**

The following was the breakdown in indication for IVF cycles performed in 2004:

Multiple factors (male and female)	18%
Male factor	17%
Diminished ovarian reserve	12%
Multiple factors (female)	12%
Unknown/idiopathic	11%
Other	8%
Ovulatory dysfunction	6%
Endometriosis	5%

○ **Male factor accounts for approximately what percentage of infertility cases?**

40%.

○ **What are normal semen parameters?**

Sperm concentration,	$\geq 20 \times 10^6$/mL.
Motility,	>50%.
Normal Forms,	>14% Kruger strict morphology.

○ **What are oligospermia, asthenospermia, and teratospermia?**

Oligozoospermia	Low concentration of sperm
Asthenozoospermia	Decreased motility
Teratozoospermia	Decreased normal forms

○ **The most severe case of male infertility is?**

Azoospermia—no sperm in ejaculate.

○ **What are the two types of azoospermia?**

Obstructive azoospermia.

Non-obstructive azoospermia—no obstruction can be found. Usually fructose is seen in the semen.

○ **What are four types of procedures used to obtain sperm from patients with obstructive azoospermia?**

TESA: Testicular sperm aspiration

PESA: Percutaneous epididymal sperm aspiration

MESA: Microepididymal sperm aspiration

TESE: Testicular biopsy

○ **What is a varicocele? How does it affect fertility?**

Dilation of the pampiniform plexus of the spermatic vein is known as a varicocele (i.e., a varicosity of the spermatic vein). Approximately 40% of men have a varicocele commonly occurring on the left side because the right spermatic vein drains into the inferior vena cava (a shorter distance). However, a severe varicocele can cause a decrease in sperm production by increasing the temperature of the left testis, which then heats up the right testis.

○ **What is ovarian reserve? How is it assessed?**

Ovarian reserve is essentially the quantity and quality of the remaining egg supply that a woman has. Women are born with approximately 2 million oocytes and do not generate any new eggs. Men constantly produce new sperm. By the age of 37, approximately 200,000 or 10% of the original egg supply remains.

The three most commonly used tests of ovarian reserve are the "Day 3 FSH level," the "Clomiphene Challenge Test," and the "Basal Antral Follicle Count." Essentially, if the pituitary is secreting comparatively high levels of FSH in order to achieve normal follicular development, this indicates a poor egg supply. The Basal Antral Follicle Count is an estimate of the number of small follicles seen without any stimulation.

○ **If elevated FSH and/or estradiol levels are found or the BAFC is low, what is the prognosis for pregnancy?**

This indicates a lower number of remaining eggs and a reduced chance of pregnancy as compared to age-matched controls. Depending on the age of the patient, the ultimate prognosis for pregnancy could be as low as <2% (for patients older than 40).

○ **How is an IVF cycle performed?**

1. Supraphysiologic doses of gonadotropins (FSH and LH) are given to stimulate the ovaries to produce multiple eggs.

2. Ultrasounds are performed to monitor the growth of the follicles containing the oocytes as well as the rising serum estradiol levels resulting from multifollicular development.

3. hCG is given to simulate an "LH surge."

4. Just prior to the time that ovulation would have occurred, the eggs are aspirated from the ovary under transvaginal ultrasound guidance and sedation anesthesia.

5. In the IVF laboratory, the oocytes are incubated with or injected with sperm.

6. Embryo development is carefully observed for the next 2 to 5 days. Using criteria such as the rate of cleavage, cell symmetry, fragmentation rate, etc, the embryologist attempts to choose the embryos with the highest probability of implantation.

7. The selected embryos are transferred into the uterus under ultrasound guidance.

8. The remainder of the embryos may be frozen for the patient's future use.

○ **How do you prevent the patient from having a spontaneous LH surge?**

One of two possible additional medications is typically given in addition to gonadotropins.

1. A GnRH agonist. The GnRH agonist is started in the mid luteal phase of the preceding cycle and will cause ovarian suppression by down regulation and desensitization of pituitary gonadotropin receptors. Once the ovaries are suppressed, the gonadotropins are administered concomitantly with the GnRH agonist until the day of hCG injection. The most widely used GnRH agonist is leuprolide acetate. The GnRH agonist basically "turns off" the pituitary.

2. A GnRH antagonist. The antagonist competes with native GnRH molecules for pituitary binding sites, thus causing an immediate suppressive action and requires a shorter administration period. The GnRH antagonist basically "blocks" the pituitary from seeing GnRH.

○ **How is multifollicular recruitment monitored?**

Recruitment is monitored with daily estradiol measurements and ultrasound.

○ **Why is hCG administered instead of LH to simulate the "LH surge"?**

Human chorionic gonadotropin is given at a dosage of 5,000 to 10,000 IU to aid in final maturation of the oocytes. hCG binds to the LH receptors, having the same effect but with a longer half-life. Recombinant LH is commercially available but would be cost-prohibitive and impractical to use to trigger ovulation.

○ **What is intracytoplasmic sperm injection (ICSI)? What is "conventional insemination"?**

A single sperm is injected into a mature oocyte. Typically this is done if the partner has a very low sperm count, low motility, or poor morphology. With conventional insemination, a microdroplet of media is placed in a Petri dish containing both the oocytes and a sample of washed sperm diluted to approximately 1 to 1.5 million/cc.

○ **How can you tell if the eggs fertilized?**

Oocytes are examined approximately 17 hours after ICSI or insemination. A normal fertilized oocyte will contain two polar bodies and two pronuclei, which will be visible under the light microscope. The presence of one polar body indicates non-fertilization (no male pronucleus) while three polar bodies suggest polyspermy (two male pronuclei).

○   **How many embryos are transferred back to the uterus?**

In general, the younger the patient and the better the prognosis, the fewer the embryos that are transferred. This is because, the older the patient, lower the likelihood that the embryo will implant and develop into a normal pregnancy.

The American Society of Reproductive Medicine guidelines recommend in general:

Under age 35	One to two
Age 35–37	Two to three
Age 38–40	Two to four
Over age 40	Three to five

○   **How can success rates for an IVF program be reported?**

Positive hCG per cycle started, per retrieval performed, or per embryo transfer performed.

Clinical pregnancy (sac seen on ultrasound) per cycle started, per retrieval performed, or per embryo transfer performed.

Positive fetal heartbeat seen on ultrasound per cycle started, per retrieval performed, or per embryo transfer performed.

Live birth per cycle started, per retrieval performed, or per embryo transfer performed.

"Success rates" will obviously differ quite a bit with positive hCG per transfer being much higher than live birth per cycle started as some pregnancies will end in early miscarriage and some cycles will be cancelled prior to embryo transfer. For this reason, it is important to define WHICH success rate is being compared.

○   **What is the SART report?**

99% of the 411+ ART programs in the USA participate in a voluntary reporting system, where the results of each ART cycle are reported to a federal registry, which is maintained by the Centers for Disease Control. The data are tabulated, audited, and posted online at www.sart.org and www.cdc.gov/ART.

○   **In 2005, the live birth rate per cycle started was approximately 28% and per embryo transfer was 34%. How is this calculated?**

In 2005, 134,260 ART cycles were initiated at these reporting clinics. Approximately 12% were cancelled prior to transfer because of low response to stimulation, concurrent illness, etc. These cycles resulted in 38,910 live births (deliveries of one or more living infants) and 52,041 infants were born. More than 1% of babies born in the USA were conceived via IVF.

○   **Approximately how many live births result in singletons, twins, and triplets?**

Singletons, 60%

Twins, 29%

Triplets or more, 5%

Unreported/miscarriage, 6%

○   **What is the age of IVF patients?**

More than two-thirds of IVF patients are 30 to 39 and 20% are older than 40.

○ **According to the 2005 National Report, what are the live birth success rates/ retrieval for women in the following age groups using their own eggs?**

<35	35–37	38–40	41–42	43	44	45	46+
40%	33%	23%	13%	4%	3.3%	1.2%	0

○ **How does frozen embryo live birth rates compare to fresh embryo live birth rates?**

Frozen embryo rates are approximately 10% lower than fresh embryo live birth rates.

○ **What is preimplantation genetic diagnosis (PGD)?**

Is a procedure available to couples whose offspring may be at risk for genetic abnormality. This technique allows couples to have their embryos screened prior to uterine transfer. In the past, the earliest detection for a genetic abnormality was late in the first trimester or early in the second trimester by chorionic villus sampling or amniocentesis. PGD helps relieve the stress involved in deciding whether or not to carry a genetically abnormal fetus to term. PGD coupled with prenatal screening could reduce the number of therapeutic abortions.

○ **How is PGD performed?**

PGD begins by using the technique of embryo biopsy. A single cell is removed from a day 3 embryo containing 6 to 8 cells. The embryo is held with gentle suction by a holding pipette and drilled with acid tyrodes by using the assisted hatching technique. Following hatching, a biopsy tool is brought in close contact with the blastomere. The blastomere is carefully removed and depending on the type of analysis will determine how to process the cell.

○ **What type of disorder can be detected by PGD?**

X-linked disorder.
Single gene defects.
Age related chromosomal aneuploidies.

○ **What are two detection techniques currently used in PGD?**

Fluorescence in situ hybridization (FISH) and polymerase chain reaction (PCR).

○ **In recessive X-linked disorders, what percent chance do males have in receiving a defective X chromosome?**

50%.

○ **Name four X-linked recessive disorders.**

Lesch–Nyhan Syndrome.
Adrenoleukodystrophy.
X-linked mental retardation.
Duchenne's muscular dystrophy.

○ **What are two single gene disorders PGD can detect?**

Cystic fibrosis.
Tay–Sachs disease.

Embryos containing a single gene defect such as cystic fibrosis or Tay–Sachs disease can be identified using the polymerase chain reaction. The PCR amplifies the embryos DNA, thus allowing for the identification of embryos containing the abnormal gene.

○ **Name three dominant disorders.**

1. Myotonic dystrophy.
2. Huntington disease.
3. Marfan syndrome.

○ **What is the definition of aneuploidy?**

Any deviation from an exact multiple of the haploid number of chromosomes, whether more or less.

○ **What are the most common aneuplodies in newborns?**

Trisomy 21.
Sex chromosome aneuploidies.
Trisomy 18.
Trisomy 13.

Studies using FISH technology have demonstrated a high occurrence of aneuploidies in women of advanced maternal age. In theory, this technique should increase the number of normal embryos for uterine replacement.

○ **Name the nine most common screened chromosomes for PGD-FISH aneuploidy testing.**

X, Y, 13, 15, 16, 17, 18, 21, 22.

○ **In mammals, sex is determined by the presence or absence of which chromosome?**

The normal Y chromosome contains a genetic region responsible for producing the testis-determining factor (TDF). Hybridization studies using DNA have shown the presence of the TDF region in XX males. In XY females, the TDF region is lacking. A translocation of a portion of the Y chromosome containing the TDF region has occurred, thus causing XX males and XY females.

○ **Can ART or PGD be used for sex selection?**

Yes, for example if a woman is a carrier for a sex linked disease such as Duchenne's muscular dystrophy, PGD may be performed using FISH to identify the sex of the embryos with the goal of transferring only female embryos.

CHAPTER 55 GnRH and GnRH Analogs

Vasiliki A. Moragianni, MD

○ **What is the olfactory placode?**

The olfactory placode is a plate of ectoderm from which the olfactory organ and GnRH neurons originate.

○ **How many cells migrated from the olfactory area will produce GnRH?**

1,000 to 3,000.

○ **What syndrome develops as a result of olfactory axons' and GnRH neurons' failure to migrate from the olfactory placode?**

Kallmann syndrome.

○ **Describe Kallmann syndrome.**

GnRH deficiency and hyposmia or anosmia. Usually inherited as an X-linked or autosomal recessive disorder with greater penetrance in males.

○ **What is GnRH and where is it produced?**

GnRH is gonadotropin releasing hormone, which is produced by the arcuate nucleus of the hypothalamus.

○ **What is the half-life of GnRH?**

2 to 4 minutes.

○ **What is the cause of the short half-life of GnRH?**

The short half-life of GnRH is a result of rapid cleavage of the bonds between amino acids 5–6, 6–7, and 9–10.

○ **What are the modes of administration of GnRH agonists?**

IV, SQ, nasal spray, sustained-release implants, and IM injections of biodegradable microspheres. The GnRH analogs cannot escape destruction if administered orally.

○ **How many GnRH receptors are in each pituitary gonadotrope?**

10,000 receptors.

○ **What is the structure of GnRH?**

GnRH is 10 amino acid decapeptide arranged in a "hair pin" loop.

○ **How is the GnRH delivered to portal circulation?**

Via an axonal pathway.

○ **Would lesions of GnRH neurons projecting outside the arcuate nucleus and median eminence cause gonadal atrophy and amenorrhea?**

No.

○ **What are the characteristics of GnRH pulsatile secretion during the follicular versus luteal phase?**

Pulsatile secretion is more frequent but lower in amplitude during the follicular phase compared the luteal phase. Lower GnRH pulse frequencies favor FSH secretion.

○ **What is the regulatory mechanism responsible for GnRH pulsatility?**

Pulsatile, rhythmic activity is an intrinsic property of GnRH neurons, although various hormones and neurotransmitters modulate that action.

○ **What is the effect of norepinephrine on GnRH pulsatile release?**

Stimulatory.

○ **What is the effect of dopamine and serotonin on GnRH pulsatile release?**

Inhibitory.

○ **What is the effect of neuropeptide Y on GnRH pulsatile release?**

Stimulatory.

○ **What is the effect of melatonin on GnRH pulsatile release?**

Inhibitory.

○ **What is the effect of endogenous opiates on GnRH pulsatile release?**

Inhibitory.

○ **Each pulse of LH measured in the peripheral blood corresponds to a hypothalamic pulse of GnRH into the portal system in a one-to-one relationship. True or False?**

True. Of note, although FSH is released with LH, FSH pulses are much more difficult to detect because the half-life of FSH is longer than the interval between GnRH pulses.

○ **What is the effect of high progesterone levels on the release of GnRH?**

Progesterone inhibits GnRH pulses at the level of the hypothalamus, and also antagonizes pituitary response to GnRH by interfering with estrogen action.

○ **What is the effect of low progesterone on GnRH pulsatile release?**

Low progesterone enhances the LH response to GnRH at the pituitary level, and allows the FSH midcycle surge.

○ **What are the two phases of GnRH therapy?**

Agonist phase.
Antagonist phase.

○ **What are the indications for GnRH agonist therapy?**

Treatment of endometriosis, uterine leiomyomas, precocious puberty, hirsutism or the prevention of menstrual bleeding in special clinical situations (e.g., in thrombocytopenic patients).
   Potential treatment also includes tumors containing GnRH receptors, such as breast, pancreatic, and ovarian.

○ **GnRH agonists can be used in the treatment of leiomyomatosis peritonealis disseminata and adenomyosis. True or False?**

True.

○ **What are the contraindications to GnRH agonist therapy?**

Pregnancy, undiagnosed abnormal uterine bleeding, breastfeeding, undiagnosed pelvic mass, reproductive tract neoplasia.

○ **What change in the circulating levels of FSH and LH is seen shortly after initiation of the GnRH agonist treatment?**

An increase in FSH and LH (flare effect).

○ **What is the duration of initial agonist phase of GnRH?**

1 to 3 weeks.

○ **What are the mechanisms that cause a hypogonadotropic, hypogonadal state after prolonged administration of GnRH antagonist?**

Desensitization, down-regulation of the receptors and secretion of biologically inactive gonadotropins.

○ **Desensitization is:**

The uncoupling of GnRH peptide/receptor complex from any intracellular actions.

○ **Down-regulation refers primarily to:**

The decrease in the number of cell surface GnRH receptors.

○ **When do desensitization and down-regulation occur?**

1 to 3 weeks after initiation of treatment.

○ **When can GnRH agonist therapy be initiated?**

Mid follicular phase to cycle day 3.

○ **What is the best time for GnRH therapy to be initiated?**

Cycle day 1 to 3.

○ **How should the GnRH therapy be monitored?**

The patient should be seen monthly. Check baseline E2, FSH and progesterone. Recheck serum E2 after 2 months of therapy. Repeat bone density if treatment ≥6 months. Appropriate testing for specific sex steroid-dependent diseases after 3 months of therapy.

○ **When does the GnRH therapy become effective in down-regulating estradiol levels?**

4 to 6 weeks. Patient should be amenorrheic by that time.

○ **What are the adverse effects of GnRH?**

Hot flashes: >75%.
Irregular (light) vaginal bleeding: 30%.
Headache, mood changes, vaginal dryness, arthralgias/myalgias: 5% to 15%.
Allergic reaction: <10%.

○ **At what estradiol level is suppression with GnRH therapy adequate?**

Less than 30 pg/mL.

○ **GnRH agonist treatment can delay the diagnosis of leiomyosarcoma. True or False?**

True. However, its incidence is extremely low, especially in premenopausal women.

○ **What percentage of women going for myomectomy will end up having hysterectomy?**

10% to 30%.

○ **What is the usefulness of GnRH therapy in fibroids?**

Reduction in size of the fibroids and improvement in symptoms by 6 to 8 weeks of therapy. It also increases the hemoglobin and hematocrit concentrations.

○ **What are the preoperative uses of a GnRH agonist?**

Before hysterectomy for stage IV endometriosis, before conservation surgery for severe endometriosis, before resection of an endometrioma, before myomectomy.

○ **Which hormones are dependent on endometrium and fibroid for growth?**

Estrogen (and perhaps progesterone for fibroids).

○ **What is the change in mean uterine volume seen with GnRH agonist treatment?**

30% to 64% decrease in mean uterine size after 3 to 6 months of treatment.

○ **When is maximal response usually noted?**

By 3 months.

○ **What is "add-back" therapy and when is it indicated in GnRH therapy?**

"Add back" refers to adding a progestational or estogen/progestin containing regimen to prevent osteoporosis. After 6 months of therapy (but this is still not a universally accepted paradigm).

○ **How long does it typically take for menses to return after cessation of GnRH agonist treatment?**

4 to 10 weeks.

○ **How long does it typically take for myoma and uterine size to return to pretreatment levels after cessation of GnRH agonist treatment?**

3 to 4 months.

○ **Why might a GnRH agonist be useful in the treatment of hyperandrogenism?**

The assumption is that the hyperandrogenism is at least in part gonadotropin-dependent, and that long-term treatment with GnRH agonists will inhibit LH and to a lesser extent FSH leading to a decline in ovarian function and consequently ovarian androgen production.

○ **Why is GnRH agonist therapy not the recommended first-line treatment for ovarian hyperandrogenism?**

GnRH agonist therapy should be considered only after failure of OCP therapy with or without spironolactone, because GnRH agonist treatment causes severe hypoestrogenism, and add-back therapy is necessary if treatment is continued for more than a few months. Also, agonist is expensive compared with OCPs, and must be given parenterally.

○ **Does the GnRH agonist therapy decrease adrenal androgen secretion?**

No.

○ **Is GnRH agonist therapy effective for treatment of pelvic pain caused by endometriosis in patients who failed treatment with NSAIDs or oral contraceptives?**

Yes.

○ **Which GnRH agonists are FDA-approved in the US for treatment of endometriosis?**

Leuprolide, nafarelin, and goserelin.

○ **What is the FDA-approved length of treatment?**

They are approved for 6 months of continuous use for endometriosis, but may be repeated or continued for an additional 6 months.

○ **Is there a difference in pain reduction using GnRH agonists with low- vs high-dose estrogen as add-back therapy for treatment of pelvic pain caused by endometriosis?**

Yes, add-back with low-dose estrogen (0.625 mg) is more effective in reducing pelvic pain than adding high-dose estrogen (1.25 mg).

○ **What are the pros and cons of evoking a mid-cycle LH surge using GnRH agonists?**

Decreased probability of ovarian hyperstimulation is a possible benefit. It is still not certain whether corpus luteum function following ovulation induction by GnRH agonists is adequate to sustain nidation and continuation of pregnancy or if pharmacological luteal support is mandatory.

○ **What percentage of bone loss occurs in women on GnRH therapy for 6 months?**

5% to 10%.

○ **How are the GnRH antagonists synthesized?**

With multiple amino acid substitutions that allow binding of the antagonist to GnRH receptor and competitive inhibition.

○ **How long does it take to produce suppression by GnRH antagonists?**

It is an immediate action resulting in therapeutic effects within 24 to 72 hours.

○ **Why is response to antagonist treatment faster than to agonist?**

Because there is no initial flare response.

○ **What are the treatment indications for use of GnRH antagonists?**

Endometriosis, prostate cancer, precocious puberty, and female infertility.

○ **What are the disadvantages of using GnRH antagonists?**

Cost, lack of potency, undesirable effects caused by histamine release.

○ **GnRH analogs currently in use have half-lives ranging:**

1.5 to 6 hours.

○ **After binding GnRH, the GnRH receptor peptide complexes do what?**

They migrate toward each other, then internalize, then are degraded and recycled to the cell surface.

○ **GnRH acts on its cell surface receptor on the gonadotrope to increase the release of LH & FSH by which mechanisms?**

Mobilization of calcium from internal sources.
Calcium influx to intracellular sites from the extracellular space.
Calmodulin binding within the cell.

○ **GnRH acts on its cell surface receptor on the gonadotrope to increase the synthesis of LH & FSH by which mechanism?**

Activation of protein kinases to achieve cytosolic protein phosphorylation.

○ **Can hirsutism be treated with GnRH on a long-term basis?**

Yes, if add-back therapy with estrogen and progestin is given.

○ **Are there differences in the isoforms of LH produced by the pituitary during GnRH treatment?**

Yes, there is a large decrease in biologically active LH compared to total immunoreactive LH and thus the ratio of bioactive to total LH is greatly reduced.

○ **What is one of the rare risks of GnRH therapy for submucous myoma?**

There is a small risk (2%) that heavy vaginal bleeding will occur usually 5 to 10 weeks later, because of hemorrhage from degenerating submucous myomata.

○ **What effect does treatment with GnRH have on menstrual bleeding?**

At least 70% of women will achieve amenorrhea; however, some women will have light intermittent bleeding or frequent spotting.

○ **What is the major disadvantage of starting GnRH treatment in the late follicular phase of the cycle?**

There is a greater tendency for a "flare effect" and a longer delay prior to down-regulation.

○ **What is the major disadvantage of starting GnRH treatment in the late luteal phase of the cycle?**

The patient may have an early pregnancy and GnRH is contraindicated in pregnancy.

CHAPTER 56
Laparoscopy and Infertility Surgery

Vasiliki A. Moragianni, MD and
Harry I. Barmat MD

○ **What are the relative contraindications to laparoscopic surgery?**

Extremes of body weight, inflammatory bowel disease, presence of large abdominal mass, and advanced intrauterine pregnancy.

○ **What is the size range of laparoscopes?**

2 to 12 mm.

○ **What are the differences between unipolar and bipolar electrocoagulation systems?**

In a unipolar system, the current passes from the generator through the instrument to a ground plate and then back to the generator.

The bipolar system uses the two insulated jaws of the instrument to carry the current to and from the generator. The tissue between the jaws completes the circuit.

○ **What is capacitive coupling?**

The ability of two conductors to transmit or receive electrical flow while separated by an insulator.

○ **True or False: Capacitive coupling occurs with bipolar electrosurgery.**

False. It only occurs in monopolar circuits.

○ **What is the disadvantage of capacitive coupling?**

The energy may be transferred to intraperitoneal tissues such as bowel and cause an inadvertent burn.

○ **How far out can lateral tissue damage occur?**

2 to 3 cm for unipolar and 1 to 2 cm for bipolar.

○ **What are the differences between cutting and coagulation currents?**

Cutting current provides a constant high-energy waveform.

The coagulation waveform creates an initial high-voltage peak that quickly dissipates and results in desiccation of the outer layer of the tissue and increased tissue resistance.

○   **Define tissue fulguration, coagulation, and desiccation.**

Fulguration means heating the tissue without contacting it. This is beneficial for superficial hemostasis with minimal tissue penetration.

Coagulation means heating the tissue to the extent that the protein loses its innate configuration and becomes solid.

Desiccation means that the liquid component of the tissue evaporates and the tissue becomes dry.

○   **The term laser is an acronym for what words?**

Light amplification by stimulated emission of radiation.

○   **What are the major types of lasers used in surgery?**

CO_2, argon, 532-nm potassium-titanyl-phosphate (KTP/532), and neodymium:yttrium-aluminum-garnet (Nd:YAG).

CO_2 is used mostly for tissue vaporization, whereas KTP and YAG mostly for coagulation.

○   **What preferentially absorbs the energy from the CO_2 laser?**

Water.

○   **What is the approximate depth of penetration of CO_2 laser?**

The depth of destruction is approximately 0.1 to 0.2 mm.

○   **How is coagulation or superficial vaporization achieved with the CO_2 laser?**

By defocusing the beam, which will increase the spot size.

○   **Since the CO_2 beam is not visible to the human eye, how does one visualize the aimed beam?**

By coupling a reddish beam of helium-neon to the invisible CO_2 beam.

○   **What are advantages of using CO_2 laser in laparoscopy?**

It cuts quickly, produces very little thermal damage, and can be used for vaporization, coagulation, and excision.

○   **What are disadvantages of using CO_2 laser in laparoscopy?**

Poor hemostasis, cumbersome equipment, too much laser plume produced, and difficulty aligning the beam and identifying the helium-neon beam.

○   **What is the depth of penetration of argon and KTP lasers?**

0.4 to 0.8 mm.

○   **What substance preferentially absorbs argon and KTP lasers?**

Hemoglobin and hemosiderin preferentially absorb these lasers.

○   **What are the advantages of using fiberoptic lasers in laparoscopy?**

Less cumbersome equipment, very accurate targeting, less plume, better hemostasis, smaller channel needed for fibers, better visualization against abdominal organs.

○   **What are disadvantages of using fiberoptic lasers in laparoscopy?**

They do not cut as well as CO_2 lasers and are less safe because of penetration of both tissue and water.

○   **What is the depth of penetration of YAG laser?**

0.6 to 4.2 mm.

○   **Why are sapphire tips used with YAG lasers?**

The artifical sapphire tip gets attached to the end of the quartz fiber and, by blocking the egress of laser energy from the fiber, absorbs most of the energy.

○   **Why is CO_2 used preferentially over nitrous oxide for achieving pneumoperitoneum?**

CO_2 is rapidly absorbed by blood and therefore less likely to lead to gas embolism.

○   **True or False: In obese patients, a more vertical angle of the Veress needle may be necessary to reach the peritoneal cavity.**

True.

○   **How do you confirm adequate hemostasis during operative laparoscopy?**

Examine the surgical site under water or without the pneumoperitoneum.

○   **What are some of the benefits of laparoscopic surgery compared to laparotomy?**

Decreased hospital utilization, recovery time, patient discomfort, and overall cost.

○   **What are alternatives to the standard umbilical insertion sites for Veress or trocar placement?**

Open laparoscopy, LUQ (beneath the costal margin of the ninth intercostal space at the edge of the lateral rectus or anterior axillary line), posterior cul-de-sac, or transfundal.

○   **Which patients may be good candidates for port placement in the LUQ?**

Patients who have undergone multiple surgeries, are known to have extensive adhesions, or in whom insufflation is not attainable in the conventional spaces.

○   **What are desired intraperitoneal pressures during laparoscopy?**

Upon entry, ≤10 mm Hg; after insufflation, ≤20 to 25 mm Hg.

○   **Describe the "hanging drop test".**

Rapid intake of the drop of fluid as well as the inability to re-aspirate the media. It suggests intraperitoneal location of the Veress needle.

○ **Which vessels can usually be identified by transillumination?**

Superficial epigastric vessels.

○ **The inferior epigastric artery is a branch of what artery?**

External iliac.

○ **When viewed from the laparoscope, the landmarks used to locate the inferior epigastric vessels are:**

The inferior epigastric vessels lie medial to the round ligament and lateral to the obliterated umbilical artery (lateral umbilical ligament).

○ **What is the urachus?**

An embryological remnant representing the original connection of the bladder to the allantois.

○ **What is the classic cardiac murmur associated with a gas embolism?**

Millwheel.

○ **What is the primary concern in a patient that reports increasing abdominal pain after laparoscopy?**

Injury to the bowel or GU tract (ureter, bladder).

○ **True or False: Hemostatic injuries to the bowel serosa do not need to be repaired.**

True.

○ **If after the initial trocal placement visualization reveals small bowel mucosa, what is your next step?**

With the trocar in place, a laparotomy is performed and the enterostomy is closed in a pursestring fashion. This may also be done laparoscopically.

○ **What bladder injuries can be managed expectantly?**

Lacerations smaller than 5 mm may heal spontaneously if a Foley catheter is maintained for 4 to 5 days postoperatively.

○ **Which test can confirm ureteral injury?**

IV indigo carmine is injected and cystoscopy should reveal dye from the ureteral orifices within 5 minutes.

○ **What test would you order on a patient who presents with a fever and right sided abdominal and flank pain two days after undergoing a laparoscopic uterosacral nerve ablation?**

Intravenous pyelogram is the procedure of choice to rule out ureteral injury.

○ **How can one prevent a postlaparoscopy incisional hernia from occurring?**

By fascial closure in ports larger than 7 mm and/or the Z-track method (trocar insertion through skin then moving trocar slightly to create a separate entry through the fascia, (i.e., not "straight-in" insertion).

○ **What is the size range of diagnostic and operative hysteroscopes?**

Diagnostic: 4 to 5 mm.

Operative: 7 to 10 mm.

○ **What is the high-viscosity distension medium used in hysteroscopy?**

Hyskon (32% dextran 70 in dextrose).

○ **What are the low-viscosity distension media used in hysteroscopy?**

Normal saline, glycine (1.5% and 2.2%), 3% sorbitol, and 5% mannitol.

○ **What is the osmolarity of these solutions?**

1.5% glycine and 3% sorbitol—hypo-osmolar.

5% mannitol and 2.2% glycine—iso-osmolar.

○ **What is the safest hysteroscopic medium?**

Normal saline (0.9% sodium chloride).

○ **What is glycine?**

It is a simple amino acid, nonhemolytic, and nonconductive.

○ **What is a dangerous fluid deficit with the use of glycine?**

A fluid deficit of ≥ 500 mL is associated with increased risk of hyponatremia and hypo-osmolality.

○ **What is the advantage of Hyskon over other media?**

It is immiscible with blood. This allows for excellent visualization, even during active bleeding.

○ **What are potential complications of Hyskon use?**

Idiosyncratic anaphylactoid reaction, hypervolemia, hyponatremia, pulmonary edema, and bleeding diathesis.

○ **What is the maximum volume of Hyskon that can be used during a single case?**

500 mL. Greater than that, the incidence of pulmonary edema has been described as high as 1.4%.

○ **What is the recurrence rate of endometriomas after surgical treatment?**

The recurrence rate is approximately 10% to 20%.

○ **What complication can arise after laparoscopic cystectomy for ruptured benign teratoma if abdominal cavity is not irrigated thoroughly?**

Severe chemical peritonitis.

○ **Name the laparoscopic procedures for chronic pelvic pain.**

LUNA (laparoscopic uterosacral nerve ablation) and presacral neurectomy.

○ **What is the term pregnancy rate following laparoscopic salpingoneostomy?**

Rates vary widely but average around 15%.

○ **What is the ectopic pregnancy rate following laparoscopic salpingoneostomy?**

Up to 40% of all pregnancies.

○ **What is the incidence of finding pelvic pathology during a laparoscopy for an infertility evaluation?**

It is reported between 25% and 75%.

○ **Does laparoscopic treatment of endometriosis increase pregnancy rates?**

This is a controversial area. In early stage disease, there is some evidence that pregnancy rates improve postoperatively.

○ **What surgical method is most effective in treating endometriosis?**

Laser ablation, sharp resection, or electrosurgical destruction have all been shown to treat endometriosis. There are insignificant data to support one modality over the other. The method of choice should be based on the surgeon's experience and training.

○ **What percentage of patients experience improvement of pelvic pain after laparoscopic ablation of early stage endometrial implants?**

Approximately 70%.

○ **What is depicted below and what surgical technique is used to correct it?**

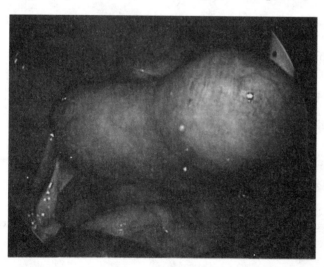

Strassman metroplasty is the classic technique used to unify the bicornuate uterus with divergent uterine horns.

○   **What surgical techniques are available to correct the uterine anomaly seen below?**

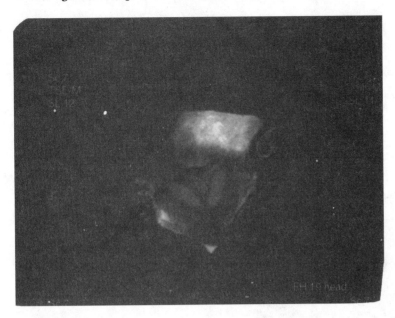

Hysteroscopic resection is the procedure of choice. A Jones metroplasty (wedge resection) is the classic abdominal procedure.

○   **What is the condition seen below?**

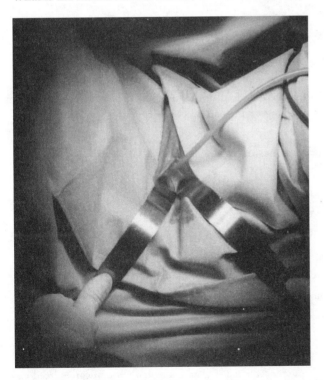

This is a longitudinal vaginal septum. Surgical removal is indicated with complaints of dyspareunia. This is also associated with duplication of the cervix and uterus.

○   **What is the agreement in determining tubal patency between laparoscopy with hydrotubation and hysterosalpingography?**

The agreement between the two methods is ~60%.

○   **Which dyes are used in chromopertubation?**

Leukomethylene blue or indigo carmine.

○   **How is proximal tubal occlusion corrected?**

With either fluoroscopic or hysteroscopic fallopian tube catheterization.

○   **Describe the technique that is used to treat the condition seen below.**

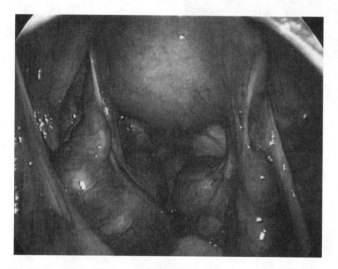

Radial incisions are made in the distal tube. The flaps are then folded back onto the tubal serosa either by heat (Bruhat technique) or sutures. Otherwise consider salpingectomy and proceed with IVF.

○   **What is the overall live birth rate following tubal reanastomosis?**

40% to 80%.

○   **What is the ectopic pregnancy rate following tubal reanastomosis?**

Approximately 5%.

○   **Under what circumstances should tubal reanastomosis not be recommended?**

Residual ampulla length of less than 4 cm, surgical interruption for more than 5 years, or interruption by cautery.

○   **What is the advantages of the da Vinci telerobotic system?**

It may help to convert a laparotomy to a laparoscopic procedure. It has an endowrist with 7 degrees freedom of motion whereas laparoscopically 4 degrees of motion. There is also three-dimensional view.

○   **What portion of the tube is being anastomosed using the da Vinci telerobotic system?**

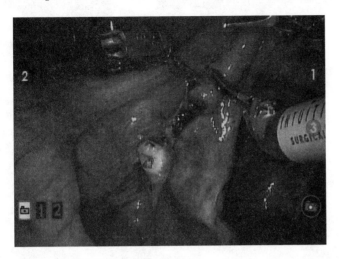

This is an isthmic-isthmic anastomosis procedure showing the grasper holding the proximal cut portion of the left fallopian tube.

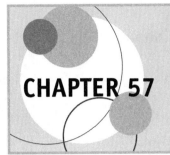

CHAPTER 57 Hyperandrogenism

Radmila Kazanegra MD and
Stephen G. Somkuti, MD, PhD

○ **What are the three sources of androgen production?**

Ovary (25%), adrenal (25%), and periphery (50%).

○ **What is the first step in adrenal steroid synthesis?**

The first step in adrenal steroid synthesis is the combination of acetyl CoA and squalene to form cholesterol, which is then converted into pregnenolone.

○ **In what disease process or syndrome is androstenedione secreted primarily by the ovary compared to normal premenopausal women who have equal production from the ovaries and adrenals?**

PCOS.

○ **What is the source of the increased androstenedione and testosterone seen in polycystic ovaries?**

Almost exclusively from the ovaries.

○ **What is the most potent circulating androgen?**

Testosterone.

○ **What are the effects of excess androgen in prepubertal boys?**

- Penile enlargement, growth of hair in androgen-dependent areas, deepening of the voice, and development of other secondary sexual characteristics.
- Increased height velocity, somatic development, and skeletal maturation.
- Premature epiphyseal fusion leading to short adult height.

○ **What are the effects of excess androgen in prepubertal girls?**

- Hirsutism, acne, and clitoromegaly (e.g., heterosexual precocious puberty).
- Increased height velocity, somatic development, and skeletal maturation.
- Premature epiphyseal fusion leading to short adult height.

○ **What are the effects of excess androgen in pubertal boys?**

Increases the rate of progression of puberty and skeletal maturation, and decreases adult height.

○ **What are the effects of excess androgen in pubertal girls?**

Virilization, primary or secondary amenorrhea, and increased skeletal maturation.

○ **What are the effects of excess androgen in adult males?**

Inhibits gonadotropin secretion that may lead to decreased testes size, testicular testosterone secretion, and spermatogenesis.

○ **What are the effects of excess androgen in adult females?**

Hirsutism, acne, male pattern baldness, menstrual irregularities, oligomenorrhea or amenorrhea, infertility.

○ **What alters sex hormone binding globulin (SHBG) concentrations?**

Increases SHBG	Decreases SHBG
Estrogens	Insulin
Oral contraceptives	Androgens
Hyperthyroidism	Liver disease
Pregnancy	Danazol

○ **True or False: The three newer progestins desogestrel, gestodene, and norgestimate decrease SHBG and increase free testosterone levels.**

False.

○ **What is cyproterone acetate ("Diane")?**

A potent progestational agent used in Europe (not available in the United States) that is usually used along with supplemental estrogen to prevent breakthrough bleeding, but also in the treatment of hirsutism. It inhibits both gonadotropin secretion and blocks the androgen receptor.

○ **How does danazol treatment (in endometriosis) result in hyperandrogenism?**

Danazol (an isoxazol derivative of 17-α ethinyltestosterone) decreases sex hormone binding globulin production and therefore elevates free testosterone levels. It also cross reacts with the androgen receptor.

○ **What happens to SHBG concentration in hyperandrogenic women with PCOS and how does it affect total and free testosterone?**

Low SHBG levels result in normal to slightly increased total testosterone and increased free testosterone.

○ **What percentage of testosterone is unbound or free in the circulation?**

1% to 2%.

○ **What percentage of circulating testosterone is bound to SHBG?**

85%.

○ **What percentage of circulating testosterone is bound loosely to albumin?**

10% to 13%.

○ **What is the immediate precursor to testosterone, and what is the enzyme that aids the conversion and is present in most tissues?**

Androstenedione, which is converted by 17-β-hydroxysteroid dehydrogenase (17-ketosteroid reductase).

○ **What are the metabolic excretory products of testosterone?**

17-ketosteroids.

○ **In ovulatory women, which ovarian cell types are involved in androstenedione (1) secretion and (2) conversion to estrone and estradiol, and which (3) hormone is directly involved in stimulating this cascade?**

(1) Theca cells; (2) granulosa cells; (3) LH.

○ **What happens to LH pulse frequency and amplitude in PCOS patients?**

They are increased.

○ **Which enzyme is involved in the conversion of androstenedione to estrogens, and what is the activity level of this enzyme in PCOS and the resulting effects?**

Aromatase, which is deceased, and as a result excessive amounts of androstenedione are secreted into the circulation, which can be converted peripherally to testosterone by the most tissues.

○ **Which hormone stimulates the granulosa cells to produce aromatase, which converts androgen to estrone and estradiol?**

FSH.

○ **True or False: The low or normal FSH levels found in PCOS patients is because of increased inhibin levels.**

False. Inhibin levels are not increased in PCOS patients.

○ **Anovulation and follicular atresia seen in PCOS patients result from:**

High androgen levels inhibiting aromatase activity and an androgen dominant microenvironment ensues in the follicle, inhibiting further maturation.

○ **What is a major marker of adrenal androgen hypersecretion and why?**

DHEA-S and DHEA, the adrenal glands have sulfokinase activity and little exist in the periphery, DHEA-S also has a long half life with minimal diurnal variation and pulsatility, also DHEA-S has minimal intrinsic androgenic activity; however, small amounts are converted to androstenedione and to testosterone (estrogen) by adrenals/ periphery and therefore with adrenal hyperandrogenism, hirsutism and virilization may exist.

○ **DHEA-S is exclusively secreted from which gland?**

Adrenal.

○ **What is the normal circulating range of DHEA-S in women?**

1.2 to 3.5 μg/mL.

○ **What enzyme is necessary for androgen to exert its effect on skin and external genitalia?**

5-alpha reductase.

○ **What active form is testosterone converted to by 5-alpha reductase?**

Dihydrotestosterone.

○ **What is the effect of IGF-1 on the enzyme 5-alpha reductase?**

5-alpha reductase activity is increased. In anovulatory patients with insulin resistance and hyperinsulinemia, this can intensify hirsutism.

○ **What is the metabolite of dihydrotestosterone that reflects 5-alpha reductase activity?**

3-alpha-androstanediol glucuronide (3α-diol G).

○ **True or False: Hirsutism indicates increased androgen activity in the skin and is directly related to increased 3α–diol G.**

True.

○ **What is the major site of androgen production in hirsute women?**

The adrenal gland.

○ **Drugs associated with hirsutism include:**

Cyclosporine, glucocorticoids, minoxidil, diazoxide, and phenytoin.

○ **True or False: Anabolic steroids used by female athletes may be a cause of hirsutism?**

True.

○ **What is the effect of estradiol on hair growth?**

Estradiol retards the rate and initiation of growth leading to finer, less pigmented, and slower growing hair.

○ **Where do the increased estrogens (slightly hyperestrogenic state) in PCOS derive from and what is a secondary serious consequence as a result?**

Increased number of multiple small follicles and most commonly from aromatization of androgens to estrogens in fat cells. Estradiol is similar in concentrations to the early follicular phase of women who normally ovulate, and estrone concentrations are high. Women with PCOS often have decreased levels of progesterone secondary to oligo- or anovulation, as a result they are at increased risk of endometrial hyperplasia, heavy menstrual bleeding, and endometrial carcinoma (as much as threefold with persistent anovulation).

○ **In women with polycystic ovarian syndrome, most estrogen is derived from:**

Extraglandular aromatization of androstenedione.

○ **Long standing amenorrhea associated with PCOS may predispose to:**

Endometrial hyperplasia and more rarely atypia and carcinoma.

○ **What are some theories driving the PCOS picture with increased ovarian androgen production?**

Increased volume of theca cells, increased LH stimulation of theca cells, potentiation of the action of LH by hyperinsulinemia, different biological activity of the beta-subunits of LH, increased LH receptor expression on thecal cells of PCOS patients, decreased FSH secretion resulting in decreased aromatase activity, leading to decreased potential estrogen production and increased androgen production as a result, and genetic predisposition.

○ **What is the relationship between hyperinsulinemia and hyperandrogenism?**

Insulin amplifies androgen production and both insulin and IGF-1 can enhance the ovarian androgen response to gonadotropin stimulation. Insulin also inhibits hepatic synthesis of SHBG and inhibits hepatic production of IGF-BP-1.

○ **What are the three phases of hair growth?**

Telogen (resting phase), anagen (active), and catagen (period of regression).

○ **What are the ovarian sources of hyperandrogenism?**

Polycystic ovarian syndrome, stromal hyperthecosis, tumors.

○ **Virilizing tumors of the ovary include:**

Sertoli–Leydig, lipoid cell, SCTAT (sex cord tumor with annular tubules), thecoma, gynandroblastoma.

○ **What is the typical age Sertoli–Leydig tumors are seen?**

Age 25 with the vast majority being benign.

○ **Virilization occurring in pregnancy should raise suspicion for:**

The presence of a luteoma, which is an exaggerated reaction of the ovarian stroma to hCG. Hyperreactio luteinalis, also a non-neoplastic condition resulting in bilateral ovarian enlargement, is more commonly seen in conditions of high hCG such as multiple gestations, fetal hydrops, hydatidiform mole, and gestational trophoblastic disease.

○ **What are the typical findings seen in stromal hyperthecosis?**

Similar to PCOS but typically more severe and long standing. Serum testosterone typically >200 ng/dL; both ovaries enlarged, and the ovary rarely responds to stimulation or suppression.

○ **What is the histologic appearance of hyperthecosis?**

Patches of luteinized theca-like cells scattered throughout ovarian stroma. This results in more intense androgenization and a greater degree of insulin resistance.

○   **What are the adrenal sources of hyperandrogenism?**

Cushing syndrome, adult onset congenital adrenal hyperplasia (CAH), tumors.

○   **An ovarian or adrenal androgen-secreting tumor should be suspected when?**

Suspect clinically by history and physical examination; sudden as opposed to gradual onset of symptoms; virilization; ovarian tumor tends to be unilateral—testosterone >150 ng/dL; adrenal tumor—DHEA-S >8 μg/dL.

○   **What percentage of DHEA and DHEA-S are produced by the testes or ovaries?**

Less than 10%.

○   **In men compared to women what is the percentage of testosterone derived from the adrenals or adrenal precursors?**

Less than 5% in men compared to 40% to 65% in women depending on the menstrual phase of the cycle.

○   **True or False: Age at onset and sex of the patient will determine the types of clinical presentation seen with adrenal hyperandrogenism?**

True, in prepubertal girls, clitoromegaly, hirsutism, and acne are seen. In pubertal girls, virilization, primary or secondary amenorrhea, and increased skeletal maturation (which could lead to premature epiphyseal fusion—decreasing adult height). In adult women, hirsutism, acne, male pattern baldness, menstrual irregularities, oligomenorrhea or amenorrhea, infertility, and possibly virilization.

○   **What are some of the causes of adrenal hyperandrogenism?**

Primary adrenal: premature adrenarche; adrenal tumors, androgen-secreting carcinomas.
ACTH-dependent causes: Congenital adrenal hyperplasia (21-hydroxylase deficiency and 11-beta-hydroxylase deficiency); ACTH-dependent Cushing syndrome; glucocorticoid resistance.
Other causes: Hyperprolactinemia, placental enzyme deficiencies (deficient in placental aromatase or sulfatase).

○   **True or False: Hyperprolactinemia may be a cause of adrenal hyperandrogenism?**

True.

○   **What is the daily dose of exogenous androgen intake (DHEA) that can cause signs of hyperandrogenism in female?**

DHEA in daily dose of 50 to 100 mg taken chronically.

○   **What is premature adrenarche?**

The appearance of pubic or axillary hair before age 8 years in girls and 9 years in boys, without other signs of puberty or virilization and without an advance in bone age.

○   **What test determines adrenal hyperandrogenism and if elevated how do you evaluate for adrenal tumors to determine adenoma versus carcinoma?**

Increased serum DHEA and DHEA-S (greater than 500 μg/dL or 13.6 μmol/L) is suggestive of adrenal tumor. Levels do not decrease in response to high-dose dexamethasone. A CT scan or MRI should be done if laboratory results are elevated. Adrenal adenomas have low signal on T-1 and T-2 weighted MRI, whereas carcinomas of the adrenals have enhanced activity on T-2 weighted images.

○ **What is the treatment of choice for adrenal tumors?**

Surgery.

○ **What is the treatment of choice for adrenal carcinomas?**

Surgical exploration followed by chemotherapy.

○ **True or False: Treatment of adrenal hyperandrogenism depends on the diagnosis.**

True, specifically adrenal tumors need surgery and adrenal carcinomas are highly malignant, with cure uncommon; glucocorticoid resistance should be treated with dexamethasone (a glucocorticoid with no intrinsic mineralocorticoid activity) and likely an androgen blocking agent (spironolactone or flutamide); CAH is treated with glucocorticoid and usually a mineralocorticoid.

○ **Adrenal sources of hyperandrogenism are best treated with?**

Low dose steroids including dexamethasone (0.25–0.5 mg/d) or prednisone (2.5–5 mg/d). However, used alone, they are not very effective.

○ **True or False: Hyperandrogenism may be seen in states of cortisol over secretion.**

True.

○ **Frequency of Cushing syndrome causes:**

Diagnosis	% of Patients
Cushing disease	68
Ectopic ACTH	12
Ectopic CRH	<1
Adrenal adenoma	10
Adrenal carcinoma	8
Micronodular/macronodular hyperplasia	1
Major depression/alcoholism	1

○ **The most likely diagnosis in a patient with amenorrhea, marked hypertension, hirsutism, decreased glucose tolerance, and elevated 24 hour urinary excretion of free cortisol is:**

Cushing syndrome.

○ **What are other signs of Cushing syndrome?**

Menstrual irregularities, progressive central obesity, skin atrophy, easy bruising, purple striae, hyperpigmentation (because of increased ACTH—usually ectopic production), fungal infections of the skin and nail (tinea versicolor), psychological changes (emotional lability, agitated depression, mild paranoia, insomnia), ophthalmologic findings, and osteoporosis.

○ **Why is osteoporosis common in Cushing syndrome?**

Because there is decreased bone formation and increased bone resorption because of decreased intestinal calcium absorption and decreased renal calcium absorption (~20% have vertebral compression fractures).

○ **What are the ophthalmologic findings and why are they concerning?**

Increased intraocular pressure in ~25% of patients, which is reversible; however, it can worsen preexisting glaucoma. As a result, glaucoma patients should not receive high-dose glucocorticoid treatment because they can have irreversible deterioration of vision suddenly. In addition, posterior subcapsular cataracts can be caused by chronic hypercortisolism.

○ **What are two screening tests for Cushing syndrome?**

Overnight dexamethasone suppression test (2 mg hs followed by 8 AM cortisol >5 mg/mL) or urinary free cortisol >250 ng/24 h or 3 times above the upper limit of normal. If the 24 h urine is equivocal, then a serum or salivary late evening cortisol may clarify the diagnosis. In addition, an 11 PM cortisol and ACTH-plasma will help determine if the diagnosis is ACTH dependent or not.

○ **What is the treatment for Cushing disease?**

Surgery or pituitary irradiation.

○ **What are the three distinct zones of the adrenal cortex and the corresponding steroids they produce?**

The outer zona glomerulosa (mineralocorticoids), the middle zona fasciculata (glucocorticoids), and the inner zona reticularis (sex steroids).

○ **Who should be screened for adult onset congenital adrenal hyperplasia?**

Hirsute patients who are young and with virilization, high androgens, strong family history of hirsutism, and those with hypertension.

○ **What enzyme converts 17-hydroxyprogesterone to 11-deoxycortisol and when deficient accounts for greater than 90% of cases of congenital adrenal hyperplasia?**

21-hydroxylase (CYP21 A2).

○ **What does 21-hydroxylase deficiency pathophysiologically cause?**

Decreased cortisol synthesis resulting in increased ACTH (corticotropin), causing adrenal stimulation leading to increased androgen production.

○ **What is the different clinical presentations/syndromes of 21-hydroxylase deficiency?**

1. *Classical form:* simple virilizing form (genital ambiguity—female infants have pseudohermaphroditism; males have normal sexual development); salt-wasting form (two-thirds of infants), may cause sexual precocity in children—if not virilized at birth and disorder is overlooked.

2. *Nonclassical form/late-onset form:* symptoms at time of puberty or soon thereafter with acne, hirsutism, menstrual irregularity, and infertility issues likely.

○ **The most common enzyme deficiency leading to hirsutism is:**

21-hydroxylase deficiency.

○ **What percentage of hirsute patients may have 21-hydroxylase enzyme deficiency?**

5%.

○ **The genetic inheritance pattern of congenital adrenal hyperplasia because of 21-hydroxylase deficiency is:**

Autosomal recessive. It is the most common autosomal recessive disorder (more common than sickle cell and cystic fibrosis).

○ **The gene coding for adrenal 21-hydroxylase activity (CYP21) is located on which chromosome?**

Short arm of chromosome 6.

○ **What percentage of Caucasian hyperandrogenic women have late-onset congenital adrenal hyperplasia?**

1% to 2%.

○ **What ethnic background predisposes one to late-onset congenital adrenal hyperplasia?**

Prevalence as follows: Ashkenazi Jews (1/27), Hispanics (1/52), Yugoslavs (1/62), Italians (1/333).

○ **The complete form of 21-hydroxylase enzyme deficiency results in a lack of what two important glucocorticoid and mineralocorticoid steroids?**

Cortisol and aldosterone.

○ **How do you screen for 21-hydroxylase deficiency for late-onset form?**

Obtain 8 AM follicular phase 17-hydroxy progesterone level. It should be less than 200 ng/dL. If it is greater than 200 ng/dL, then an ACTH stimulation test should be performed by high dose (250 μg); most patients' results exceed 1500 ng/dL (43 nmol/L); if borderline results—genotyping should be done.

○ **What is the treatment for congenital adrenal hyperplasia?**

A glucocorticoid and usually a mineralocorticoid.

○ **Other rare enzyme deficiencies that result in hirsutism include:**

3β-hydroxysteroid dehydrogenase (3β-HSD); 11β-hydroxylase deficiency.

○ **How can a 3β-HSD enzyme defect be diagnosed?**

By performing an ACTH stimulation test and finding an elevated 17-hydroxypregnenolone to 17-hydroxyprogesterone ratio (usually >6.0). You will also see an increase in DHEA-S levels. There is now gene sequence testing available as well.

○ **How do you diagnose an 11β-hydroxylase enzyme deficiency?**

Presence of hypertension and an elevated serum DOC (11-deoxycorticosterone).

○ **What is the most common cause of ambiguous genitalia in girls?**

21-hydroxylase deficiency congenital adrenal hyperplasia. Prenatal diagnosis and treatment can prevent formation of ambiguous genitalia.

○ **Between what gestational weeks do exposure to androgen excess results in female sexual ambiguity?**

Between gestation weeks 7 and 12.

○ **What is the serum hormonal LH and testosterone pattern in patients with complete androgen insensitivity (testicular feminization)?**

Increased testosterone and normal LH.

○ **Which chromosome is the gene for the androgen receptor located on?**

The X chromosome. Defects may result in incomplete masculinization of males.

○ **The diagnosis of PCOS requires the presence of:**

Any two of the following three criteria: (1) Oligomenorrhea and/or anovulation; (2) clinical or biochemical signs of hyperandrogenism (free testosterone is most sensitive); (3) polycystic ovaries by U/S (12 or more follicles in each ovary, 2 to 9 mm in diameter; and/or greater than 10 mL ovarian volume per ovary [0.5 × length × width × thickness]). *Note:* other etiologies, such as CAH, androgen secreting tumor, Cushing syndrome, etc., must be excluded.

○ **What are the definitions of amenorrhea and oligomenorrhea?**

Amenorrhea is no menstrual periods for 3 consecutive months or more.
Oligomenorrhea is less than 9 menstrual periods per year.

○ **Define hirsutism.**

Excess terminal and thick pigmented body hair in a male distribution, commonly on upper lip, chin, periareolar area, midsternum, along the linea alba of the lower abdomen.

○ **What percentage of women with PCOS have hirsutism?**

70%.

○ **Do Asian women with PCOS typically have hirsutism?**

No.

○ **Other features of PCOS often include:**

Polycystic appearing ovaries, increased body weight, elevated LH:FSH ratios (>2–3), elevated bioactive LH, insulin resistance.

○ **What lipid abnormalities are typically found in PCOS patients?**

Decreased high-density lipoprotein cholesterol, increased triglycerides.

○ **What test should be ordered in suspected diagnosis of PCOS and why?**

Fasting blood sugar or oral glucose tolerance test to rule out type 2 diabetes (FBS > 125/OGTT > 199) or impaired glucose tolerance (FBS 101–125/OGTT 140–199); free testosterone, if not clinically hyperandrogenic to help with diagnosis; total testosterone, if with hirsutism, to help rule out adrenal or ovarian androgen secreting tumor (>200 concern for ovarian tumor—pelvic U/S; >500–800 concern for adrenal tumor—CT scan or MRI); DHEA-S, if with hirsutism, to rule out adrenal source with CAH or tumor; 17-OH progesterone, if with hirsutism, to rule out CAH (5% of PCOS with hirsutism); prolactin, if with hirsutism, (hyperprolactinemia can cause hirsutism); TSH to rule out thyroid disease.

○ **What percentage of obese women with PCOS develop impaired glucose tolerance or NIDDM by the time they are 40 years old?**

20%.

○ **What is the normal range of total serum testosterone in women?**

Between 20 and 80 ng/dL.

○ **What range of total serum testosterone is typically seen in PCOS patients?**

Just above normal, typically less than 100 ng/dL.

○ **Patients with PCOS typically present with:**

Androgen excess, dysfunctional bleeding, increased body weight, amenorrhea or infertility.

○ **What are the abnormal feedback signals that may result in anovulation in the PCOS patient?**

Estradiol levels may not fall low enough to allow sufficient FSH response for the initial growth stimulus of oocytes. This may result from excess estrogen production because of peripheral conversion in adipose cells of androgens (principally androstenedione) to estrogens. The levels of estradiol may also be inadequate to induce the ovulatory surge of LH.

○ **What happens to the surface area of the ovary in PCOS?**

It typically doubles and the volume may increase up to 2.5-fold.

○ **Histologically, the PCOS ovary is characterized by:**

Multiple atretic and cystic follicles, a thickened tunica (outermost layer), a fivefold increase in stroma.

○ **True or False: Weight loss in the obese PCOS patient may improve hyperandrogenism and anovulation.**

True, this may be our most effective yet most difficult to achieve approach.

○ **An effective pharmacological treatment of ovulatory dysfunction in the infertile PCOS patient is:**

Clomiphene citrate.

○ **What percentage of PCOS patients placed on clomiphene citrate will ovulate?**

80%, with pregnancy rates being approximately 40% to 60%.

○ **The spontaneous abortion rate in PCOS patients is increased and may be as high as:**

50%.

○ **What effects may the insulin-sensitizing agent metformin have in obese women with PCOS?**

It has been reported to lower serum insulin, decrease serum free testosterone, increase serum sex hormone binding globulin levels, and decrease ovarian 17α-hydroxylase and 17,20 lyase activity. However, further studies remain to be done to confirm the clinical utility of metformin in this population of women. The weight loss experienced in these women may also account for the observed effects.

○ **What is metformin?**

An insulin-sensitizing agent that has been used "off label" in hyperandrogenic women with elevated insulin levels to restore menstrual cyclicity and ovulatory function. It does not cause hypoglycemia. It is an FDA category B drug, which has been studied for use with prevention of spontaneous abortions in PCOS patients (one study showed 6 SABs out of 68 pregnant PCOS patients on metformin versus 13 SABs out of 31 pregnancies in PCOS patients not on metformin). Metformin has also been considered for use in prevention of gestational diabetes, preliminary findings look hopeful. Metformin does cross the placenta and is excreted in breast milk.

○ **What are metformin's mechanisms of action?**

(1) To suppress hepatic glucose output; (2) to decrease intestinal absorption of glucose; (3) to increase insulin-mediated glucose utilization in peripheral tissues; (4) to have an antilipolytic effect that decreases fatty acid concentrations, as a result decreasing gluconeogenesis.

○ **What is the therapeutic effects of combined OCPs?**

(1) Decreased LH secretion, resulting in a decrease in ovarian androgen production; (2) increased hepatic production of SHBG, resulting in decreased free testosterone; (3) decreased adrenal androgen secretion; (4) regular menses, resulting in prevention of endometrial hyperplasia.

○ **Why should a birth control method always be used with spironolactone?**

Because it can cause antiandrogen effects on a fetus preventing normal external genitalia in a male fetus.

○ **For women who desire pregnancy and have PCOS with infertility, what would be some management options?**

(1) Weight loss and diet modification, (2) Clomid, (3) metformin and combined Clomid/metformin.

○ **How should metformin be dosed and what are some contraindications?**

Because of GI side effects, the dose should be increased slowly to a maximum of 2000 mg qd with 1 to 2 weeks elapsing between increases in doses. Contraindications: avoid in renal insufficiency, CHF, sepsis; it should be stopped prior to IV contrast; should not be given with cimetidine as it competes for renal clearance; creatinine should be checked prior to starting metformin (and should be less than 1.4) and make sure normal fluid intake.

○ **What surgical treatments are available for PCOS/hirsutism?**

Historically, wedge resection was used, now in disfavor because of postoperative adhesions. Laparoscopic YAG laser drilling of the ovary has been used with some success in otherwise medically refractory patients to induce ovulation. Laparoscopic ovarian diathermy (electrocautery) was compared to gonadotropin therapy in two randomized controlled trials, resulting in similar success rates ($\sim$55% pregnancy rates), with lower multiple gestation rates.

○ **When should surgical treatments be used?**

When the only cause of infertility is PCOS and additional tubal factors, endometriosis, and oligospermic male partners have been excluded. Then the pregnancy rates are 80% to 87% compared to 14% to 29%. In addition,

Clomid and metformin should first be attempted, BMI should be less than 30, and in women with an increased LH concentration of greater then 10 IU/L.

○ **What are the possible treatments of hirsutism?**

- Hair removal and weight losshow structurer came to know about the 2 levels?
- Vaniqa (eflornithine hydrochloride cream 13.9%)
- OCP
- Androgen receptor-competitive inhibitors
  - Spironolactone
  - Flutamide
  - Finasteride
  - Cyproterone acetate
- Gonadotropin-releasing hormone agonist
- Glucocorticoid therapy
- Insulin-lowering agents
- Combined therapy with an estrogen-progestin contraceptive, metformin plus flutamide

○ **What is the mechanism of action of spironolactone?**

It blocks the effects of androgens in the periphery at the receptor and has a suppressive effect on enzymes important in the biosynthesis of androgens.

○ **What is the recommended dose of spironolactone for the treatment of hirsutism?**

100 to 200 mg/d.

○ **What is the new specific 5-alpha reductase inhibitor that may prove useful in treating hirsutism?**

Finasteride.

○ **What is the medication used for hirsutism and prostate cancer that is an androgen receptor blocker and has side effects of green urine, skin and scalp dryness?**

Flutamide.

○ **What is the minimum period of treatment necessary to see clinical improvement in hirsutism?**

3 to 6 months.

○ **What is leptin?**

A protein hormone produced by adipocytes that increases general metabolism. Abnormalities may contribute the metabolic disturbances resulting in infertility in PCOS patients.

○ **What is the mechanism of action of testolactone?**

Inhibits conversion of androgens to estrogens.

○ **True or False: Hyperandrogenic women are at increased risk for cardiovascular disease and development of adult onset diabetes.**

True.

○ **Define android obesity.**

A waist:hip ratio greater than 0.85. It is more metabolically active and results in higher free fatty acid concentrations leading to hyperglycemia.

○ **What is "HAIR-AN" syndrome?**

Hyperandrogenism, insulin resistance, acanthosis nigricans.

○ **What is acanthosis nigricans?**

Grey-brown, velvety, occasionally verrucous discoloration of the skin (neck, groin, axillae) associated with hyperinsulinemia. It is characterized histologically by papillomatosis and hyperkeratosis.

○ **What are the three types of hair, which are most affected by androgens?**

Lanugo, vellus, and terminal (most affected).

○ **What is hypertrichosis?**

Excess terminal or vellus hair in areas not androgen dependent.

○ **What drugs may cause hypertrichosis as an adverse effect?**

Phenytoin, penicillamine, diazoxide, minoxidil, **or** cyclosporine.

○ **What medical conditions may be associated with hypertrichosis?**

Hypothyroidism, anorexia nervosa, malnutrition, porphyria, and dermatomyositis.

○ **Is there a place for gonadotropin-releasing hormone agonist therapy in the treatment of hirsutism?**

Yes, typically, in the HAIR-AN patient, or hyperthecosis patient that has been resistant to conventional first-line therapies. Regimen consists of low-dose add-back using HRT or OCPs to avoid hypoestrogenism.

○ **Hair loss after pregnancy is explained by:**

The anagen phase of hair growth, which is prolonged by estrogens and increases the absolute number of hair follicles in this phase. Once the high estrogen levels end, many hair follicles enter telogen simultaneously, and are shed as new hairs begin to grow.

○ **What is the Ferriman–Gallway score?**

A grading system (1–4), scoring amount of hair growth and the location. This then can be used to follow objectively and quantitate hair growth.

CHAPTER 58
Disorders of Prolactin Secretion

Stephanie J. Estes, MD

○ **What are the causes of hyperprolactinemia?**

Pituitary disease (most common 50%)

- Prolactinomas
- Lymphocytic hypophysitis
- Empty sella syndrome
- Cushing disease
- Growth hormone secreting tumors

Hypothalamic disease (rare)

- Craniopharyngiomas, meningiomas, sarcoidosis, metastasis of other tumors
- Vascular
- Pituitary stalk section

Neurologic

- Chest wall lesions (chest trauma, herpes zoster; with neural mechanism similar to suckling)
- Spinal cord lesions
- Breast stimulation

Medications

- Phenothiazines
- Tricyclic antidepressants, SSRIs
- Narcotics
- Centrally acting antihypertensive agents (methyldopa, reserpine)
- Verapamil (unknown mechanism; does not occur with other Ca channel blockers)
- Oral contraceptive pills
- Antiemetics (metoclopramide)

Idiopathic hyperprolactinemia

Decreased clearance of prolactin

- End-stage renal disease
- Big prolactin = macroprolactinemia (prolactin circulates in large aggregates)

Other

- Pregnancy
- Hypothyroidism
- Cirrhosis
- Adrenal insufficiency

○ **What is the predominant physiologic prolactin inhibitory factor?**

Dopamine.

○ **What are other prolactin inhibitory factors?**

GnRH-associated protein.

GABA.

○ **Name five prolactin releasing "factors".**

Serotonin.

TRH (thyrotropin-releasing hormone).

VIP (vasoactive intestinal peptide).

Opioid peptides.

PRLrP (prolactin-releasing peptide).

Estrogens and the hormonal milieu of pregnancy.

GHRH (growth hormone-releasing hormone).

GnRH (gonadotropin-releasing hormone).

○ **What is the most common pituitary tumor?**

Prolactin secreting adenoma.

○ **How does elevated prolactin cause amenorrhea?**

Prolactin inhibits the pulsatile secretion of GnRH.

○ **What conclusions can be made based on prolactin serum levels?**

- Greater than 15 to 20 ng/mL considered abnormal by most laboratories.
- Slightly increased values (21–40 ng/mL) should be rechecked as it may reflect response to physiologic stimuli rather than true hyperprolactinemia.
- 20 to 200 ng/mL can be found in any patient with hyperprolactinemia.
- >200 ng/mL usually indicates presence of lactotroph macroadenoma (= more than 1 cm in diameter).
- >1000 ng/mL suggestive of macroadenomas greater then 2 cm in diameter.

○ **What is the most common cause of mildly elevated prolactin levels?**

Stress.

○ **If a prolactin level is mildly elevated, what instructions are important for the patient to know when obtaining her repeat prolactin laboratory testing?**

Optimal time to obtain a prolactin level is 11 AM. Patient should not have recently awakened, had recent breast stimulation, exercise or a meal.

○ **True or False: Symptoms of hyperprolactinemia correlate with its severity.**

True

- Severe hyperprolactinemia (>100 ng/mL): typically associated with overt hypogonadism, subnormal estradiol levels and its consequences (i.e., amenorrhea, hot flushes, vaginal dryness).

- Moderate hyperprolactinemia (50–100 ng/mL) usually causes amenorrhea or oligomenorrhea.
- Mild hyperprolactinemia (20–50 ng/mL) may cause only insufficient progesterone secretion and thus short luteal phase. Even without menstrual abnormalities, these levels of prolactin are associated with infertility.

○ **What is the association between hyperprolactinemia and galactorrhea?**

Premenopausal women: most patients with hyperprolactinemia do not have galactorrhea; most patients who have galactorrhea have normal prolactin levels.

Postmenopausal women: as they are markedly hypoestrogenemic, the galactorrhea is rare. In this group of patients, hyperprolactinemia is recognized only when adenoma becomes so large that causes headache or visual disturbances.

○ **What percentage of women with high prolactin levels have galactorrhea?**

33%.

○ **What are the physiologic stimuli that might slightly increase serum prolactin levels?**

Sleep, strenuous exercise, occasionally emotional or physical stress, intense breast stimulation, high protein meals.

○ **What occurs to the prolactin concentration in pregnant women?**

It increases from the normal range (10–25 ng/mL) to 200 to 400 ng/mL, as estrogen suppresses the hypothalamic dopamine.

○ **What are the physiologic prolactin concentrations after delivery and in response to suckling?**

Basal rate is high comparing to nonpregnant state and may further increase in response to suckling (up to few hundreds ng/mL). Over 4 to 12 weeks, the prolactin level decreases to normal and there is no longer a rapid release of prolactin with each suckling episode.

○ **Does breast examination or nipple stimulation increase prolactin secretion in nonlactating women?**

No. The magnitude of the increase in prolactin level is directly proportional to the degree of preexisting lactotroph hyperplasia caused by estrogen.

○ **Can prolactin adenomas secrete other hormones?**

Yes. Approximately 10% secrete growth hormone as well.

○ **Can other pituitary hormone levels be affected by a mass lesion in the area of sella turcica?**

Yes. Thus, levels of all pituitary hormones should be checked in such situation.

○ **Are lactotroph adenomas more frequent with multiple endocrine neoplasia type 1?**

Yes. Prolactinomas occur in 20%.

○ **Are lactotroph tumors benign in nature?**

In most cases, yes; but rare tumors can be malignant and metastasize.

○ **What is the natural history of microadenomas?**

Studies with 4 to 6 years of follow-up show that 95% of microadenomas do not enlarge.

○ **What is the treatment for hyperprolactinemia?**

Dopamine agonists are the first line of treatment as they decrease hyperprolactinemia and the size and secretion of most lactotroph adenomas.

○ **What is the rationale for treatment of hyperprolactinemia?**

Existing or impending neurologic symptoms because of the size of lactotroph adenoma.

Endocrine effects of hypogonadism: in women infertility, oligomenorrhea or amenorrhea, hypoestrogenemia (which may lead to osteoporosis); in men decreased libido and energy, impotence, loss of sexual hair, osteoporosis, possibly loss of muscle mass.

Usually galactorrhea is not sufficiently bothersome to require treatment.

○ **Which dopamine agonists are available for the treatment of hyperprolactinemia?**

Cabergoline—used once or twice weekly, probably more effective and less nauseating than bromocriptine, effective in patients resistant to bromocriptine as well.

Bromocriptine—used at least twice a day. It has been on the market for more than 20 years, which makes it a safe choice for pregnant patients.

Pergolide—no longer recommended as it has been shown to cause valvular heart disease.

Quinoglide, bromocriptine depo—are still being studied.

○ **When can one expect prolactin level to fall after initiation of dopamine agonist therapy?**

Usually it happens within 2 to 3 weeks.

○ **Dopamine agonists restore ovulation in what percentage of cases?**

90%.

○ **What percentage have cessation of galactorrhea after bromocriptine therapy?**

50% to 60% have cessation, 75% have reduction in galactorrhea. Thus, cessation of galactorrhea is slower and may not occur as frequently as resumption of ovulation/menses.

○ **When can one expect decrease in size of adenoma after initiation of dopamine agonist therapy?**

It is always preceded by fall in prolactin levels. One may see tumor shrinking after 6 weeks, though usually it is observed within 6 months.

○ **When can one expect improvement in visual symptoms after initiation of dopamine agonist therapy?**

Patient should be reassessed within 1 month, although improvement may occur within 24 to 72 hours.

○ **What are the side effects of therapy with dopamine agonists?**

Most common is nausea. Others include postural hypotension, headache, dizziness, constipation, fatigue. Less common are vomiting, nasal congestion, depression, Raynaud phenomenon. Rare ones are cardiovascular events.

○ **How can side effects of dopamine agonists be minimized?**

Start with half dose, take it with food, give medication at bedtime, then add second dose in the morning after the patient is tolerating the night dose. In women, nausea can be avoided by vaginal administration.

○ **What is the regimen for bromocriptine therapy?**

Start at 1.25 mg after dinner or at bedtime for 1 week, then increase to 1.25 mg twice a day. After 1 month, evaluate for side effects and prolactin levels. May increase the dose up to 5 mg bid. The dose that results in normal serum prolactin level should be continued.

○ **What is the regimen for cabergoline therapy?**

Start with 0.25 mg twice a week (FDA-approved dose) or 0.5 mg once a week. May increase the dose gradually up to 1.5 mg 2 to 3 times a week.

○ **What is the definition of a microadenoma? Of a macroadenoma?**

Microadenoma is less than 10 mm in diameter.
Macroadenoma is 10 mm in diameter or greater.

○ **What percentage of hyperprolactinemic women achieve pregnancy with dopamine agonist therapy?**

80%.

○ **What group of patients with prolactin adenomas should undergo surgery?**

Patients with symptoms of hyperprolactinemia that did not respond to medical therapy, patients with adenomas that do not shrink during therapy or patients with giant lactotroph adenomas (>3 cm) wishing to become pregnant.

○ **What is the best single predictor of persistent cure of prolactin adenoma with surgery?**

Serum prolactin concentration of 5 ng/mL or less on the first postoperative day.

○ **What is the role of radiation therapy in patients with lactotroph adenomas?**

It decreases the size and secretion of adenoma but it occurs slowly and prolactin may be elevated many years after treatment. Radiation is limited to patients after the debulking surgery of very large macroadenomas. With this treatment, there is 50% chance of loss of anterior pituitary hormone secretion during subsequent 10 years.

○ **Is there a place for estrogen therapy in patients with hyperprolactinemia?**

There is a narrow group of patients that may benefit from estrogen therapy—patients with lactotroph microadenomas causing hyperprolactinemia and hypogonadism, not responding or not tolerating dopamine agonist treatment; patients with hyperprolactinemia and amenorrhea because of antipsychotic agents. In such patients, prolactin levels should be monitored regularly as there is a small risk of increasing the size of adenoma.

○ **What are the risks of complications of microadenomas versus macroadenomas during pregnancy?**

The risk is small for microadenomas at approximately 5% to 6% level, whereas for macroadenomas it might be as high as 36%. Complications are—increase in adenoma size, headache, visual impairment, diabetes insipidus.

○ **What is the treatment of lactotroph microadenomas before and during pregnancy?**

Treatment is with dopamine agonists, bromocriptine is the preferred medication as there is long history of its safe usage during pregnancy. The goal is to decrease prolactin level to normal before conception (patient should attempt pregnancy after a few months of normal menses and prolactin levels) and stop the medication once pregnancy is confirmed. Medication may be restarted (and is effective) if complications arise.

○ **Is the management of patients with macroadenomas any different from those with lactotroph microadenomas before and during pregnancy?**

Patients with a macroadenoma and those with evidence of compression of optic chiasm should be treated with transsphenoidal surgery with possible postoperative radiation before pregnancy. If complications arise during pregnancy, the treatment of choice is bromocriptine. If the adenoma does not respond to medical therapy and vision is severely impaired, patients undergo surgery in the second trimester or after delivery if it is diagnosed in the third trimester. Pregnancy should be discouraged in patients not responsive to medical therapy. Follow-up depends on size of adenoma and complications.

○ **What therapeutic options should be considered in patients desiring pregnancy but not responding to dopamine agonists?**

Transsphenoidal surgery or ovulation induction.

○ **May patients with prolactin adenomas breastfeed? Does this depend on the size of tumor?**

It is safe to breastfeed with a microadenoma or if there is an asymptomatic macroadenoma. Symptomatic patients with macroadenomas should be treated. If patients are receiving dopamine agonists, nursing should be stopped.

○ **Do patients with microadenomas or macroadenomas have increased incidence of spontaneous miscarriage or other complications of pregnancy?**

No.

○ **When may treatment with dopamine agonists for hyperprolactinemia be stopped?**

After 1 year, the dose can be decreased. If the prolactin levels have been normal for 2 years and there is no evidence of adenoma on MRI, then cessation of therapy can be considered. Prolactin level should be checked periodically as there is a significant rate of recurrence (24%–85% recurrence rate depending on the cause and study during 4–5 years of follow-up).

○ **What is the treatment of hyperprolactinemia secondary to hypothyroidism?**

Thyroid hormones only.

○ **Does the decidual endometrium have any endocrine function?**

Yes, the secretion of prolactin.

○ **During pregnancy, what areas contribute to prolactin secretion?**

The uterus, maternal and fetal pituitaries.

○ **Is the decidual secretion of prolactin affected by dopamine agonist treatment?**

No.

○ **What area is typically being invaded in patients with prolactin levels >2000?**

Cavernous sinuses.

○ **How frequently do prolactin levels need to be followed in a patient with a macroadenoma?**

Every 3 months until stable.

○ **When treating macroadenomas, is it necessary to check frequent (every 3 month) MRIs?**

No. Serum prolactin can be followed alone. MRI should be obtained 6 months after treatment.

○ **What is the classic visual field impairment seen in patients with macroadenomas?**

Bitemporal hemianopsia.

○ **What is the empty sella syndrome?**

A syndrome associated with the incomplete development of the sellar diaphragm that allows the subarachnoid space into the fossa of the pituitary.

○ **Does the empty sella syndrome progress eventually resulting in pituitary failure?**

No.

○ **What is Sheehan syndrome?**

Panhypopituitarism following infarction and necrosis of the pituitary secondary to postpartum hemorrhage.

○ **How does the hypothalamus maintain suppression of the pituitary prolactin secretion?**

The hypothalamus delivers a prolactin inhibiting factor through the portal circulation.

○ **How does suckling affect prolactin secretion?**

Suckling inhibits the production of prolactin inhibiting factor.

○ **How does dopamine suppress prolactin?**

Dopamine binds lactotroph cells and blocks prolactin secretion.

○ **If medication is the cause of galactorrhea, will discontinuation of the medication resolve the galactorrhea?**

Yes, usually within 3 to 6 months.

○ **How is hypothyroidism associated with galactorrhea?**

Excess TRH is released and acts as prolactin releasing factor, stimulating prolactin release from the pituitary.

○ **Can excessive estrogen lead to galactorrhea?**

Yes, estrogen can suppress the hypothalamus reducing the production of prolactin inhibiting factor.

○ **Can prolonged suckling stimulate release of prolactin and subsequent galactorrhea from a nonpregnant patient?**

Yes.

○   **Can mild hirsutism occur with ovulatory dysfunction caused by hyperprolactenemia?**
Yes.

○   **Can breast implants lead to galactorrhea in women with normal levels of prolactin?**
Yes, because of the stimulation of the sensory afferent nerves.

○   **Do normal ovulatory menstrual periods occur in women with hyperprolactinemia if they are given exogenous GnRH?**
Yes.

○   **What are the most common tumors associated with delay in pubertal development?**
Prolactinomas and craniopharyngiomas.

○   **What is the most common symptom patients report with intrasellar expansion?**
Headache.

○   **Can primary hypothyroidism appear similar to a pituitary tumor in imaging studies?**
Yes, because of the hypertrophy of the thyrotrophs.

○   **Is galactorrhea more suspicious for malignancy if produced from a single alveolar duct?**
Yes.

○   **What is the "hook effect," when interpreting prolactin levels?**
In the presence of a macroadenoma, markedly elevated prolactin levels (5000 ng/mL) can appear as mildly elevated levels (20–200 ng/mL), which is from the hook effect. This occurs because both the capture and signal antibodies in the sandwich immunoassays are saturated giving an artificially low result. Repeat the test with a 1:1000 dilution to evaluate the true prolactin level.

CHAPTER 59

Miscarriage, Recurrent Miscarriage, and Pregnancy Termination

Namitta Kattal, MD

○ **What is the definition of miscarriage?**

Involuntary termination of pregnancy before 20 weeks of gestation (dated from LMP) or below a fetal weight of 500 g.

○ **What is "habitual abortion" or recurrent pregnancy loss?**

Three or more consecutive SABs.

○ **What percentage of pregnancies end in spontaneous abortion?**

12% to 15% of clinically recognized pregnancies end in SAB.

○ **What is the incidence of two or more consecutive spontaneous abortions?**

0.4% to 2%.

○ **What is the risk of subsequent spontaneous abortion in a patient with three consecutive miscarriages?**

30% to 45%.

○ **What is the risk of subsequent spontaneous abortion in a patient with three consecutive miscarriages and with at least one liveborn?**

30%.

○ **Name three independent risk factors for spontaneous abortion.**

Increasing parity, maternal age, and paternal age.

○ **What are the causes of recurrent SAB?**

Genetic, anatomic, immunologic, inherited thrombophilias, infectious, endocrine, environmental.

○ **What is the prevalence of major chromosomal abnormalities being present in either partner of a couple with two or more pregnancy losses?**

In 4% to 8% of couples with recurrent pregnancy loss, one or the other partner may have a chromosomal abnormality.

○ **What is the most common single type of karyotypic abnormality present in spontaneous abortion?**

Aneuploidy, especially trisomies.

○ **What percentage of first trimester spontaneous abortions have karyotypic abnormalities?**

50%.

○ **What percentage of second trimester spontaneous abortions have karyotypic abnormalities?**

30%.

○ **What percentage of stillbirths have karyotypic abnormalities?**

3%.

○ **What are the most common types of abnormal karyotypes found?**

Trisomy (50%), monosomy 45,X (20%), triploidy (10%), and structural abnormalities (5%).

○ **What is the most common single chromosomal abnormality?**

45,X.

○ **What is the occurrence of uterine anomalies in those with repeated abortion?**

6% to 7%.

○ **What is the most common uterine anomaly?**

Septate uterus.

○ **What is the etiology of uterine anomalies?**

Müllerian ducts fusion defects that occur between 6 and 10 weeks in fetal development.

○ **Name some causes of cervical incompetence.**

Vigorous D&C, cervical conization, laceration of the cervix, or congenital.

○ **Is the prevalence of urinary tract anomalies increased in patients with all uterine malformations?**

Only for those with unicornuate/bicornuate uterus or uterus didelphys, NOT in those with septate uterus.

○ **What is the approximate incidence of spontaneous abortion associated with the unicornuate uterus?**

50%.

○ **What is the spontaneous abortion rate for those with either a septate or a bicornuate uterus?**

65% and 30% to 40%, respectively.

○ **What is the spontaneous abortion rate following surgical correction of bicornuate and septate uteri?**

It decreases to 15%.

○ **What effect does DES (diethylstilbestrol) have on exposed patients who are able to conceive?**

It may have an increased spontaneous abortion rate, preterm labor and delivery, as well as an increase in the ectopic pregnancy rate.

○ **What is the fetal survival rate in patients with cervical incompetence who receive a cerclage?**

From 20% to 80%.

○ **What percentage of habitual aborters have corpus luteal defects?**

30% to 40%.

○ **What percentage of recurrent aborters have abnormal placentation?**

6%. Most are of the circumvallate type.

○ **What percentage of habitual aborters conceive post myomectomy?**

Approximately 50%.

○ **Name three endocrinologic abnormalities associated with spontaneous abortion.**

Thyroid diseases (both hyper and hypo), uncontrolled diabetes mellitus, and luteal phase defect.

○ **Name two organisms associated with spontaneous abortion.**

Mycoplasma and *Ureaplasma*. Other infections implicated in early fetal loss include *Chlamydia*, *Toxoplasma gondii*, *Listeria*, herpes, and cytomegalovirus.

○ **Name tests for evaluation of fetal loss caused by antiphospholipid syndrome.**

Lupus anticoagulant and anticardiolipin antibody.

○ **What is the effect of smoking on the abortion rate?**

Those who smoke more than 14 cigarettes daily have a 1.7 times greater chance of abortion.

○ **What is the risk of abortion in those women who have more than 2 drinks/day of alcohol?**

A twofold greater abortion risk.

○ **Does caffeine influence fertility?**

>300 mg caffeine (three cups) may be associated with decreased chance of conception and a twofold miscarriage risk.

○ **What effect will 5 rads have on the abortion rate?**

Irradiation of less than 5 rads will have no effect.

○ **What percentage of intrauterine adhesions are caused by spontaneous and induced abortions?**

Two-thirds.

○ **Does hyperglycemia affect miscarriage rates?**

Yes, studies suggest that achieving euglycemia may lower the miscarriage rate.

○ **What androgens have been associated with miscarriage rates?**

Androstenedione, testosterone.

○ **Patients experiencing spontaneous, recurrent abortion would benefit from what established testing?**

Category	Recommended Tests	Other Tests
Genetic	Karyotype, both parents	
Anatomic	HSG or sonohysterogram or hysteroscopy	MRI as indicated
Immunologic	Lupus anticoagulant Anticardiolipin antibody	
Thrombophilias	Factor V Leiden Prothrombin gene mutation Activated protein C resistance Homocysteine MTHFR* Protein C Protein S Antithrombin III	
Endocrine	TSH, fasting blood glucose, HbA$_{1c}$ Prolactin	
Infectious	If symptomatic	Ureaplasma, mycoplasma cultures
Environmental	History	

*Methylenetetrahydrofolate reductase

○ **When is the appropriate time to do such a workup?**

After three spontaneous abortions or in women older than 35 after two spontaneous abortions.

○ **What is the risk of ectopic pregnancy in those experiencing repetitive spontaneous abortion?**

A fourfold increased risk.

○ **What is the miscarriage rate, if embryonic cardiac activity is seen sonographically at 6 weeks gestation? If seen at 8 weeks?**

6% to 8% and 2% to 3%, respectively.

○ **What is the occurrence of threatened miscarriage and what percentage results in abortion?**

Threatened miscarriage occurs in 30% to 40% of human gestations leading to abortion in half of these.

○ **How many weeks after fetal death with retained products of conception may consumptive coagulopathy with hypofibrinogenemia occur?**

5 weeks.

○ **What percentage of spontaneous abortions become infected?**

1% to 2%.

○ **What is the risk of death from abortion?**

0.6/100,000 for elective abortions.

○ **Menstrual extraction is used to terminate pregnancies at what gestational age?**

5 to 6 weeks.

○ **Suction or vacuum curettage is used to terminate pregnancies at what gestational age?**

7 to 13 weeks.

○ **D&E is defined as termination of pregnancy at what gestational age?**

13 weeks or greater.

○ **Are prophylactic antibiotics recommended for pregnancy termination?**

ACOG recommends use of 100 mg doxycycline prior to procedure followed by 200 mg postoperative or metronidazole 500 mg bid for 5 days.

○ **What is the most common cause of postabortal pain, bleeding, and low-grade fever?**

Retained gestational tissue or clot (27.7/100,000 induced abortions).

○ **What is the optimal management for postabortal pain, bleeding, and fever?**

Oral antibiotics and ergot medications followed by repeat uterine evacuation performed under local anesthesia in an ambulatory center, if retained products are suspected.

○ **How effective is RU 486 when used with misoprostol in first trimester medical pregnancy termination?**

97% had successful pregnancy termination, if given by 49 days from the last menstrual cycle.

○ **How effective is methotrexate when used with misoprostol in first trimester medical pregnancy termination?**

96% had successful pregnancy termination, if given by 63 days from the last menstrual cycle.

○ **What agent is commonly used for multifetal, selective reduction to prevent cases of extreme prematurity?**

Intracardiac KCl (0.05–3 mL).

○ **What percentage of abortions are performed within the first 12 weeks of pregnancy?**

90%.

○ **Why is local anesthesia preferable to general anesthesia with pregnancy termination?**

General anesthesia is associated with greater risk of perforation, visceral injury, hemorrhage, and death.

○ **What morbid events can occur with the use of local anesthetics?**

Convulsions, syncope, and fever have been associated with the use of local anesthetics.

○ **What is the risk of surgical perforation in the first trimester patient?**

9.4/100,000 induced abortions.

○ **Which country has the highest abortion rate among all Western Nations?**

The United States of America.

○ **Suction curettage accounts for what percentage of all abortion procedures?**

75%.

○ **What is the predominate method of abortion beyond the first trimester?**

Dilatation and evacuation.

○ **Name two methods used to induce contractions to perform abortion in the second trimester.**

Installation of hypertonic solution and prostaglandin induction.

○ **What are two important determinants of abortion complication?**

Gestational age and method of abortion chosen.

○ **What are the associated causes of hemorrhage after pregnancy termination?**

Uterine atony, a low-lying implantation site, a pregnancy of more advanced gestational age, or perforation.

○   **What percentage of pregnancy terminations are done in the first trimester?**

In 1990, approximately 88% were done in the first trimester, 11% between 13 and 20 weeks, and 1% were done at 21 weeks or greater.

○   **Which groups of medical agents have been found extremely useful for pregnancy termination?**

Prostaglandin E2 (dinoprostone) and prostaglandin E1 (misoprostol) as well as the antiprogestin RU 486 (mifepristone) and the antimetabolite methotrexate have been very useful for this purpose.

○   **RU 486 is an analog of which steroid used frequently in oral contraceptive pill formulations?**

Norethindrone.

○   **Under what conditions is hysterotomy indicated?**

Failed abortion when uterine anomaly is suspected.

○   **Which landmark Supreme Court decision concludes that the state may not interfere with the practice of abortion in the first trimester?**

Roe vs Wade.

○   **What percentage of abortions are obtained by married women?**

25%.

○   **What effect does *Laminaria japonicum* have on the morbidity associated with forcible dilation during D&E?**

Fivefold reduction in cervical laceration.

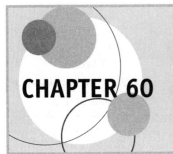

CHAPTER 60

Family Planning and Sterilization

Rachael Cohen, DO and Namita Kattal, MD

○ **What are the failure rates of different contraceptive methods during first year of their use in the United States?**

Method	Percent of Women with Pregnancy		Percent of Women Continuing Use at 1 Year
	Typical	**Lowest Expected**	
No method	85	85	
Spermicides	29	18	42
Withdrawal	27	4	43
Periodic abstinence			
Calendar	25	9	
Ovulation method	25	3	
Symptothermal	25	2	
Postovulation	25	1	
Cervical cap with spermicide			
Parous	32	26	46
Nulliparous	16	9	57
Diaphragm with spermicide	16	6	57
Condom			
Female	21	5	49
Male	15	2	53

(continued)

| Method | Percent of Women with Pregnancy | | Percent of Women Continuing Use at 1 Year |
	Typical	Lowest Expected	
Pill			68
Combined	7.6	0.1	
Progestin only	3	0.5	
Ortho Evra patch	8	0.3	68
NuvaRing	8	0.3	68
Depo-Provera	0.3	0.3	56
IUD			
Copper T	0.8	0.6	78
Levonorgestrel	0.1	0.1	100
Sterilization			
Female	0.4	0.2	100
Male	0.15	0.10	100

○ **What are the methods to measure the contraceptive efficacy?**

Pearl index and life table analysis.

○ **True or False: Failure rates increase with duration of use with most contraceptive methods.**

False. Failure rates actually decline with duration of use. The Pearl index is based on the number of unintended pregnancies per 100 women per year and therefore fails to accurately compare methods at various durations of exposure. This limitation is overcome by using the method of life table analysis, which gives the failure rate for each month of use.

○ **What are the recommendations following vasectomy?**

Alternate forms of contraception are recommended until 2 semen samples show no sperm.

○ **What is the pregnancy rate after vasectomy reversal?**

70% to 80%. However, the prospect of pregnancy decreases with time elapsed from vasectomy decreasing to 30% after 10 years.

○ **What are the most common adverse effects of vasectomy?**

Hematomas and infection.

○   **Does vasectomy increases the risk for prostate cancer?**

Current data do not support an association between prostate cancer and vasectomy. Therefore, screening for prostate cancer should be no different in men who had a vasectomy.

○   **Describe the 10-year cumulative failure rates for female tubal sterilization.**

Unipolar coagulation, 0.75%

Postpartum tubal excision, 0.75%

Silastic/Falope-Ring, 1.77%

Interval partial salpingectomy, 2.01%

Bipolar coagulation, 2.48%

Hulka–Clemens clip, 3.65%

○   **What is the tubal sterilization technique with lowest failure rate?**

Postpartum partial salpingectomy has the lowest failure rate.

○   **What is the mortality rate of tubal sterilization?**

Mortality rates in the United States have been calculated as 1 to 4 deaths per 100,000 procedures.

○   **Describe the different methods of postpartum or interval mini-laparotomy tubal sterilization.**

Modified Pomeroy's—Ligation at the base of a loop of isthmic portion of tube followed by excision of the knuckle of tube.

Modified Parkland's—Excision of segment of isthmic portion of tube after separate ligation of cut ends.

Irving—Double ligate and sever tubes. Bury proximal stump into uterus and put distal stump into mesosalpinx.

Uchida—Inject mesenteric part of tube with saline. Divide muscular part of tube/excise 3 to 5 cm. Bury proximal tube and exteriorize or excise distal tube.

Fimbriectomy—Excision of fimbria of tube.

○   **Which method is associated with increased risk for ectopic pregnancy after tubal sterilization?**

Bipolar tubal coagulation.

○   **How long after tubal sterilization does the risk of ectopic pregnancy increase?**

Ectopic pregnancies following tubal ligation are more likely to occur 3 or more years after sterilization, rather than immediately after and continues to increase for at least 10 years after surgery.

○   **Does the patients' age at the time of sterilization determine the risk for ectopic pregnancy after tubal sterilization?**

Yes. Except for postpartum partial salpingectomy, the chance of ectopic pregnancy is greater for women sterilized before age 30 years than for women sterilized at age 30 or older.

○   **True or False: Women who undergo tubal sterilization are more likely to have menstrual abnormalities.**

False. Current evidence indicates that tubal sterilization does not cause menstrual abnormalities.

○ **How many sterilized women will eventually undergo tubal reanastomosis?**

2 per 1000 sterilized women.

○ **What determines the pregnancy rates after tubal reanastomosis?**

Pregnancy rates correlate with the length of the remaining tube; a length of 4 cm or more is optimal.

○ **What is ESSURE?**

ESSURE is a method of transcervical/hysteroscopic permanent sterilization that causes tubal blockage by encouraging local tissue growth with polyester fibers. An attached outer-coiled spring is released that molds to the shape of interstitial portion of each fallopian tube.

○ **What are the advantages of ESSURE?**

ESSURE can be done in the physician's office without the need for conscious/general anesthesia. It is a transcervical approach with no incision required and may be preferred for obese women, women with abdominal adhesions, and women with risk factors for general anesthesia.

○ **What is the follow-up post ESSURE?**

Hysterosalpingogram must be done 3 months post procedure to ensure complete tubal blockage. The couple must use another form of contraception in the interim.

○ **What is the effectiveness of ESSURE?**

99.74% effective after 4 years.

NATURAL METHODS

○ **What are the four fertility awareness based methods of contraception?**

Calendar charting, basal body temperature charting, cervical mucus charting, and sympto-thermal charting.

○ **Why is the sympto-thermal method of natural family planning more effective than the others?**

Because it relies on several indices to determine the fertile period (calendar, mucus, and temperature).

○ **Does pre-ejaculate contain sperm?**

No. It is fluid produced by local glands. However, a previous ejaculate may leave sperm hidden within the urethral lining.

HORMONAL CONTRACEPTION

○ **Are combined oral contraceptives (COCs) contraindicated in patients with a history of benign breast disease or a family history of breast cancer?**

No.

○ **What positive test prevents women with lupus from taking COC?**

Positive antiphospholipid antibodies.

○ **At what age should women stop using COCs?**

Women without medical problems who are nonsmokers should discontinue the use of COC after the age of 50 to 55 years.

○ **Should COCs be prescribed to women with diabetes and/or hypertension?**

Patients who are compliant with follow-up and management of their hypertension and diabetes may be started on a trial of COC, provided they have no comorbidities.

○ **Is depression a contraindication for COCs?**

No, as symptoms are not exacerbated by these medicines.

○ **Should COCs be discontinued prior to major surgery?**

It is suggested that oral contraceptives be discontinued approximately 6 weeks prior to any major surgery. If they are continued, heparin prophylaxis should be provided.

○ **Can women with dyslipidemia use COCs?**

Yes, provided that their disease is well controlled. The parameters for poor disease control include LDL >160 mg/mL, triglycerides >250 mg/d, or comorbidities of the disease. The patients who meet criteria should be started on a low-dose estrogen pill.

○ **Should patients on depot-medroxyprogesterone acetate (DMPA) be assessed for bone mineral density?**

No. At this time, the short-term data do not support the need for DXA for patients on DMPA.

○ **Name the conditions where progestin-only methods may be more appropriate than combination contraceptives.**

The conditions include migraine headaches, smokers, obesity, hypertension, history of thromboembolism, SLE, CAD, CHF, sickle cell disease, and cerebrovascular disease.

○ **True or False: Women taking medications that accelerate the metabolism of estrogens should probably be started on a 50-microgram pill.**

True.

○ **Which anticonvulsants may decrease the effectiveness of combined oral contraceptives?**

Barbiturates, carbamazepine, felbamate, phenytoin, topiramate, and vigabatrin.

○ **What are the regimens available for emergency contraception?**

The two most commonly used oral emergency contraception regimens are the progestin-only regimen that consists of a total of 1.5 mg levonorgestrel (Plan B), and the combined estrogen-progestin regimen that consists of two doses, each containing 100 μg of ethinyl estradiol plus 0.5 mg of levonorgestrel taken 12 hours apart.

○ **How long after exposure can emergency oral contraceptives be given?**

Up to 120 hours. It is most effective if initiated in 12 to 24 hours.

○   **What is the most common side effect of oral contraceptives when used for emergency contraception?**

Nausea. It occurs in 50% to 70% of those treated. Up to 22% may vomit.

○   **When should the woman prescribed emergency oral contraceptives expect her menses?**

Within a few days of her normal menses. It may be a few days early or late.

○   **What to do when pills are missed?**

Scenario	What to do?	Backup Method Needed?
1 pill is missed	Take pill as soon as possible and resume schedule	None needed
2 pills missed in the first 2 weeks	Take 2 pills on each of the next 2 days and finish pack	Need for backup method minimal but recommended for 7 days
2 pills missed in the third week	Start new pack or if Sunday start- take one pill until Sunday and start new pack	Start immediately and continue for 7 days
More than 2 active pills are missed at any time	Start new pack or if Sunday start- take one pill until Sunday and start new pack	Start immediately and continue for 7 days

○   **How much is menstrual blood flow decreased by pill use?**

By 60% or more. This results in less iron deficiency anemia.

○   **By how much is the incidence of functional cysts reduced by pill use?**

80% to 90%. Oral contraceptives suppress FSH and LH ovarian stimulation.

○   **For the treatment of PMS are monophasic or triphasic pills better?**

Probably monophasic. All low-dose combination pills may result in decrease in anxiety, headaches, and fluid retention.

○   **For women using oral contraceptives for 4 years or less, what is their reduction in risk of ovarian cancer?**

30%. For 12 or more years of use, the risk is decreased by 80%.

○   **For women using oral contraceptives for at least 2 years, what is the reduction in risk of endometrial cancer?**

40%. This increases to 60% for 4 or more years of use.

○   **In lactating women, how soon after delivery can combination oral contraceptive pills be started?**

Combination oral contraceptive may be started once milk production is well established. Progestin only pills, however, are a better choice because they are not associated with decreased milk production.

○ **In nonlactating postpartum women, when should combination pills be started?**

After 4 weeks postpartum. This avoids the immediate postpartum hypercoagulable state.

○ **Among nonlactating postpartum women, when does the first ovulation occur?**

On average after 45 days. Few first ovulations are followed by a normal luteal phase.

○ **How effective is breast feeding alone in preventing pregnancy?**

98% for the first 6 months in women who have not resumed their menses.

○ **Are women more likely to gain or lose weight with oral contraceptive use?**

Both are equally likely. Rarely do pills cause a gain of 10 pounds or more.

○ **How does vitamin C (1-g dose) affect the oral contraceptive user?**

It increases the amount of ethinyl estradiol absorbed and increases serum levels by up to 50%. Intermittent use may cause spotting when the vitamin is stopped.

○ **What is NuvaRing?**

It is a combined hormonal contraceptive. The ring is placed in the vagina for 3 weeks and then removed for a week to allow withdrawal bleeding.

○ **How does NuvaRing work?**

NuvaRing releases 15 μg ethinyl estradiol and 120 μg etonogestrel daily.

○ **Is it necessary to remove NuvaRing for sexual intercourse?**

No. The ring should not be removed for sexual intercourse. However, if the ring is displaced outside the vagina during intercourse, it may be rinsed and should be placed back in the vagina within 3 hours.

○ **How does the transdermal contraceptive patch work?**

Ortho Evra patches deliver 20 μg of ethinyl estradiol and 150 μg of norelgestromin daily. The patch is changed once a week for 3 weeks, followed by 1 week of no patch.

○ **What is the most frequent reason to discontinue the patch?**

Reaction at the application site is the leading cause to stop using the patch.

○ **Is the patch more effective than oral contraceptive pills (OCP)?**

No. The efficacy of these methods is similar. However, the efficacy may decrease in women with weight >90 kg.

○ **What should be recommended if the patch becomes detached?**

A partially detached patch for less than 24 hours duration should be reattached. For longer detachment, a new patch should be applied and 7-day backup contraception should be provided.

○ **True or False: The transdermal patch has a better compliance than OCP?**

True.

○ **What is the Seasonale pill?**

A 91-day extended cycle OCP. It consists of 84 active pills followed by 7 inactive pills providing 4 withdrawal bleeds per year.

○ **What is the hormonal component of Seasonale?**

The pill contains 30 μg of ethinyl estradiol and 150 μg of levonorgestrel.

○ **What is Seasonique and how does it differ from Seasonale?**

Seasonique is also a 91-day extended cycle OCP. It consists of 84 active pills followed by 7 pills containing 10 mg of ethinyl estradiol.

○ **Is the efficacy of Seasonale pill comparable to conventional OCPs?**

Yes. The Seasonale pill has similar effectiveness to 28-day cycle combined OCPs.

○ **Is the breakthrough bleeding more frequent with the Seasonale pill?**

Yes. Compared to traditional combined OCP, women who take Seasonale have more unplanned bleeding. However, it decreases after the fourth cycle.

○ **Do the side effects increase with Seasonale?**

No. The side effects and contraindications of Seasonale are similar to other combined OCPs.

○ **How does Depo-Provera work?**

It inhibits ovulation by suppressing FSH and LH levels and eliminating the LH surge.

○ **What is the effect of progestin on the uterus?**

It results in a shallow atrophic endometrium and a thick cervical mucus. These both result in decreased sperm transport.

○ **What is Implanon?**

Implanon is a progestin containing implant, which protects against pregnancy for 3 years.

○ **When should Implanon be inserted to minimize pregnancy risk?**

Within 5 days of the onset of menstruation or 3 to 4 weeks after delivery.

○ **What is the "grace" period with Depo-Provera?**

2 weeks. A 150-mg injection actually provides more than 3 months protection.

○ **What is the average weight gain per year with the use of Depo-Provera?**

2 to 5 pounds. Norplant users gain just less than 1 pound per year.

○ **What is the expected period of time for return of fertility after Depo-Provera?**

6 months to 1 year.

○ **In progestin-only pill users, which women are at the greatest risk of pregnancy?**

Those, whose menstrual cycles prior to pill use were ovulatory and whose cycles are least disturbed.

BARRIER METHODS

○ **Do all condoms protect against all sexually transmitted diseases?**

No. Skin condoms may permit the passage of viruses.

○ **What is the method failure rate of the condom?**

3% versus actual use rates of approximately 12%. Method failure implies perfect use.

○ **Are spermicidal condoms as effective as a condom plus intravaginal spermicide?**

No. The dose delivered by a lubricated condom is much less than intravaginal spermicide.

○ **What is the rate of pregnancy after a condom breaks?**

Approximately 1 per 23 breaks. Rates of breakage are approximately 1 to 2 per 100 condoms used.

○ **What lubricants increase breakage?**

Oil-based lubricants such as Vaseline, baby oil, and lotions.

○ **What are the two components of spermicides?**

Base or carrier (foam, cream, jelly, film, suppository, tablet) and spermicidal chemical.

○ **How do spermicides work?**

They are surfactants that destroy the sperm cell membrane.

○ **How much time does it take for spermicidal suppositories to be effective?**

10 to 15 minutes versus 5 minutes for film.

○ **How quickly can sperm enter the cervical canal?**

As soon as 15 seconds after ejaculation.

○ **Does spermicide have any non-contraceptive benefits?**

Yes. It provides protection against gonorrhea and *Chlamydia*. The risk reduction is greatest, when used with a mechanical barrier.

○ **Can oil-based products be used with female condoms?**

Yes. The polyurethane is stronger than latex and is less susceptible to deterioration.

○ **After insertion, how long does the diaphragm provide effective contraception?**

A diaphragm should be left in place for 6 hours following intercourse. For longer intervals, additional spermicide is recommended.

○ **How much spermicide should be used with the cervical cap?**

The dome should be one-third full. Additional spermicide is not necessary for up to 48 hours.

○ **Are female condoms, diaphragms, and caps equally effective for nulliparous and parous women?**

For nulliparous women, yes. For parous women, the cap is less effective.

○ **How frequently should women using cervical caps have Pap smears?**

The FDA recommends a Pap after 3 months of use. Otherwise, women using vaginal barriers, need no special follow-up.

IUD

○ **What percentage of women use IUD?**

Less than 2% of women using contraception.

○ **Who are the candidates for an IUD?**

Candidates for intrauterine device use:

- Multiparous and nulliparous women at low risk for STDs.
- Women who desire long-term reversible contraception.
- Women with the following medical conditions:
  - Diabetes.
  - Thromboembolism.
  - Menorrhagia/dysmenorrheal—levonorgestrel only preferred.
  - Breastfeeding—copper only till 4 to 6 weeks postpartum.
  - Breast cancer—copper only.
  - Liver disease—copper only.

○ **What are the contraindications to intrauterine device use?**

- Pregnancy.
- Pelvic inflammatory disease (current or within the past 3 months).
- Sexually transmitted diseases (current).
- Puerperal or postabortion sepsis (current or within the past 3 months).
- Purulent cervicitis.
- Abnormal vaginal bleeding.
- Malignancy of the genital tract.
- Known uterine anomalies or fibroids distorting the cavity in a way incompatible with intrauterine device (IUD) insertion.
- Allergy to any component of the IUD or Wilson disease (for copper-containing IUDs).

○ **Is routine screening for STDs (e.g., gonorrhea and *Chlamydia*) required before insertion of an IUD?**

Current data do not support routine screening in women at low risk for STDs.

○ **Is antibiotic prophylaxis before IUD insertion recommended?**

Routine use of prophylactic antibiotics at the time of IUD insertion confers little benefit.

○ **When should an IUD be removed in a menopausal woman?**

At least 1 year after the cessation of menses.

○ **If *Actinomyces* is found on a Pap smear of an IUD user what should be done?**

First a culture to confirm the diagnosis. If confirmed, the infection should be treated. The IUD does not have to be removed.

○ **What is the mean menstrual blood loss associated with the copper IUD use?**

70 to 80 mL. This compares to 35 mL for a normal menstrual cycle.

○ **With the progesterone-releasing IUD, what is the mean menstrual blood loss?**

25 mL per cycle.

○ **What is the risk of ectopic pregnancy in a woman using an IUD compared to a woman using other forms of contraception or no contraception?**

Because the possibility of pregnancy is reduced, the overall risk of ectopic pregnancy with a failed IUD is only 5%. However, if pregnancy does occur with an IUD in place, the chances of it being an ectopic are higher than in those who use other forms of contraception or none at all.

○ **Which method of reversible contraception has the highest 1-year continuation rate?**

The IUD. This is because discontinuation necessitates a visit to a health care facility to discontinue use.

○ **When is a woman using an IUD at the greatest risk for PID?**

At insertion and in the first 3 months of use.

○ **What is the rate of IUD expulsion?**

2% to 10% in the first year.

○ **When should the IUD be inserted in the postpartum period?**

Within the first 10 minutes after the placenta delivers, or at 6 to 8 weeks. If the IUD is inserted 1 to 2 days after delivery, the risk of expulsion increases.

○ **For postcoital contraception, when should the IUD be inserted?**

Within 6 days of unprotected intercourse.

○ **What is the incidence of uterine perforation with IUD insertion?**

1/1,000. The string may still be visible in the os.

CHAPTER 61 Reproductive Toxicology

Emese Zsiros, MD

○ **A 21-year-old female requests counseling because she was taking birth control pills without knowing she was pregnant. Should she abort the pregnancy?**

Extensive epidemiological studies have revealed no increased risk of birth defects in children of women who have used oral contraceptives prior to pregnancy. It is recommended that for any woman who has missed two consecutive periods, pregnancy should be ruled out before continuing oral contraceptive use. If the woman has not adhered to the prescribed dosing schedule, the possibility of pregnancy should be considered at the time of the first missed period. Oral contraceptive use should be discontinued if pregnancy is confirmed.

○ **Your dermatologist colleague wishes to prescribe tetracycline to a pregnant lady for her severe acne. What do you advise him?**

Tetracycline is contraindicated in the last half of the pregnancy and in childhood to the age of 8 years, because it might cause permanent discoloration of the teeth (yellow-grey-brown) and enamel hypoplasia. This adverse reaction is more common in long-term use and in repeated short-term therapy.

There are no adequate and well-controlled studies in pregnant women regarding the topical use of tetracycline solutions; however, animal studies have shown no harm to the fetus with topical applications.

○ **What is the current recommendation for treating epilepsy during pregnancy?**

According to studies, 90% of the pregnant women on antiepileptic medication deliver normal infants. Antiepileptic drugs (AEDs) should not be discontinued in patient in whom the drug is administered to prevent major seizures, because of the strong possibility of precipitating status epilepticus. All commonly used AEDs have been associated with congenital malformations, although some of the newer anticonvulsants have not been used in large enough numbers to have meaningful data. In general, AED polypharmacy and higher blood levels of AEDs are associated with the increased incidence of birth defects in infants born to women with epilepsy. A single anti-convulsant at the lowest possible dose for efficacy is recommended whenever possible.

○ **Is the antiepileptic phenytoin (Dilantin) safe in pregnancy?**

Children of women receiving phenytoin can develop fetal hydantoin syndrome. This consists of prenatal growth deficiency, microcephaly, mental retardation, nail and digit hypoplasia, and mid-facial abnormalities.

Some of the AEDs' side effects are related to folate deficiency. Phenytoin, carbamazepine, barbiturates, and valproate are linked to folate malabsorption or they interfere with folate metabolism. Thus, folic acid supplementation (at a minimum dosage of 0.4 mg daily) is especially important prior to conception, during pregnancy, and throughout childbearing years in these women to reduce the adverse effects of these drugs.

○ **What are the risks of amphetamine use during pregnancy?**

Infants born to mothers dependent on amphetamines have an increased risk of premature delivery and low birth weight. Also, these infants may experience symptoms of withdrawal as demonstrated by dysphoria, including agitation, and significant lassitude. However, there is no known association with structural abnormalities.

○ **Are all social and illicit drugs associated with increased rates of placental abruption?**

No. Only cocaine and smoking are known to cause increased rates of placental abruption. Alcohol, coffee, heroin, marijuana, and amphetamines have no such association.

○ **Does amphetamine use in pregnancy cause congenital abnormalities?**

Amphetamine use in pregnancy has not been associated with congenital abnormalities; however, its use correlates to a reduction in birth weight, prematurity, postpartum hemorrhage, and retained placenta. Babies born to amphetamine users can have an increase in jitteriness, drowsiness, and respiratory distress, suggesting an amphetamine withdrawal syndrome. Because of anorectic impact of the drug, amphetamines may severely affect maternal nutrition prior and during pregnancy also.

○ **Your 28-year-old pregnant patient expresses concerns about the ultrasound examination you have prescribed. How do you counsel her?**

There is no documented effect on patients and their fetuses with the use of current ultrasound techniques. High-level ultrasound energy could potentially cause harm to the fetus by two mechanisms—thermal damage and cavitation. However, these effects are not seen at the low levels of ultrasound energy used during diagnostic studies.

○ **What is pica?**

Pica is an appetite for nonnutritive substances (e.g., coal, soil, chalk, paper etc.) or an abnormal appetite for things that may be considered foods, such as food ingredients (e.g., flour, raw potato, starch). Symptoms must persist for more than one month, it is not part of a culturally sanctioned practice, and does not occur exclusively during the course of another mental disorder (e.g., schizophrenia). In children aged 18 months to 2 years, the ingestion and mouthing of nonnutritive substances is common and is not considered to be pathologic. The condition's name comes from the Latin word for the magpie, a bird which is reputed to eat almost anything. Pica is seen in all ages, particularly in pregnant women and small children, especially among children who are developmentally disabled, where it is the most common eating disorder.

○ **Should pregnant anesthetists and nurses be allowed to administer anesthetic agents?**

Yes, provided there is adequate ventilation and a functioning gas scavenger system in the operating room so that any possible fumes or vapors are quickly dissipated to the outside environment.

○ **Is lithium use for manic depression indicted in pregnancy?**

Early studies described a condition associated with lithium use in the first trimester known as Ebstein's anomaly. The tricuspid value is abnormal and has only 2 leaflets. Thus, many women using this drug terminated their pregnancies. Later studies have shown that, although there is an association between the drug and the cardiac lesion, it is very rare and does not warrant routine pregnancy termination. Lithium is a category D drug.

○ **What immunizations are contraindicated during pregnancy?**

In general, live virus vaccines are contraindicated during pregnancy. These include measles, mumps, rubella, varicella, and yellow fever. On the other hand, all toxoids, immunoglobulins, and killed virus vaccines are considered safe in pregnancy and should not be withheld, if indicated.

○ **What is the current recommendation for giving influenza vaccine to pregnant women?**

The influenza vaccine is an inactivated live vaccine and so far no risks from immunization have been described. According to the current American College of Obstetricians and Gynecologists (ACOG) guidelines all women who are pregnant in the second and third trimester during the flu season (October–March) and women at high risk for pulmonary complications regardless of the trimester should receive the influenza vaccination.

○ **Is breast feeding a contraindication to immunization?**

Breast feeding is not a contraindication to immunizations. Live and inactivated vaccines and toxoids can all be given during this time.

○ **What factors affect the ability of a drug or a chemical to cross the placenta and reach the embryo?**

These include molecular weight, lipid solubility, degree of ionization, protein binding. Compounds with low molecular weight, high lipid affinity, low degree of ionization, and low protein binding affinity will cross the placenta with ease and rapidity.

○ **What other factors affect the quantitative aspect of placental transport?**

These are placental blood flow, the pH gradient between the maternal and fetal serum and tissues, and placental metabolism of the chemical or drug.

○ **What criteria are necessary to establish that a drug or chemical exposure causes congenital abnormalities?**

1. Epidemiologic studies should consistently display an adverse association in exposed individuals.
2. Secular trends consistently display a relationship between the incidence of a particular malformation and human exposures.
3. An animal model mimics the human malformation at clinically comparable exposures.
4. The teratogenic effects should increase in relation to the dose.
5. The observed teratogenic effect should be consistent with biologic and scientific principles of occurrence.

○ **What are the baseline congenital anomaly risks in the general population?**

Regardless of family history or teratogenic exposure, the background risk for major congenital anomalies is 3% to 5%. These include abnormalities that, if uncorrected, affect the health of the individual. Some examples are pyloric stenosis, cleft lip and palate, and neural tube defects. The background rate for minor congenital anomalies is 7% to 10%. These include strabismus, polydactyly, misshapen ears, etc. If uncorrected, they do not significantly affect the health of the individual.

○ **Who is more susceptible to carbon monoxide (CO) poisoning, a mother or her fetus?**

The fetus. CO causes toxicity by asphyxiation. It binds to hemoglobin to form carboxyhemoglobin (COHb). Fetal COHb levels tend to be 10% to 15% higher than maternal levels. If a woman has a significant enough exposure to cause unconsciousness, more than 50% of fetuses will die in utero and many of the remainder suffer from significant impairment.

○ **How do you treat a patient with suspected CO poisoning?**

High dose O_2 displaces CO from Hb and causes it to diffuse out of tissues. Hyperbaric oxygen therapy will more significantly reduce the half-life of CO in the blood stream and it is the treatment of choice when available. The half-life of CO in maternal blood is approximately 230 minutes and it is longer in the fetus. The half-life is reduced to 90 minutes with 100% O_2 and can be safely reduced to less than 30 minutes with hyperbaric oxygen therapy.

○   **What maternal blood level of lead is toxic to her fetus?**

Maternal blood lead levels as low as 10 μg/mL have been linked to neurobehavioral disturbances in their offspring. The CDC has defined blood levels greater than 25 μg/mL as elevated, because this is when toxic effects are seen in adults, but the fetus appears to be more susceptible to lead poisoning.

○   **What effect does lead have on the human body?**

Lead can affect multiple organ systems and may cause death in adults when blood concentrations exceed 300 μg/mL. The central nervous system, GI tract, kidneys, joints, and reproductive systems may all be affected. Studies vary whether lead causes structural malformations in exposed fetuses, but one researcher found increased numbers of cranial and cardiovascular anomalies as well as stillbirths in exposed fetuses. It is clear that lead causes learning disabilities and other behavioral disturbances.

○   **Which women today are most at risk for mercury poisoning?**

Fish-eaters. The only real human exposure to organic mercury is through consumption of fish. Fetuses are more susceptible to toxic effects of mercury than their maternal hosts, so extra care must be taken when working with pregnant patients. Large exposures to methylmercury have resulted in infants with microcephaly, mental retardation, cerebral palsy, and blindness.

○   **What advice do you give pregnant women about fish consumption?**

According to the US Food and Drug Administration (FDA) and the Environmental Protection Agency (EPA), a pregnant woman can safely eat up to 12 ounces (two average meals) a week of a variety of fish and shellfish. Nearly all fish contain trace amounts of methylmercury, which are not harmful to humans. However, long-lived, larger fish that feed on other fish accumulate the highest levels of methylmercury and pose the greatest risk to people who eat them regularly. Hence, pregnant and nursing women and also young children should not eat the following fish:

Shark.

Swordfish.

King mackerel.

Tilefish.

○   **What recommendations would you make to a woman who requires a magnetic resonance imaging (MRI) study during pregnancy?**

MRI has not been shown to be harmful in pregnancy. However, based on a lack of evidence that supports the safety of MRI during pregnancy, the National Radiological Protection Board has recommended that women in the first three months of pregnancy be excluded from MRI examinations. There is insufficient evidence to recommend termination of pregnancy after an inadvertent first trimester exposure.

○   **What is the time of gestation during which a fetus is most susceptible to the effects of ionizing radiation?**

The fetus is most susceptible to radiation between 8 and 15 weeks of gestation. Before 8 weeks , if the exposure does not result in a spontaneous abortion, the fetus will be unaffected. Between 16 and 25 weeks postfertilization, the fetus is less vulnerable to radiation effects. After the 26 weeks of pregnancy, the radiation sensitivity of the unborn baby is similar to that of a newborn.

○   **How would a significant radiation exposure affect a fetus?**

Doses of greater than 100 rads (cGy) have been associated with microcephaly, which may or may not be associated with mental retardation. Growth retardation is also seen in exposed fetuses. From epidemiologic and animal studies, it does not appear that exposures of less than 10 rads could affect a pregnancy at any gestational age.

○ **Does radiation from diagnostic studies present a risk to pregnant women?**

Aside from the emotional distress induced by this exposure, probably not. Authorities have stated that the risk of teratogenesis with exposures of less than 5 rads is minuscule. The following table presents radiation doses presented to the uterus by various radiographic procedures.

Study	View	Dose/Study (mrad)
Chest	AP and lateral	0.05
Abdomen	AP and lateral	125–25
IVP		1000
Upper GI series		50
Barium enema		2–4 rads
CT abdomen		2.5 rads

○ **How much radiation does a ventilation-perfusion (V-Q) scan deliver to a fetus?**

Technetium used in the perfusion scan is bound to macro aggregated albumin, which is sequestered in the lung: exposure to the fetus is limited to 40 mrad. Xenon is used during the ventilation scan and only delivers 10 mrad to the fetus. Therefore, the fetus is only exposed to 50 mrad, which is 1/100 the minimum dose of radiation hypothesized to be teratogenic. In general, radionuclide imaging delivers small amounts of radiation to the uterus and may be used during pregnancy.

○ **How does thalidomide affect the developing fetus?**

Thalidomide is a sedative, hypnotic, and anti-inflammatory medication, which was chiefly sold and prescribed during the late 1950s and early 1960s to pregnant women, as an antiemetic to combat morning sickness and as an aid to help them sleep. It was sold from 1957 to 1961 in almost fifty countries under at least forty names, including Distaval, Talimol, Nibrol, Sedimide, Quietoplex, Contergan, Neurosedyn, and Softenon. From 1956 to 1962, approximately 10,000 children were born with severe malformations, approximately 5,000 survived beyond childhood. Malformations were amelia (absence of limbs), phocomelia (short limbs), hypoplasticity of the bones, absence of bones, external ear abnormalities, facial palsy, eye abnormalities, and congenital heart defects. The medication never received approval for sale in the United States, but 2.5 million tablets had been given to more than 1,200 American doctors during Richardson-Merrell's "investigation," and nearly 20,000 patients received thalidomide tablets, including several hundred pregnant women. In the end, 17 American children were born with thalidomide-related deformities.

○ **What is the mechanism behind thalidomide-induced teratogenesis?**

The mechanism of action of thalidomide is not fully understood. Thalidomide possesses immunomodulatory, anti-inflammatory and anti-angiogenic properties. Available data from in vitro studies and clinical trials suggest that the immunologic effects of this compound can vary substantially under different conditions, but may be related to suppression of excessive tumor necrosis factor-alpha (TNF-α) production and down-modulation of selected cell surface adhesion molecules involved in leukocyte migration. Thalidomide is racemic—it contains both left- and right-handed isomers in equal amounts. One enantiomer is effective against morning sickness. The other is teratogenic and causes birth defects.

○ **Is thalidomide still on the market in some countries?**

Yes, thalidomide (Thalomid) is currently used in three countries: Mexico, Brazil, and the United States. The current indication for thalidomide use is erythema nodosum leprosum (ENL), a severe and debilitating complication of leprosy (Hansen disease). In 2006, thalidomide was approved by the Food and Drug Administration (FDA) for use in combination with dexamethasone for the treatment of newly diagnosed multiple myelomas. Thalidomide, along with another new drug, bortezomib, is changing the landscape of multiple myeloma treatment, such that toxic stem cell transplants may no longer be the standard treatment for this incurable malignancy. Effective contraception must be used for at least 4 weeks before beginning thalidomide therapy, during thalidomide therapy, and for 4 weeks following discontinuation of thalidomide therapy.

○ **Many women have purchased protective devices to guard against radiation emitted by video display terminals, VDT (e.g., computer screens). Do they need them?**

No. VDTs do not produce ionizing radiation. Prospective studies have not demonstrated an increased risk of miscarriages in exposed workers.

○ **Is working as a medical resident harmful during pregnancy?**

Overall, residency training has not been shown to cause spontaneous abortion, preterm birth, or low birth weight. However, in one study when women worked more than 100 hours/week, preterm births were increased. Mild preeclampsia, which was not associated with adverse pregnancy outcome, was also increased in women residents.

○ **To which toxins is a ceramic artist or a painter exposed?**

Ceramic artists and painters may be exposed to lead and other heavy metals. Kilns emit toxic gases including carbon monoxide. In general, you would not know what their exposures are at work or at home if you do not ask!

○ **In which occupation do workers face the greatest risk of job-related violence?**

In a 1996 report, OSHA stated that more assaults occur against health care workers and social workers than in any other industry. Pregnancy does not offer any protection against violence.

○ **How does pregnancy affect an individual's susceptibility to toxins?**

The physiologic changes that occur during pregnancy modify their susceptibility to toxins.

1. Increased ventilation enhances absorption of toxic gases.
2. Progesterone decreases gut motility and may enhance absorption of certain agents.
3. Hypoalbuminuria results in decreased serum protein binding and thus increased bioavailability of protein-bound toxins.
4. Increased GFR may increase clearance of some agents.
5. Increased blood volume and body fat results in increased distribution and sequestration.

○ **What is the primary problem facing women who become pregnant while living at high altitude (>1600 m)?**

Intrauterine growth restriction. The average birth weight decreases by 100 grams per 100 meters of elevation for term pregnancies. Smoking appears to exacerbate the effects of high altitude on fetal growth. As far as traveling, it seems probable that a 2-week visit to moderate altitude (less than 3000 meters) is unlikely to affect the final birth weight of a baby.

○ **How would you counsel a woman exposed to dioxin during the first trimester of pregnancy?**

Studies in animals have demonstrated that dioxin may be a potent teratogen. But women exposed to dioxin following accidental exposures have not demonstrated an increase in congenital malformations. Therefore, there is no evidence to suggest that she terminate her pregnancy, but a targeted ultrasound examination during pregnancy would be prudent. Dioxin has been postulated to exert at least some of its biological effect by acting as an antiestrogen or "endocrine disrupter".

○ **Which substances have specific standards based at least in part on reproductive toxicities in the occupational safety and health act (OSHA)?**

Only lead, dibromochloropropane (DBCP), and ethylene oxide have standards based on reproductive effects. Use of DBCP was discontinued in 1981. Many other substances have demonstrated reproductive toxicity but were not addressed by OSHA.

○ **What are the major reproductive hazards facing pregnant health care worker?**

Working with antineoplastic drugs in improperly ventilated areas has been associated with increased risk of pregnancy loss and congenital anomalies. Anesthetic agents may increase the risk of pregnancy loss, but do not appear to increase malformation rates. Infectious diseases such as hepatitis and HIV pose a risk to workers and their fetuses. Chemical sterilants widely used in operating rooms, pharmacies, and laboratories may have reproductive toxicity. Lastly, the stress on residents imposed by long working hours may increase the risk of preterm delivery and preeclampsia.

○ **How does cocaine adversely affect pregnancy?**

Cocaine is especially toxic during pregnancy. The most common complication caused by cocaine during pregnancy is abruptio placentae, which may result in fetal death. In addition, brain anomalies, intestinal atresia, and limb reduction defects have been described. Investigators have also reported increases in congenital heart defects in exposed infants. Cocaine may cause these effects by vasoconstriction and subsequent infarction.

○ **Methadone is as bad for pregnancy as cocaine. True or False?**

False. One study compared cocaine-abusing women to women being treated with methadone and found a much higher complication rate in the cocaine-abuse group. Methadone is not thought to be a teratogen, although its safe use in pregnancy has not been established.

○ **What is fetal alcohol syndrome?**

Infants suffer from intrauterine growth restriction, mental retardation, and develop characteristic facies, which consists of short palpebral fissures, a flat midface, a thin upper lip, and hypoplastic philtrum. Alcohol abuse is the most common preventable cause of mental retardation during pregnancy.

○ **At what time during gestation is the fetus most susceptible to alcohol toxicity?**

Probably in the second and third trimesters. In a study of 60 women, those who were heavy drinkers but stopped after the first trimester had children with normal mentation and behavioral patterns.

○ **In general, during which time of pregnancy is the fetus most susceptible to teratogens?**

During the embryonic period, this lasts from 2 to 8 weeks postconception. This is the time of organogenesis.

○ **Is the hot tub dangerous to pregnancy?**

The American College of Obstetricians and Gynecologists (ACOG) states that becoming overheated in a hot tub is not recommended during pregnancy. ACOG also recommends that pregnant women never let their core body temperature rise more than 102.2°F. Hot tubs are often factory programmed to maintain a water temperature of approximately 104°F, and at this temperature it takes only 10 to 20 minutes to raise the body temperature to 102°F or higher. If pregnant women whishes to use the hot tub, then its temperature should be lowered, and she should not spend more than 10 minutes in the warm water.

○ **Describe the pattern of congenital malformations caused by isotretinoin (Accutane).**

Affected offspring develop severe ear defects, cardiovascular anomalies (conotruncal malformations), CNS defects, and disturbances in development of the thymus. Another retinoid, vitamin A when ingested in quantities greater than 10,000 IU/day has also been shown to increase the incidence of cranioneurofacial anomalies in exposed fetuses. Beta-carotene (a vitamin A precursor) is safe in pregnancy.

○ **What is the fetal trimethadione syndrome?**

Fetuses have intrauterine growth restriction (IUGR). Affected infants have typical facial anomalies with a short upturned nose; a low, broad nasal bridge; prominent forehead; an up slant of the eyebrow; and a poorly developed overlapping helix of the external ear. They also develop cardiac septal defects as well as mental retardation and behavioral disturbances.

○ **What are the major adverse effects of smoking during pregnancy?**

The Surgeon General warns women of the dangers of smoking on every pack they buy. Smoking causes intrauterine growth restriction and increases the incidence of preterm delivery in a dose-dependent manner. The incidence of placenta previa, abruptio placentae, and spontaneous abortion also appears to be increased in smokers.

○ **Which is potentially more harmful in pregnancy, smoking or caffeine?**

Of the two, cigarette smoking is by far more potentially harmful. Studies about the effects of caffeine on pregnancy report conflicting results. Of the studies that do show that caffeine is harmful to pregnancy, the effects seem to be most significant when caffeine intake is greater than 300 mg/day (approximately 3 cups of coffee per day). Caffeine may be associated with IUGR when consumed in these quantities.

○ **What are the fetal toxic effects of the agents listed in the left hand column?**

Benzodiazepines	Orofacial clefting
Lithium	Epstein's anomaly
Valproic acid	Neural tube defects
DES	Vaginal adenosis, uterine malformations
ACE inhibitors	Renal dysplasia

○ **What is folate toxicity in pregnancy?**

Actually, it is a lack of folate, which is important during fetal development. Folate deficiency is associated with neural tube defects (i.e., spina bifida, anencephaly). Women of reproductive age should ingest 0.4 mL of folate per day. If they have had a child with neural tube defect in the past, they should take 4 mg of folate daily periconceptionally.

○ **What are the special concerns of flying during pregnancy?**

The American College of Obstetricians and Gynecologists (ACOG) recommends women not to fly after their 36th week of pregnancy. Airlines have their own flight restrictions for pregnant women, which can vary according to whether she is flying domestically or internationally. Most airlines would not take pregnant women past 32 to 36 weeks, even on short-haul flights of two hours, and most of the travel insurance would not cover her late in pregnancy, usually from around 32 weeks. There is no evidence to suggest that air travel is riskier for pregnant women, the biggest risks result from cramped seating, dehydration, and the development of deep vein thrombosis.

○ **What is the neonatal abstinence syndrome, and what agents cause it?**

It is caused by maternal heroin addiction or maternal methadone treatment during pregnancy. It results from neonatal withdrawal and consists of tremulousness, hyper-reflexia, high pitch cry, sneezing, sleepiness, tachypnea, yawning, sweating, fever and seizures. The onset of symptoms is at birth.

○ **What are the categories of fetal development defects?**

There are malformations, disruptions, and deformations.

○ **What are these malformations, disruptions, and deformations?**

A *malformation* is a defect that results from a developmental process, which has been abnormal from the beginning of conception at very early in the life of the embryo. Its impact may be seen in a single or in multiple developmental regions. A *disruption* is a developmental defect that results from an intrinsic or extrinsic factor that interferes with the originally normal development process. In the absence of the effects of this factor, the development would have been normal. It cannot be inherited. A *deformation* is an abnormal form, shape, or position of a part of the body because of the effect of mechanical force acting on that area during development.

○ **What are the differences between a sequence, syndrome, and association?**

A *sequence* is multiple anomalies resulting from a single known of presumed malformation, deformation, or disruption. A *syndrome* is multiple anomalies because of a single malformation. An *association* is the occurrence of multiple anomalies associated with a known or unknown malformation in two or more persons.

○ **What steps are required to assess a person's risk for an adverse reproductive outcome?**

The first step is identifying whether the agent can cause a defect, and if so, the type of defect caused. The next step is characterization of the hazard to assess the critical amount of an exposure needed to produce the result being studied. Thirdly, the degree, type, and timing of the exposure are identified. Finally, how likely is it that the defect resulted from the exposure being studied and not from other internal or external causes or from chance.

○ **What are the hazardous effects of rubella vaccination during embryogenesis?**

Even though the vaccine contains live attenuated virus, there are no known cases of congenital rubella syndrome (malformations of the heart and CNS, deafness, cataracts, mental retardation) as a consequence of inadvertent vaccination during early pregnancy. However, to be safe, all women receiving the vaccine should be advised to postpone pregnancy for 3 months.

○ **Is varicella infection during pregnancy innocuous?**

No. Varicella (chicken pox) is a known teratogen. Maternal infection in the first half of pregnancy results in congenital varicella syndrome in 1% to 5% of cases. This syndrome consists of CNS and skeletal abnormalities and mental retardation. Maternal varicella infection late in pregnancy (within 5 days before and after delivery) may result in chickenpox skin lesions, pneumonia, and other complications. Approximately 30% of infected children develop disseminated disease.

○ **What does the word *teratogenesis* mean?**

Teratogenesis is a medical term, literally meaning *monster-birth*, which derives from teratology, the study of the frequency, causation, and development of congenital malformations—misleadingly called *birth defects*. Teratogenesis has gained a more specific usage for the development of abnormal cell masses during fetal growth, causing physical defects in the fetus. The study of teratogenesis is called teratology.

○ **What are Wilson's general principles of teratology?**

The six principles of teratology provide a framework for understanding how structural or functional teratogens act. These principles were developed by James G. Wilson and are as follows:

1. Susceptibility to teratogenesis depends on the genotype of the conceptus and the manner in which this interacts with environmental factors.
2. Susceptibility to teratogenic agents varies with the developmental stage at the time of exposure.
3. Teratogenic agents act in specific ways (mechanisms) on developing cells and tissues to initiate abnormal embryogenesis (pathogenesis).
4. The final manifestations of abnormal development are death, malformation, growth retardation, and functional disorder.
5. The access of adverse environmental influences to developing tissue depends on the nature of the influences (agent).
6. Manifestations of deviant development increase in degree as dosage increases from the no-effect to the totally lethal level.

○ **What are the three general categories of epidemiologic studies?**

These are descriptive, analytic, and experimental. The *descriptive* category includes case reports, descriptive studies, and surveillance programs. The *analytic* category includes ecologic studies, cross-sectional studies, case control studies, and cohort studies. The *experimental* category includes clinical trials.

○ **What are the adverse reproductive outcomes associated with occupational and environmental exposure?**

These include infertility, single gene defects, chromosome abnormalities, spontaneous abortions, congenital malformation, intrauterine growth restriction, perinatal deaths, developmental disabilities, behavioral disorders, and malignancies.

○ **What is "recall bias"?**

Women with an adverse pregnancy outcome such as spontaneous abortion, fetal or neonatal demise, or a congenital malformation are more likely to recall exposure to environmental or occupational or infectious agents. On the other hand, those with satisfactory pregnancy outcomes tend to forget such exposures.

○ **What is "selection bias"?**

When studying a particular outcome or teratogenic agent, there are potential problems that can affect the interpretation of reported results. Some examples are (i) inaccurate or incomplete information about single or multiple exposures and confounding exposures; (ii) incomplete, inaccurate, or absent survey responses; (iii) not validating the reproductive history; (iv) recall bias; (v) inaccurate methods of data collection; (vi) investigators' bias toward one of the possible outcomes of a study.

○ **What are the drug labeling categories for use during pregnancy?**

The FDA lists five categories of labeling. *Category A*: safe for use in pregnancy. *Category B*: animal studies have demonstrated the drug's safety and human studies do not reveal any adverse fetal effects. *Category C:* the drug is a known animal teratogen, but no data are available about human use; or there are no data in either humans or animals. *Category D:* there is positive evidence of human fetal toxicity but benefits in selected situations makes use of the drug acceptable despite its risks. *Category X:* the drug is a definite human and animal teratogen and should not be used in pregnancy.

○ **Is the spermicide nonoxynol-9 a teratogen?**

No. Recent literature demonstrates that vaginal spermicide use before or during pregnancy is not associated with increased rates of pregnancy loss or abnormal offspring.

○ **Is ingestion of large amounts of vitamins safe during pregnancy?**

No. Even though increased amount of most vitamins are encouraged and also considered safe during pregnancy, there are some that can become teratogenic when taken in large amounts. These include *vitamin A*, which in normal doses is not a teratogen. However, if amounts equal to or greater than 25,000 IU are ingested during pregnancy, it causes craniofacial and cardiac anomalies and mental retardation.

○ **What should you tell the patient who is thinking about starting an isotretinoin treatment for her acne?**

Patients who are taking isotretinoin treatment, even for short periods of time, have an extremely high risk that severe birth defect will result if pregnancy occurs during the therapy. Abnormalities of the face, eyes, ears, skull, central nervous system, cardiovascular system, thymus, and parathyroid glands have been reported. There is an increased risk of spontaneous abortions and premature birth also.

Thus, she must have negative results from two pregnancy tests before her first prescription, and she needs to have pregnancy tests every month during treatment and also at the end of treatment and one month after stopping treatment.

○ **What happens if pregnancy does occur during the treatment of a female patient who is taking isotretinoin capsules (Accutane)?**

Accutane must be discontinued immediately and the patient referred to an obstetrician-gynecologist who is experienced in reproductive toxicology for further evaluation.

○ **How long should the female patient who is taking isotretinoin capsules (Accutane) avoid getting pregnant?**

Before prescribing Accutane, the patient must sign that she understands that she must not get pregnant 1 month before, during the entire time of her treatment, and for 1 month after the end of her treatment with isotretinoin. She must avoid sexual intercourse completely, or she must use two separate, effective forms of birth control at the same time.

○ **What is the iPLEDGE?**

iPLEDGE is a new risk-management program created by the manufacturers of isotretinoin, in March 2006. iPLEDGE is a comprehensive distribution system that includes mandatory registration of patients, healthcare providers, pharmacies, and wholesalers. It allows real-time linkage of pregnancy-test results for verification prior to the dispensing of isotretinoin. Although the challenges of implementing a closed distribution system for a very widely used medication have been extensive, the potential public health benefits from preventing fetal exposure to isotretinoin are substantial.

○ **Is topical tretinoin (Retin-A Micro microsphere, 0.1% and 0.04%) also teratogenic?**

Retin-A Micro is a pregnancy category C drug. There are no adequate and well-controlled studies in pregnant women regarding the teratogenic effect of Retin-A Micro; however, topical tretinoin has been shown to be fetotoxic, resulting in skeletal variations and increased intrauterine death in rats and rabbits when applied at higher doses. Thus, this only should be used during pregnancy if the potential benefit justifies the potential risk to the fetus.

○ **Is it safe to use topical tretinoin (Retin-A Micro) in nursing mothers?**

So far no study has been conducted to evaluate whether this drug is excreted in human milk. Because many drugs are excreted in human milk, caution should be exercised when Retin-A Micro is administered to a nursing woman.

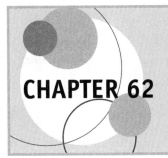

CHAPTER 62

Epidemiology and Clinical Biostatistics

Jerry Cohen, MPH

○ **Define epidemiology.**

Epidemiology is the study of the distribution and determinants of disease in human populations.

○ **What is descriptive epidemiology and analytic epidemiology?**

Descriptive epidemiology includes activities related to characterizing the distribution of diseases in a population. Analytic epidemiology is related to identifying possible causes for the occurrence of disease.

○ **How is epidemiology applied to obstetrics and gynecology?**

Epidemiology can be used for descriptive purposes, such as surveillance of the occurrence (incidence) of a particular illness. It can also be used for analytic purposes, such as studying risk factors for disease development. Epidemiologic methods can be used to assess the performance of diagnostic tests. Epidemiology can be used to study the progression or natural history of a disease. Epidemiology can be used to study prognostic factors, which are determinants of the progression of a disease. Epidemiology can be used to evaluate treatments for a disease.

○ **What does the phrase "sentinel cases" refer to?**

The first few affected patients identified in a disease outbreak are referred to as sentinel cases.

○ **Define epidemic.**

An epidemic is a sudden and great increase in the occurrence of a disease within a population.

○ **Define pandemic.**

A pandemic is a rapidly emerging disease outbreak that affects a wide range of a geographically distributed population.

○ **How are patterns of disease occurrence characterized?**

Patterns of disease are characterized by person, place, and time.

○ **What is disease surveillance?**

Disease surveillance refers to monitoring patterns of disease occurrence in a population.

○ **How is the number of newly diagnosed cases per year for a disease determined?**

Numbers of newly diagnosed cases are affected by (1) the frequency with which the disease occurs, (2) how the disease is defined, (3) the size of the population from which cases develop, and (4) completeness of case reporting.

○ **What is the incidence rate?**

It is the measure of how fast disease occurs.

○ **What are risk factors?**

Associations between characteristics that accompany disease can occur by coincidence, or by cause–effect relationships. Risk factors are attributes or agents suspected to be related to the occurrence of a particular disease.

○ **What is the difference between an epidemiologic case and control?**

Persons affected by a disease are referred to as cases, and unaffected, comparison persons are known as controls.

○ **What is a case–control study?**

A case–control study is an observational study in which subjects are sampled based on the presence (case) or absence (controls) of a disease of interest. Information is collected about earlier exposure to risk factors of interest.

○ **Define bias.**

Bias is a nonrandom error in a study that leads to a skewed result.

○ **How can bias be averted?**

Bias can be circumvented by using a cohort study design. Cohort studies are observational, in which subjects are sampled based on the presence (exposed) or absence (unexposed) for a risk factor of interest. These subjects are followed over time for the development of a disease outcome of interest.

○ **What is the purpose of diagnostic testing?**

In epidemiology, the purpose of diagnostic testing is to obtain objective evidence of the presence or absence of a particular condition. This is done in a given population through the process of screening.

○ **What is meant by the phrase "natural history" of an illness?**

Natural history of an illness is the progression of a disease through successful stages, often used to describe the course of an illness for which no effective treatment is available.

○ **Define case fatality.**

It is a way of characterizing the natural history of an illness. It is represented as the percentage of patients with a disease who die within a specified observation period.

○ **What is the term used for the time duration from diagnosis to death?**

Survival time. The median survival time is the duration of time from diagnosis to death that is exceeded by 50% of subjects with a particular disease.

○ **What types of measures are used to describe disease occurrence?**

Risk is the likelihood or probability that a person will contract a disease. A simple formula for calculating this is as follows:

$$R = A/N,$$

where R is risk, A is the number of *newly* affected persons, and N is the number of unaffected persons under observation.

Prevalence indicates the percentage of existing cases of the disease of interest in a population. It can be calculated as follows:

$$P = C/N,$$

where P is prevalence, C is the number of *existing* affected cases, and N is the number of persons in the population.

Incidence rate measures how rapid newly affected cases of the disease of interest develop. It can be calculated as follows:

$$IR = A/PT,$$

where IR is incidence rate, A is the count of new cases of the disease in a population, and PT is the measure of net time that persons in the population at risk for developing the disease is observed. PT is also known as person-time.

○ **How is "survival" defined in epidemiologic terms?**

Survival is the likelihood of remaining alive for a specified period of time after the diagnosis of a particular disease. It can be estimated as follows:

$$S = A - D/A,$$

where S is survival, A is the number of newly diagnosed patients under observation, and D is the number of deaths observed in a specified period of time. It can be expressed as a decimal or converted to the corresponding percentage.

○ **What is a "case fatality"?**

The probability for a disease to cause the death of an affected patient is referred to as a case fatality. Case fatalities are estimated in the following way:

$$CF = D/A,$$

where CF is case fatality, D is the number of deaths, and A is the number of diagnosed patients. The resulting estimate can be left as a proportion or multiplied by 100 to convert it to a percentage.

○ **What three questions should be asked when trying to characterize the nonrandom occurrence of disease?**

Who gets the disease?

Where does the disease occur?

When does the disease occur?

In epidemiologic terms who, where, and when, are known respectively as **person**, **place**, and **time**.

○ **What is age adjustment?**

Age adjustment takes summary rates for various populations and removes differences in age distributions, so that the adjusted rate is independent, of any confounding factor.

○ **How do you define premature death?**

Premature death measures the years of potential life lost to a particular disease.

○ **What is SEER?**

SEER is an acronym for Surveillance, Epidemiology, and End Results program. It is a population-based registry utilized and managed by the US National Cancer Institute as one way of monitoring the incidence of cancer by geographic area.

○ **Define disease outbreak.**

Epidemic occurring suddenly, within a specific geographic area.

○ **What does it take for a disease outbreak to occur?**

A pathogen of sufficient quantity, a susceptible population, and a mode of transmission.

○ **Define attack rate of a disease outbreak.**

It is the number of persons affected by the disease among the persons at risk for the disease. It is calculated as follows:

$$\text{Attack rate (AR)} = \frac{\text{Number new cases}}{\text{Persons at risk}} \times 100.$$

○ **What are the two primary modes of transmission of a disease outbreak?**

Disease can be spread *person to person* and by *common sources of exposure* (contact with a risk factor originating in a shared environment of people).

○ **When should a disease outbreak be investigated?**

Consideration should be given to the number and severity of affected persons, an unknown cause, and public health concerns.

○ **What is the sensitivity of a diagnostic test?**

Sensitivity is the likelihood that someone with a disease of interest will have positive test results.

○ **What is the specificity of a diagnostic test?**

Specificity is the likelihood that someone *not* having a disease of interest will have negative test results.

○ **What does positive predictive value measure?**

Positive predictive value (PPV) measures the likelihood of having a disease of interest in those persons with diagnostic test results that are positive.

○ **What does a negative predictive value refer to?**

Negative predictive value (NPV) is the likelihood of *not* having a disease of interest in those persons with diagnostic test results that are negative.

○ **How are likelihood ratios used?**

They can be used to measure the extent to which the likelihood of the disease of interest is changed by the results of a diagnostic test.

○ **What does ROC refer to?**

Receiver operating characteristic. In diagnostic testing, it is a plot of true-positives on the *y*-axis, versus the false-positives on the *x*-axis. The ROC curve is used to evaluate the properties of a diagnostic test.

○ **Why is disease screening performed?**

It is done in order to detect a disease of interest at an earlier stage than would occur through routine methods.

○ **What is an error in a screening process called?**

Lead-time bias occurs when people with disease appear to live longer as a result of early recognition of the disease because they were detected through a screening process.

○ **What is length-time bias in screening processes?**

It is an error in the evaluation of a screening process. It can happen when those with a particular disease detected by screening appear to live longer simply because they have more slowly progressing disease.

○ **What is a nomogram?**

A nomogram is a graphical scale that can assist in determining positive and negative predictive values (the post-test probability of disease) to be determined from the likelihood ratios of a diagnostic test and from the prevalence of a disease (pre-test probability of disease) in a population.

BIOSTATISTICS

○ **Define biostatistics.**

Biostatistics is the application of study design and statistical analysis in research medicine.

○ **What are the two types of study designs in medical research?**

One type is where subjects are observed, and the other where studies of an intervention are observed.

○ **What is an observational study?**

A study *not* involving intervention.

○ **Describe the various types of observation studies?**

An observational study may be forward-looking (cohort), backward-looking (case–control), or looking at simultaneous events (cross-sectional). Cohort studies generally provide stronger evidence than the two other designs.

Cohort—an observational study composed of two groups of people; one group having a risk factor or who have been exposed to something, and the other group who do not have the risk factor or exposure. Both groups are followed prospectively through time to learn how many in each set develop the outcome or consequences of interest.

Case–control—type of study that includes patients who have the outcome or disease of interest, and control subjects who do not have the outcome or disease.

Cross-sectional—an observational study that examines a characteristic in a set of subjects at one point in time.

○ **Describe intervention studies?**

These types of studies are called experiments. They provide stronger evidence than observational studies.

○ **What is bias?**

Bias is an error related to the ways the targeted and sampled populations differ; sometimes called measurement error, it threatens the validity of a study.

○ **What is a Type I error?**

A Type I error results if a true null hypothesis is rejected or if a difference is concluded when no actual difference exists. Also known as an alpha (α) error.

○ **What is a Type II error?**

A Type II error results if a false null hypothesis is not rejected or if a difference is not detected when a difference exists. Also known as a beta (β) error.

○ **What are variables?**

Variables are characteristics of interest in a study that have recorded value(s) for each patient in the study. Variables can be either independent or dependant. An independent variable is also known as the explanatory or predictor variable. A dependent variable refers to an outcome in a study.

○ **Describe a nominal variable.**

Nominal variables allow for only *qualitative* classification. That is, they can be measured only in terms of whether the individual items belong to some distinctively different category, but we cannot quantify or even rank order the category.

Nominal data can be measured as proportions, percentages, ratios, and rates. Characteristics measured on a nominal scale do not have numerical values but are frequencies of occurrence.

○ **What is a binary observation?**

It is a nominal measure that has only two outcomes (an example: amenorrhea: yes or no).

○ **Describe an ordinal.**

Ordinal variables allow us to rank order the measured items, but still do not allow us to say how much more.

○ **What are the two basic features of relations between variables?**

Magnitude and reliability. Reliability refers to how probable it is that a similar relation would be found if the experiment were replicated with other samples drawn from the same population.

○ **What is a box plot?**

A box plot is a graph that displays both the frequencies and distributions of observations. It is useful for comparing two distributions. It is also called a "box and whisker" plot.

○ **Define frequency distribution.**

It is a list of values that occurs along with the frequency of occurrence. It can be displayed as a graph or table.

○ **What is "statistical significance" (p value)?**

The statistical significance of a result is the probability that the observed relationship (e.g., between variables) or a difference (e.g., between means) in a sample, occurred by pure chance ("luck of the draw"), and that in the population from which the sample was drawn, no such relationship or differences exist.

The higher the p value, the *less* we can believe that the observed relation between variables in the sample is a reliable indicator of the relation between the respective variables in the population.

Typically, results that yield $p \leq 0.05$ are considered borderline statistically significant but remember that this level of significance still involves a probability of error (5%). Results that are significant at the $p = 0.01$ level are commonly considered statistically significant, and $p \leq 0.005$ or $p \leq 0.001$ levels are often called "highly" significant.

○ **What is meant by a null hypothesis?**

It represents the hypothesis being tested about a population. Null means "no difference", and refers to a situation in which no difference exists (e.g., between the means in a treatment group and a control group).

○ **What is the chi-square test (χ^2)?**

It is a test to determine whether factors or characteristics are independent or not associated with each other. A chi-square distribution is used to analyze counts in frequency tables.

○ **Define confidence interval.**

The interval calculated from sample data that has a given probability that the unknown parameter, such as a mean or proportion is contained within the interval. Confidence intervals are usually expressed as 90%, 95%, or 99%.

○ **What is meant by the effect size?**

It is the magnitude of difference or relationship. It is used to determine sample sizes for studies, and for combining results across studies as in meta-analysis work.

○ **What is the t test?**

The statistical test for comparing a mean with a norm, or for comparing two means with small sample sizes.

○ **What is the difference between clinical and statistical significance?**

A clinically important finding is a conclusion that has possible implications for patient care. A statistically significant finding is a conclusion that there is evidence against the null hypothesis.

○ **What is relative risk?**

Relative risk (RR) is the ratio of the incidence of a given disease in exposed or at-risk population to the incidence of the disease in unexposed persons. It is calculated in cohort or prospective studies.

○ **What is a control event rate (CER)?**

The number of subjects in a control group who develop the outcome being studied.

○ **What is an experimental event rate (EER)?**

The number of subjects in the experimental or treatment group who develop the outcome being studied.

○ **Define relative risk reduction.**

Relative risk reduction (RRR) is the reduction in risk with a new therapy; it is the absolute value of the difference between experimental event rate (EER) and the control event rate (CER) divided by the control event rate.

○ **Define absolute risk reduction.**

Reduction in risk *with* a new therapy compared with the risk *without* a new therapy. It is the absolute value of the difference between the experimental event rate (EER) and the control event rate (CER).

○ **Define absolute risk increase.**

Increase in risk *with* a new therapy compared with the risk *without* the new therapy.

○ **What is meant by a hazard ratio?**

Ratio of risk for an outcome (such as osteoporosis) occurring at any time in one group compared with another group.

○ **What does ANOVA stand for?**

ANOVA stands for analysis of variance. It is a statistical procedure that determines whether any differences exist between two or more groups of subjects on one or more variables.

○ **Describe the Fisher's exact test.**

It is a statistical test for 2×2 contingency tables. A contingency table is used to display counts, or frequencies for two or more nominal or quantitative variables. The Fisher's exact test is used when the sample size is too small to use the chi-square test.

○ **What is the Mantel–Haenszel test?**

A statistical test of two or more 2×2 tables. It is used to compare survival distributions or to control for confounding factors.

○ **What is meant by the phrase "central tendency"?**

Index, or summary numbers that describe the middle of a distribution.

○ **What does NNH stand for?**

NNH stands for number needed to harm. Number of patients that need to be treated with a proposed therapy in order to cause one undesirable outcome.

○ **What does NNT stand for?**

NNT stands for number of patients needed to be treated with a proposed therapy in order to prevent or cure one person. It is the reciprocal of the absolute risk reduction (1/ARR).